Mechanical Ventilation Amid the COVID-19 Pandemic

Amir A. Hakimi • Thomas E. Milner
Govind R. Rajan • Brian J-F Wong

Editors

Mechanical Ventilation Amid the COVID-19 Pandemic

A Guide for Physicians and Engineers

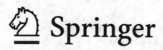

Editors
Amir A. Hakimi
Otolaryngology – Head and Neck Surgery
Medstar Georgetown University Hospital
Washington D.C., WA, USA

Govind R. Rajan
Anesthesiology & Critical Care Medicine
University of California, Irvine
Orange, CA, USA

Thomas E. Milner
Beckman Laser Institute and Medical Clinic
Irvine, CA, USA

Brian J-F Wong
Otolaryngology – Head and Neck Surgery
University of California, Irvine
Orange, CA, USA

ISBN 978-3-030-87980-8   ISBN 978-3-030-87978-5   (eBook)
https://doi.org/10.1007/978-3-030-87978-5

© The Editor(s) (if applicable) and The Author(s), under exclusive license to Springer Nature Switzerland AG 2022
This work is subject to copyright. All rights are solely and exclusively licensed by the Publisher, whether the whole or part of the material is concerned, specifically the rights of translation, reprinting, reuse of illustrations, recitation, broadcasting, reproduction on microfilms or in any other physical way, and transmission or information storage and retrieval, electronic adaptation, computer software, or by similar or dissimilar methodology now known or hereafter developed.
The use of general descriptive names, registered names, trademarks, service marks, etc. in this publication does not imply, even in the absence of a specific statement, that such names are exempt from the relevant protective laws and regulations and therefore free for general use.
The publisher, the authors and the editors are safe to assume that the advice and information in this book are believed to be true and accurate at the date of publication. Neither the publisher nor the authors or the editors give a warranty, expressed or implied, with respect to the material contained herein or for any errors or omissions that may have been made. The publisher remains neutral with regard to jurisdictional claims in published maps and institutional affiliations.

This Springer imprint is published by the registered company Springer Nature Switzerland AG
The registered company address is: Gewerbestrasse 11, 6330 Cham, Switzerland

Preface

The surge in COVID-19 cases leading to hospitalizations around the world quickly depleted hospital resources and reserves, forcing physicians to make extremely difficult life-or-death decisions on ventilator allocation between patients. Leaders in academia and industry have developed numerous ventilator support systems using both consumer- and industry-grade hardware to sustain life and to provide intermediate respiratory relief for hospitalized patients. This book is the first of its kind to discuss the respiratory pathophysiology underlying COVID-19, explain pulmonary and ventilator mechanics, provide and evaluate a repository of innovative emergency resuscitators conceived amid the pandemic, and explain both hardware and software components necessary to develop an inexpensive emergency resuscitator. The book serves both as a historical record of the collaborative and innovative response to the anticipated ventilator shortage during the COVID-19 pandemic and as a guide for physicians, engineers, and DIY-ers interested in developing emergency resuscitator devices.

Several mechanisms for these transitory emergency resuscitators or "bridge ventilators" have been proposed including automatic compression of resuscitation bags through various mechanical and pneumatic means, repurposing CPAP and BiPAP devices to function as ventilators, and noninvasive ventilation through oxygen helmets, snorkel masks, and more. Herein, the authors explore and appraise the functionality of each unique approach. Additionally, expert leaders behind several emergency ventilator designs provide a detailed review of resuscitation bag and motor mechanics and impart insight on their ventilator models. This resource provides a thorough framework for basic ventilatory support and guides readers toward developing their own bridge ventilators through evidence-based expert recommendations. We also encourage readers to go to our website www.bli.uci.edu/hvc or scan the QR code below to access supplemental videos and posts.

Washington, DC, USA   Amir A. Hakimi
Irvine, CA, USA   Thomas E. Milner
Orange, CA, USA   Govind R. Rajan
Orange, CA, USA   Brian J.-F. Wong

Contents

About the Editors

Amir A. Hakimi, MD is a resident in the Department of Otolaryngology-Head and Neck Surgery at MedStar Georgetown University Hospital. He received his Bachelor of Science degree in Neuroscience at the University of California, Los Angeles. He then graduated from Chicago Medical School at Rosalind Franklin University of Medicine and Science. During medical school, he became involved in clinical and translational research under the mentorship of Dr. Brian Wong. Dr. Hakimi has published numerous articles in peer-reviewed scientific journals, and he has developed a medical application for the iPhone to expedite the diagnosis of ocular injury.

Thomas E. Milner, PhD is Director of the Beckman Laser Institute and Medical Clinic and Professor of Biomedical Engineering and Surgery at the University of California, Irvine. He received his bachelor's and master's degrees from the Colorado School of Mines and his Ph.D. from the University of Arizona. Dr. Milner's research interests are in the fields of optical based therapeutics and diagnostic imaging, biomedical optics sensors, and optical tomography. He has published more than 180 journal articles, holds 55 issued US patents, and has started two technology companies. Dr. Milner is a fellow of the National Academy of Inventors, the American Institute for Medical and Biological Engineering, and the American Society for Lasers in Medicine and Surgery.

Govind R. Rajan, MBBS is an anesthesiologist in Orange, CA, and is affiliated with the UC Irvine Medical Center. He received his medical degree from Maulana Azad Medical College and has been in practice for 29 years. He also speaks multiple languages, including Hindi. He specializes in critical care medicine.

Brian J.-F. Wong, MD, PhD is Professor and Director of the Division of Facial Plastic Surgery in the Department of Otolaryngology-Head and Neck Surgery at the University of California Irvine Medical Center. Dr. Wong's clinical practice is based at both the UC Irvine Medical Center and the Beckman Laser Institute and Medical Clinic. He graduated summa cum laude with a bachelor's degree in biomedical engineering from the University of Southern California and earned his medical degree from Johns Hopkins University. He also studied engineering at Oxford University as a Rotary Foundation Scholar and medical physics at the University of Amsterdam. Dr. Wong's research interests are in the field of biomedical engineering, with specific interests in medical device development and laser applications in medicine. He has more than 100 publications, and his research is funded by the National Institutes of Health, the Department of Defense, and the Health Science Partners.

Chapter 1
Establishment of the Bridge Ventilator Consortium

Amir A. Hakimi, Thomas E. Milner, Govind Rajan, and Brian J. F. Wong

The Bridge Ventilator Consortium (BVC) serves as a multidisciplinary organization linking industry, academia, government, nonprofit organizations, and community members who have voluntarily partnered to develop breathing devices for use if ICUs run short of conventional ventilators. Within days, we were able to recruit a motivated team of physicians, engineers, scientists, legal advisors, respiratory therapists, and manufacturers among others to combat the pandemic. There was a lot to learn about ventilators prior to delving into production. Our team

A. A. Hakimi (✉)
Department of Otolaryngology – Head and Neck Surgery, Medstar Georgetown University Hospital, Washington, DC, USA

Beckman Laser Institute & Medical Clinic, University of California – Irvine, Orange, CA, USA
e-mail: amir.a.hakimi@medstar.net

T. E. Milner
Beckman Laser Institute & Medical Clinic, University of California – Irvine, Orange, CA, USA

G. Rajan
Department of Anesthesiology and Perioperative Care, University of California – Irvine, Orange, CA, USA
e-mail: grajan@hs.uci.edu

B. J. F. Wong
Beckman Laser Institute & Medical Clinic, University of California – Irvine, Orange, CA, USA

Department of Otolaryngology – Head & Neck Surgery, University of California – Irvine, Orange, CA, USA

Department of Biomedical Engineering, University of California – Irvine, Irvine, CA, USA
e-mail: bjwong@uci.edu

© The Author(s), under exclusive license to Springer Nature Switzerland AG 2022
A. A. Hakimi et al. (eds.), *Mechanical Ventilation Amid the COVID-19 Pandemic*,
https://doi.org/10.1007/978-3-030-87978-5_1

meetings intertwined the medical knowledge of anesthesiologists, critical care physicians, and respiratory therapists with the technical prowess of engineers from all backgrounds.

Our daily teleconference meetings were open forum, allowing participants worldwide to learn and contribute to this cause. Many individual groups within our team successfully developed emergency resuscitators, several of whom received or are in the process of receiving emergency use authorization from the United States Food and Drug Administration. The purpose of this textbook is to help guide readers toward a similar path in emergency resuscitator development. Experts from the BVC team have come together in this textbook to highlight the most essential medical, engineering, and regulatory concepts that we have learned throughout this process.

There is no doubt that improvements in the cost, availability, and function of ventilators are eminent. The need for ventilators and emergency resuscitators expands beyond the COVID-19 pandemic as many countries have long suffered a shortage of these lifesaving devices. It is our hope that the information in this textbook helps promote future works to advance ventilatory care.

Conflicts of Interest The authors have no relevant conflicts of interest to disclose.

Funding This work was not funded.

Part I
Lung Physiology and Ventilator Basics

Chapter 2
An Overview of Lung Anatomy and Physiology

Karen Katrivesis, Jennifer Elia, Brent Etiz, Keaton Cooley-Rieders, Sina Hosseinian, and Sean Melucci

Lung Anatomy

At the most basic level, normal human anatomy consists of two lungs. Each lung is divided into different lobes by separations known as fissures. The left lung consists of a superior and inferior lobe, separated by the oblique fissure located at the T4–5 vertebral level. The right lung is divided into superior, middle, and inferior lobes by the oblique and horizontal fissures. The right lung is larger and heavier, but also shorter and wider than the left lung. This is due to the diaphragm extending higher on the right and the heart bulging more to the left. The left and right lungs have different anatomical features. One of the most prominent features of the left lung is the cardiac notch which is an indentation on the anterior margin that allows for the leftward bulging of the heart. The right lung has vasculature grooves which allow for the passage of the superior and inferior vena cava.

Each lung has an apex, three surfaces, and three borders. The apex of the lung is the most superior aspect, ascending above the first rib into the root of the neck. The lung also has three surfaces: the costal surface, which is adjacent to the sternum and ribs; the mediastinal surface, which is found medially to the mediastinum and posteriorly to the vertebrae; and the diaphragmatic surface, which rests on the convex dome of the diaphragm. Each lung has an anterior, posterior, and inferior border.

The mediastinal surface includes the hilum of the lung, the medial aspect where structures enter and exit the lung. These structures form the root of the lung which has different orientations of structures for the left and right lungs. The most notable

K. Katrivesis (✉) · J. Elia
Department of Anesthesiology, Division of Critical Care Medicine, University of California, Irvine, CA, USA
e-mail: kkatrive@hs.uci.edu; jelia@hs.uci.edu

B. Etiz · K. Cooley-Rieders · S. Hosseinian · S. Melucci
Irvine School of Medicine, University of California, Irvine, CA, USA

© The Author(s), under exclusive license to Springer Nature Switzerland AG 2022
A. A. Hakimi et al. (eds.), *Mechanical Ventilation Amid the COVID-19 Pandemic*,
https://doi.org/10.1007/978-3-030-87978-5_2

difference is the location of the main bronchus. In the left lung, the main bronchus is located inferior to the pulmonary arteries. In the right lung, the main bronchus is located posterior to the pulmonary arteries.

Both lungs are enclosed by a serous pleural sac that consists of two continuous layers of membranes, the visceral and parietal layers. Together, these layers are known as the pleurae. The visceral pleura fully covers the lungs and adheres to all its surfaces. The parietal pleura lines the pulmonary cavities, providing support for the lungs by adhering to the thoracic wall, mediastinum, and diaphragm. At rest, the inferior boundary of the lungs is at vertebral level T10, whereas during inhalation, the inferior boundary is at T12, the boundary of the pulmonary cavity. The pleural cavity contains two recesses: the costodiaphragmatic recess and the costomediastinal recess. The costodiaphragmatic recess is a bilateral recess that is bound by the lung superiorly and by the diaphragm inferiorly. The costomediastinal recess is a lateral recess that is located posterior to the sternum [1].

Trachea and Bronchi

The trachea, commonly referred to as the windpipe, is the airway that leads from the larynx to the large airways of the lungs known as the bronchi. Beginning at vertebral level C6, the trachea extends inferiorly to the carina, where it then bifurcates into the left and right main bronchi. The trachea is a tough airway surrounded by C-shaped cartilage rings.

The main bronchi extend inferolaterally and enter the lung at the hilum. It is one of the structures that form the root of the lung. The opposing sides of the bronchi have differing features. The right bronchus is wider, shorter, and more vertical than the left main bronchus. These bronchi branch into secondary bronchi: two secondary bronchi on the left and three on the right. Each secondary bronchus then divides into several tertiary bronchi that supply the bronchopulmonary segments. The right lung contains ten bronchopulmonary segments to supply three lobes. The left lung contains nine bronchopulmonary segments to supply two lobes.

Tertiary bronchi continue within the lung, dividing into smaller and smaller airways, termed as bronchioles. The tertiary bronchi continue as 20–25 generations of conducting bronchioles and terminal bronchioles. This represents the end of the conducting component of the airway. Terminal bronchioles extend as respiratory bronchioles, followed by alveolar ducts, sacs, and finally the alveoli, the main respiratory component of the lung.

Pulmonary Neurovasculature

Pulmonary arteries carry poorly oxygenated blood from the heart to the lung for oxygenation. They enter the lung at the hilum, descend to the main bronchi, and divide into several lobar and segmental arteries in a pattern similar to the main bronchi. This ultimately allows for a branch to go into each lobe and segment of the lung. There are two pulmonary veins in each lung that carry oxygenated blood back to the heart to then be circulated to the rest of the body.

The innervation of the lungs and pleura is rather simple. Both are innervated by autonomic fibers derived from the pulmonary plexus. The pulmonary plexus consists of the vagus nerve (cranial nerve X) and fibers from the sympathetic trunk. The vagus nerve supplies parasympathetic fibers whereas the sympathetic trunk supplies sympathetic fibers. Parasympathetic innervation will dilate the pulmonary vessels, constrict the bronchioles, and excite glandular secretions. Sympathetic innervation will constrict the pulmonary vessels, dilate the bronchioles, and inhibit glandular secretions [2].

Lung Mechanics

Before discussing lung mechanics, we must first discuss pressure and how it is measured. It is commonplace in lung mechanics for units of pressure to be measured in cmH_2O. Historically, physiologists conducted experiments by applying air pressure to the lungs using columns of water. A column of water 50 cm high produces a pressure of 50 cmH_2O. 1033 cmH_2O is equal to one standard atmosphere, or to 760 mmHg. It is standard practice in lung mechanics and clinical settings to report pressures relative to atmospheric pressure. Thus, atmospheric pressure is equal to 0 cmH_2O.

There are four locations where air pressure is determined. First is alveolar pressure (P_{alv}) which is the pressure inside the alveolar regions. Second is the pressure at the airway opening (P_{ao}). Third is the pressure inside the chamber but outside the lung, the pleural pressure (P_{pl}). Fourth is the pressure outside of the system, or barometric pressure (P_B).

Much of what we know now about static lung mechanics is a result of physiology experiments conducted in the last century. Lungs removed from autopsies were studied by suspending them in a humidified chamber. The airways were connected to a pressure gauge and a syringe was used to inflate and deflate the lungs. An open pipe was placed in the chamber so that the chamber was always equal to atmospheric pressure. In one particular experiment, researchers discovered that the resting lung volume is roughly 1/5th of the total lung capacity. This experiment demonstrated that this volume, termed the residual volume (RV), is typically observed in normal human lungs. The pressure of lungs at rest is roughly measured at 2 cmH_2O [3].

Another important experiment was conducted in a similar manner. In this case, a syringe was placed on the pipe so that it is no longer completely open to the atmosphere. When the pressure is advanced to +5 cmH_2O, the lungs are at roughly 50% of the total lung capacity. This volume is referred to as the functional residual capacity (FRC). Since we are discussing static lung mechanics, there is no flow of air. As a result, the pressure in the airway and the alveolar pressure are the same value. In a human body, this is referred to as the mouth pressure.

If we were to continue to inflate the lungs to its maximum capacity, or the total lung capacity (TLC), the pressure would reach +25 cmH$_2$O. Further pressure on the system would not result in additional air inflation to the lungs but may result in rupturing of the lungs. In this scenario, a constant pressure must be applied to the syringe to keep it at +25 cmH$_2$O. If the syringe was let go, or disconnected, air will be expelled rapidly until the lung is approximately 1/10th of the total lung capacity. So, to maintain a given lung volume, there must be pressure continuously applied. As a result, researchers concluded that the lung generates an opposing pressure, termed the elastic recoil of the lung, which is working to expel air [3]. The elastic recoil is always acting to expel air from the lung at any lung volume.

In the previous experiments, the syringe and pressure gauge were connected to the airways. Although useful, these experiments failed to provide an accurate representation of lung mechanics in humans, as the pressure differential is not derived in such a manner. To account for this, researchers removed the gauge and syringe from the airways and instead attached them to the pipe that invaded the chamber, representing our pleural cavity. In this case, as in the case of a normal respiratory system, the airways and alveoli are open to the atmosphere. By pulling on the syringe, we create a negative pressure inside the chamber, and the lungs inflate. A chamber or pleural pressure of −2 cmH$_2$O would cause the lung volume to be approximately 1/5th of the total lung capacity [3].

Notice the similarities between this and the previous experiment. At total lung capacity in the first example, the pressure gauge read +25 cmH$_2$O, as that was the pressure being applied directly to the airway. In this example, the gauge would read −25 cmH$_2$O, as this subatmospheric pressure in the chamber still causes the lungs to fully inflate. An important note is that the elastic recoil of the lungs is the same in both experiments, and is +25 cmH$_2$O, as the elastic recoil is always positive.

These experiments set the basis for discussion of lung mechanics in the thoracic cavity. We previously discussed the FRC including that it corresponds to roughly ½ of the total lung inflation and is approximately +5 cmH$_2$O if one were to measure the pressure inside the lung, or −5 cmH$_2$O if one were to measure the pressure inside the pleural cavity. For our purposes, we will refer to pressure as pleural or chamber pressures, as is commonplace in literature. In a clinical setting, FRC is defined as the volume of air in the lungs at the resting expiratory level. In simple terms, it is the volume of the lungs when the glottis (vocal cords), or the airway to the atmosphere, is open and there is no airflow or effort to breathe. It is also the lung volume at the end of a quiet breath. Although muscular effort is required to inhale, no effort is required to exhale back to FRC, because the elastic recoil of the lungs does all the work. Thus, the pressure in the pleural cavity, at rest, is at −5 cmH$_2$O [3].

If the pleural region is sealed and intact, the respiratory system is stable at FRC. If air is introduced into the pleural space, the integrity of the system is compromised, and the pleural space is no longer at −5 cmH$_2$O, but now equal to atmospheric pressure. This causes the lung to deflate and collapse. Clinically, this is known as a pneumothorax.

Compliance and Elastance

To understand the basic physiology of the lungs, key biophysical concepts inter-twining lung anatomy and mechanics must be outlined. Two of these concepts, which are inversely related, include compliance and elastance. Compliance refers to the propensity of the anatomic structure, in this case both the lung and the chest wall, to allow expansion of volume to accommodate pressure changes. Elastance, on the other hand, refers to the propensity of the lungs or chest wall to return to rest-ing volume after being expanded. Mathematically, compliance can be represented by change in lung volume (DV) divided by the change in pressure (DP), while elas-tance can be represented by the reciprocal, DP divided by DV. Both of them must work in tandem for both the chest wall and the lungs themselves to maintain optimal inflation and deflation for adequate gas exchange [4]. Deviations to this lead to com-mon lung pathologies, including restrictive interstitial lung diseases with reduced lung compliance and chronic obstructive pulmonary disease with diminished lung elastance [5].

Airway Resistance and Drive Pressure

The next key factor affecting the amount of air that enters the lung during inspira-tion and exits the lung during exhalation is airway resistance. As discussed earlier in the chapter, the airway progresses from the trachea down to the individual alveolar air sacs where gas exchange ultimately occurs. As air travels through this pathway, it experiences resistance to flow. For simplicity, this resistance can be represented through modeling of airflow as laminar flow. With that assumption, resistance to flow at a specific point along the airway can be modeled with the following param-eters: air viscosity (m), length of the airway (L), and radius of the airway (r), with the overall resistance equation, $R = \dfrac{8\,\mathrm{mL}}{\neq r^4}$.

Using this model at specific points in the airway, it is clear that smaller diameter bronchioles have a much larger resistance to airflow than the larger diameter bron-chi or trachea. However, as air travels down the airway, the trachea splits into two bronchi which continually branch further eventually leading to terminal bronchioles and ultimately alveoli. As the airway splits, it becomes a parallel resistance circuit leading to an overall decrease in resistance at the terminal small airways compared to the large airways (trachea, bronchi). Furthermore, when looking at inspiration versus expiration, the overall diameter of the airways is increased during inspiration compared to expiration, so the overall airway resistance is greater during exhala-tion [6].

Lastly, a key aspect of ventilation includes the drive pressure, which is the pres-sure gradient that provides the force behind the airflow during inspiration and expi-ration. Using the concepts discussed earlier, the drive pressure can be described by the ratio between the tidal volume, which is the volume of air that goes into and out of the lung during a normal breathing cycle, and the overall compliance of the respiratory system, assuming a static overall compliance. This concept is key, because it attempts to quantify the pressure gradient needed to produce adequate volume expansion of the lungs. The ability to model and calculate this value can be used to guide therapy for patients. This will be useful later when mechanical ventilation strategies are discussed [7].

Work of Breathing

In normal physiology, to create the drive pressure needed to achieve the tidal volume, energy is required via adenosine triphosphate (ATP) to create mechanical changes through respiratory muscles moving the chest wall and the diaphragm. The amount of energy required for both inspiration and expiration can be quantified as work of breathing, expressed in units of energy (joules). To understand this in terms of respiratory physiology, the units can be manipulated to describe the energy expended in terms of a product of pressure and volume. Looking at the inspiratory work of breathing, several components discussed earlier are involved. First, work must be done to overcome the elastance or elastic recoil of both the chest wall and the lung. Second, work must be done to overcome the overall resistance from both the lung and chest wall tissue, as well as the airway resistance described above. The overall work for inspiration is the sum of these different components. As properties including elastance and resistance change, the work necessary to produce a specific tidal volume changes as well. This remains true when looking at the expiratory work of breathing. Overall, the drive pressure is generated through the contraction of respiratory muscles, which occurs using ATP created mainly from the metabolic pathway oxidative phosphorylation. Understanding the concept of the work of breathing will be necessary in subsequent chapters [8].

Gas Exchange

At the most fundamental level, the main function of the respiratory system is the exchange of oxygen (O_2) and carbon dioxide (CO_2) in a process known as gas exchange. As these gases are constantly produced and consumed during bodily reactions, there must be an efficient system for this exchange to occur. In the human body, gas exchange occurs in two predominant areas—the lungs and the peripheral tissues. The lungs provide the first location for gas exchange in a process known as ventilation while the peripheral tissues provide the second location for gas exchange in a process called oxygenation. The goal for the respiratory system is to bring atmospheric O_2 into the lungs for eventual distribution to the cells for cellular respiration. At the same time, these cells must rid themselves of their gaseous waste product, CO_2, for removal via the lungs. Thus, the respiratory system functions as a circuit, bringing O_2 into the body while removing CO_2. We will begin our discussion of gas exchange by exploring the concepts of ventilation and oxygenation. Ventilation is the process of bringing O_2 from the atmosphere into the lungs whereas oxygenation is the uptake of O_2 in the lungs followed by O_2 delivery to the body. Oxygenation is the process that delivers oxygenated blood from our pulmonary and systemic circulation to the peripheral tissues.

Ventilation

Ventilation is a topic central to lung physiology that brings together foundational concepts of chemistry and physics. Simplistically, ventilation is the movement of gases in and out of the lungs. The impact of this seemingly simple process influences a number of systems, best understood beginning with blood flow to the lungs, following it as it interfaces with alveoli, and finally finishes at the tissue level in the body. Air enters the body via the upper respiratory tract which includes the nasal cavities, pharynx, and larynx. Along the upper respiratory tract, the air is humidified by mucus in the airway and heated from the blood traveling in adjacent blood vessels. Beyond the upper airway, the air continues into the lower respiratory tract which contains the trachea, bronchi, bronchioles, and alveoli. The upper airway, trachea, and bronchi predominantly function in the conduction of air and do not play a major role in gas exchange. Alternatively, the respiratory bronchioles and alveoli of the lower respiratory tract play a major role in gas exchange.

Once the now humidified and heated air reaches the terminal portions of the lower respiratory tract, it diffuses across the lung's air-filled sacs called alveoli. Each human lung contains roughly 150 million alveoli whose compact shape and distribution allow for roughly 50–75 m^2 of surface area for gas exchange. The alveolar epithelium is composed of simple squamous epithelium that enables efficient diffusion of gases. On the basal lamina of the alveoli, there is a very thin membrane (varying from 0.2 mm to 2.2 mm in thickness) known as the respiratory membrane. It is across this membrane that the O_2 diffuses from alveoli to the pulmonary capillaries. The alveolar respiratory membrane is separated from the pulmonary capillaries by only a tiny interstitial space, providing an advantageously small distance for gaseous diffusion into the capillary blood. CO_2 diffuses out of the pulmonary capillaries into the airway and is removed from the body via the respiratory tract [3].

Perfusion

Cardiac output from the heart is a mostly parallel circuit with equal quantities of blood delivered to both the systemic and pulmonary circulations. The delivery of blood and its "perfusion" to the lungs differ from that of systemic circulation in a number of ways.

First, the pressures within the pulmonary vasculature are low, with average systolic of 25 mmHg, diastolic of 8 mmHg, and mean of 15 mmHg, denoted with the syntax 25/8 (15). These numbers are approximately 1/4 to 1/5 that of systemic circulation [9]. Additionally, unlike systemic circulation where the majority of pressure loss in the system occurs at an arteriole level, instead in pulmonary vessels, this loss occurs directly at the capillary bed [10].

Also unique to pulmonary perfusion is its "capacitance" or ability to handle increases in cardiac output without a proportional increase in pressure. For example, during exercise, flow to lungs can increase 4–5 times that of baseline with relatively unchanged pressures. Systemic circulation significantly contrasts this, with increases in systolic pressure in excess of 50% during exercise. Consequently, when comparing both circulations, pulmonary resistance can be as much as ten times lower than that of systemic [9].

The capacitance of the pulmonary circuit can partly be described by a phenomenon where areas of the lungs, at rest, are unequally perfused. During times of increased cardiac output, recruitment of additional alveoli to participate in gas exchange as well as dilation of blood vessels occurs which is reflected in a large drop in resistance. "West zones" dividing the lung into base or 1, midportion or 2, and apex or 3 help describe the relationship between alveolar and arterial pressure with the result of lung bases being preferentially perfused (Fig. 2.1) [11].

Finally, a remnant of fetal physiology also has large impacts on lung perfusion. In utero, O_2 levels are much lower than those seen after birth and this results in vasoconstriction of pulmonary vasculature [11]. Aptly named "hypoxic

Fig. 2.1 Alveolar pressure (P_A) and arterial pressure (P_a) differences between the West zones of the lung

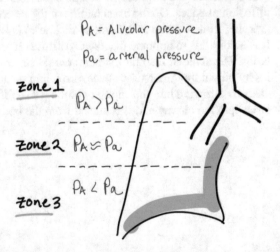

vasoconstriction," this mechanism persists beyond the womb. Alveoli not participating in gas exchange, for example during airway obstruction or external compression by a pneumothorax, experience lower levels of O_2, vasoconstriction of nearby vessels, and subsequently blood flow redirected towards areas of active gas exchange [12].

Dead Space

Understanding that areas of lung perfusion and ventilation are unequal brings up an important concept of ventilation called "dead space." Areas that are well ventilated, but poorly perfused, are central to this concept. Three types of dead space exist: physiologic, anatomical, and device related (Fig. 2.2).

Physiologic dead space is best seen at the apex of the lung or West zone 1. At rest these areas receive adequate movement of gases in and out of alveoli, however with minimal blood flow. This is normal physiology and varies based on cardiac output as previously described. The ratio of dead space to perfused alveoli can be calculated by the formula:

$$\frac{Dead\,space}{Perfused} = \frac{\left(Alveolar\,partial\,pressure\,carbon\,dioxide\right) - \left(Exhaled\,partial\,pressure\,carbon\,dioxide\right)}{\left(Arterial\,partial\,pressure\,carbon\,dioxide\right)}$$

Because it is nearly impossible to measure the partial pressure of CO_2 at the alveolar level, the arterial partial pressure of CO_2 is substituted instead [13].

Anatomical dead space exists within the airways where gases are transmitted from the atmosphere to alveoli but no gas exchange occurs. This includes all the volume from the trachea to the terminal bronchioles. The amount of anatomical

Fig. 2.2 Dead space may exist as related to the device, patient anatomy, or patient physiology

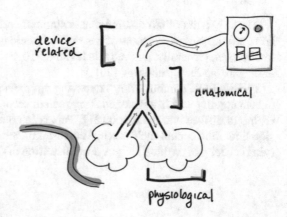

dead space is based on sex and height, and can be estimated at 1 mL/kg of ideal body weight [14].

Lastly, device- or apparatus-related dead space can exist. Mechanical ventilation requires tubes for delivering gases which exist outside of the body. These tubes contain a volume of gas that is considered dead space. This volume is generally clinically insignificant; however, it can become a problem with long circuits or small patients [15, 16].

Shunt

A related concept representing the opposite of "dead space" is "shunt" where blood travels from pulmonary to systemic circulations without gas exchange. This can occur within the lung where blood bypasses beyond areas of ventilated alveoli [17]. Additionally, blood can be "shunted" from pulmonary to systemic circulations at extrapulmonary locations which are seen in utero and congenital heart disease [18]. However, this extrapulmonary shunt physiology is complex and beyond the scope of this chapter.

A-a Gradient

As blood interfaces at the alveolar/endothelial basement membrane, gas exchange occurs. This process is primarily driven by diffusion. The volume of gas diffused is based on a number of factors including area, properties of gas, carrying capacity of blood/hemoglobin content, membrane thickness, and difference in partial pressures of gas from alveoli (Pa_{Alv}) to arterial (Pa_{Art}). These factors can be summarized in the following relationship [19]:

$$\text{Volume gas} = \frac{\text{Area} \times \text{Gas properties} \times \text{Hemoglobin content}}{\text{Thickness}} \times \left(Pa_{Alv} - Pa_{Art} \right)$$

The only part of this equation that is clinically relevant is the difference in alveolar to arterial partial pressures of gas or "A-a gradient" and their relative relationship to diffusion. Generally, this value is less than 10, but when elevated it can be helpful in diagnosing lung pathology [20].

For example, administering increasing amounts of O_2 to a patient with substantial shunt will result in a widened A-a gradient secondary to the relatively small area O_2 has to diffuse into the blood [21]. This is in contrast to instances where a diffusion limitation occurs such as with increased membrane thickness or decreased carrying capacity of the blood where administration of O_2 narrows the A-a gradient [22].

V/Q Mismatch

An additional cause of an increased A-a gradient that narrows with O_2 administration is "V/Q mismatch" or ventilation/perfusion mismatch [23]. Simplistically, this physiological condition represents areas of imbalanced ventilation and perfusion. This occurs under normal circumstances, described in previous sections by "West zones" where bases or zone 1 receives more perfusion than ventilation and apices or zone 3 experiences more ventilation than perfusion [24]. With approximately 4 L/min of ventilation and 5 L/min of perfusion to the lungs, the overall average V/Q ratio is 0.8 [25].

Pathologically this overall lung ratio can be decreased in instances of reduced ventilation such as obstructive lung disease, or increased with reduced pulmonary blood flow seen in pulmonary emboli [26].

Carbon Dioxide

The most important gas that diffuses at the alveolar/endothelial membrane and is central to ventilation is CO_2. This by-product of cellular respiration is used as a surrogate for the adequacy of ventilation, and its interaction with water is unique in that it contributes significantly to maintaining normal body pH.

The solubility of CO_2 into water is represented by the formula from Henry's law [27]:

$$\text{Dissolved carbon dioxide} = 0.0301\, mM\,/\,\text{mmHg} \times \text{Partial pressure of carbon dioxide}$$

With a normal partial pressure of this gas ranging from 35 to 45 mmHg, the total amount diffused in water is very small at approximately 1.2 mM.

However, CO_2 undergoes chemical change with water into the unstable intermediate of carbonic acid and then stable product bicarbonate, a weak acid. This reaction is represented in the equation $CO_2 + H_2O \rightleftharpoons H_2CO_3 \rightleftharpoons H^+ + HCO3^-$. As a weak acid, bicarbonate obeys the principles of the Henderson-Hasselbalch equation with its relationship to pH explained in the formula [28]

$$pH = 6.1 + \log\left[\frac{HCO3-}{Pa_{CO2} \times 0.0301}\right]$$

Using this formula, at physiologic pH of 7.4 with a partial pressure of CO_2 of 40 mmHg, approximately 24 mM of bicarbonate is soluble in water.

With this conversion to bicarbonate, a nearly 20 times increase in the capacity of water to carry CO_2 is seen beyond that of just dissolved gas. The acid base properties of this reaction also allow for relatively large amounts of CO_2 in the form of bicarbonate to be transported with small changes in pH. However, these small changes become clinically significant as normal physiologic pH is tightly regulated between 7.35 and 7.45 [29]. Increases in the partial pressure of CO_2 beyond 45 mmHg can lower pH beyond physiological limits. The opposite is also true with decreases in the partial pressure of this gas to less than 35 mmHg, increasing pH to values outside of physiological limits.

The rate at which CO_2 is eliminated via ventilation is represented by the alveolar ventilation equation, which is a derivation of the ideal gas law. In this equation, minute ventilation, volume of CO_2, and partial pressure of CO_2 are related to each other in the following formula [30]:

$$\text{Minute ventilation} = \frac{\text{Volume } CO_2}{\text{Pa}_{CO_2}} \times K \text{, where } K \text{ equals 863 at a body tempera-}$$

ture of 37 °C and 1 atmosphere.

The inverse relationship between minute ventilation and partial pressure of CO_2 is clinically useful in adjusting ventilation to match CO_2 production. For example, to halve a given partial pressure of CO_2, minute ventilation would have to double [31].

Bohr Effect

Emphasizing its importance to ventilation, the impacts of CO_2 extend beyond those of its influence on acid-base balance, and its clinical use to assess the adequacy of ventilation. At the tissue level, this gas has significant effects on the availability of O_2. The Bohr effect describes the elegant relationship between increasing levels of CO_2 and increased availability of O_2 gas that can be used in cellular respiration (Fig. 2.3) [32].

The mechanism of this process is a result of changes to the oxygen-hemoglobin dissociation curve, discussed in the below section. CO_2 reversibly interacts with the

Fig. 2.3 Graphical representation of the Bohr effect

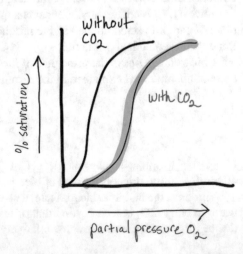

protein structure of hemoglobin, decreasing its affinity to O_2. This effectively shifts the overall oxygen-hemoglobin dissociation curve to the right [32].

The effect of this interaction is twofold. At the tissue level where CO_2 levels are high, it causes O_2 molecules to be "released" from hemoglobin. This stands in contrast to the conditions at the alveolar level where CO_2 gas is rapidly removed, increasing the affinity of hemoglobin to O_2. The overall net effect is an increase in the efficiency of oxygen transport to tissues [32].

O_2 Delivery to Tissues

Once in the blood, O_2 is carried in two forms: dissolved O_2 and O_2 that is reversibly bound to hemoglobin. During its journey to the tissues, dissolved O_2 accounts for roughly 2% of the total O_2 content in the blood while the remaining 98% of O_2 is reversibly bound to hemoglobin. Hemoglobin is a globular protein that contains four subunits. Each hemoglobin subunit is able to bind and transport one molecule of O_2 for a total of four molecules of O_2 per hemoglobin molecule. As we will go on to later explore, O_2 is able to dissociate from the hemoglobin molecule under different conditions. This dissociated O_2 is what exerts the partial pressure of O_2 within the blood, leading to important implications for O_2 delivery and gas exchange within the peripheral tissues.

The amount of dissolved O_2 in the blood abides by Henry's law regarding the concentrations of dissolved gases. In the context of blood as a solution, Henry's law states

$$Cx = Px \times \text{Solubility}$$

where Cx = concentration of dissolved gas (mL gas/100 mL blood), Px = partial pressure of gas (mmHg), and solubility = solubility of gas in blood (mL gas/100 mL blood per mmHg).

Henry's law demonstrates that the concentration of dissolved gas is directly proportional to the partial pressure of the gas and the solubility of the gas in the blood. The dissolved O_2 is solely responsible for exerting the partial pressure of O_2 in the blood. The partial pressure of O_2 is a crucial factor when it comes to establishing the gradient for oxygen's eventual exchange in the lungs and peripheral tissues.

Similar to the lungs, the capillaries within the peripheral tissues have thin membranes that allow for the rapid and efficient exchange of gases. O_2, bound to hemoglobin within the blood, is released for utilization by O_2-deprived tissues. At the same time, CO_2 is rapidly diffused from the peripheral tissues back into the capillaries for eventual removal by the lungs. In both ventilation and oxygenation, gas exchange occurs as a result of the underlying properties and laws that drive the movement of gases. We will now explore the underlying forces that drive the process of gas exchange.

The diffusion of O_2 and CO_2 in gas exchange is driven primarily by Fick's law for the diffusion of gases. Fick's law defines how the volume of gas transferred per unit time is affected by factors such as the diffusion coefficient of a specific gas, surface area for diffusion, partial pressure difference, and thickness of the membrane and it is represented by the following equation:

$$\dot{V}x = \frac{(D \times A \times \Delta P)}{\Delta x}$$

where $\dot{V}_x$ = volume of gas transferred per unit time, D = diffusion coefficient of the gas, A = surface area, ΔP = partial pressure difference of the gas, and Δx = membrane thickness.

This law states that the volume of gas transferred per unit of time is directly proportional to the diffusion coefficient of the gas, surface area available for diffusion, and partial pressure difference of the gas. Conversely, the volume of gas transferred per unit of time is inversely proportional to the thickness of the membrane. The main driving force for the volume of gas transferred per unit time is the partial pressure difference of the gas across the membrane. As previously mentioned, the partial pressure of O_2 in the blood is exerted by the amount of freely dissolved, non-bound O_2 in the blood. In the context of O_2 diffusion in the lungs and peripheral tissues, the larger the gradient of partial pressure of O_2 across the membrane, the larger the volume of gas transferred per unit time.

Haldane Effect

The removal of CO_2 from the tissues is another key component of gas exchange. CO_2 exists in the body in three forms: dissolved CO_2, carbaminohemoglobin (CO_2 bound to hemoglobin), or bicarbonate. As mentioned previously, CO_2 binds to hemoglobin as carbaminohemoglobin at a site different from O_2 and decreases hemoglobin's affinity for O_2. This effect is known as the Bohr effect. Alternatively, O_2 affects hemoglobin's affinity for CO_2 in a process known as the Haldane effect. When less O_2 is bound to hemoglobin, the affinity for CO_2 is increased. The Bohr and Haldane effects operate in tandem at the peripheral tissues. As the amount of CO_2 increases, hemoglobin's affinity for O_2 decreases (Bohr effect), and as the amount of O_2 on hemoglobin decreases, hemoglobin increases its affinity for CO_2. At the molecular level, the Bohr and Haldane effects lead to an efficient system for delivery of O_2 with concurrent removal of CO_2.

Oxyhemoglobin Dissociation Curve

The O_2-hemoglobin dissociation curve demonstrates how hemoglobin saturation with O_2 varies with changes in the pressure of O_2. As mentioned previously, hemoglobin is a globular protein with four subunits, each of which can bind one molecule of O_2 for a total of four molecules of O_2 per molecule of hemoglobin.

The sigmoid shape of the O_2-hemoglobin dissociation curve demonstrates an important concept related to the hemoglobin molecule called positive cooperativity. The hemoglobin molecule is structured in such a way that its affinity for a molecule of O_2 increases as each molecule binds. This means that as the first molecule of O_2 binds to hemoglobin, there is a stronger affinity for a second molecule of O_2 to bind, and so on.

The curve also demonstrates why O_2 has a preference for binding to hemoglobin in the lungs and a preference for dissociating in the peripheral tissues. As you move from right to left along the curve, the hemoglobin saturation percent increases as the partial pressure of oxygen (PO_2) increases. The systemic arterial blood has a PO_2 of roughly 100 mmHg which correlates to 100% hemoglobin saturation. As the pulmonary capillary blood also has a PO_2 of 100 mmHg, hemoglobin becomes nearly 100% saturated with O_2 in the lungs. Alternatively, in the peripheral tissues, mixed venous blood has a PO_2 of roughly 40 mm Hg meaning that the hemoglobin saturation will be lower as demonstrated by the curve and the O_2 will have a higher propensity to be off-loaded. Let us now explore how changes in certain factors lead to shifts with the O_2-hemoglobin dissociation curve.

There are four main factors that tend to shift the O_2-hemoglobin dissociation curve to the right or the left. These factors are P_{CO2}, pH, temperature, and 2,3-diphosphoglycerate (2,3-DPG). Shifts of the curve to the right demonstrate a decreased affinity for O_2 to hemoglobin. When tissues are in highly metabolic states, they produce CO_2 as waste, leading to a subsequent drop in the pH of that area. CO_2 binds to hemoglobin at a site different from O_2. As previously described, the binding of CO_2 to hemoglobin leads to increased O_2 dissociation from hemoglobin and this is known as the Bohr effect. Additionally, metabolic tissues produce heat, leading to an increase in temperature. This increase in temperature leads to a decrease in oxygen's affinity for hemoglobin, leading to an increase in O_2 dissociation from hemoglobin. The increased CO_2, decreased pH, and increased temperature indicate that tissues are utilizing O_2 through metabolic cellular respiration. As a result, more O_2 is needed and the O_2-hemoglobin dissociation curve shifts to the right. Lastly, 2,3-DPG indicates hypoxic tissue as it is a by-product of glycolysis. Rates of glycolysis increase during anaerobic conditions leading to an increase in the production of 2,3-DPG. When 2,3-DPG binds to hemoglobin, it decreases the affinity for O_2 to hemoglobin and leads to a subsequent off-loading of O_2 in these hypoxic tissues. Shifts in the O_2-hemoglobin dissociation curve to the left demonstrate an increased affinity for O_2 binding and are caused by the same factors described above. These factors shift the curve to the left for the exact opposite contextual reason that shifts the curve to the right.

Hypoxemia vs. Hypoxia

Hypoxemia and hypoxia both refer to lack of O_2. However, hypoxemia is more specifically decreased arterial PO_2 while hypoxia is decreased O_2 at the tissue level. As mentioned previously, O_2 contained in atmospheric air travels through the respiratory tract to the alveoli where it is diffused into the pulmonary capillaries. Hypoxemia is defined as decreased arterial PO_2, indicating either an issue with the actual inspiration of O_2 or an issue somewhere along the respiratory tract. Causes of hypoxemia include high altitude, hypoventilation, diffusion defects across the membranes, ventilation/perfusion (V/Q) defect, and right-to-left shunts.

Approximately, 2% of O_2 in the blood is found as dissolved O_2. This dissolved O_2 is able to exert a partial pressure known as PaO_2. The remaining 98% of O_2 is bound to hemoglobin. The percentage of hemoglobin sites that are saturated is known as the SaO_2. O_2 content in the blood, denoted by CaO_2, is calculated by adding the amount of dissolved O_2 with the amount of O_2 bound to hemoglobin. CaO_2 can be better represented by the following equation:

$$CaO_2 = \left(Hb \times 1.34 \frac{ml\,O_2}{gm\,Hb} * SaO_2 \right) + \left(PaO_2 \times 0.003\,ml\,O_2\,/\,mmHg\,/\,dl \right)$$

where Hb = hemoglobin, 1.34 = oxygen-combining capacity, SaO_2 = oxygen saturation, PaO_2 = partial pressure of arterial oxygen, and 0.003 = solubility coefficient of oxygen at body temperature.

Lastly, O_2 delivery (D_{O2}) is calculated using cardiac output and O_2 content of the blood (CaO_2). It is represented by the following equation:

$$D_{O2} = Q \times CaO_2$$

where DO_2 = oxygen delivery in mL/min, Q = cardiac output in L/min, and CaO_2 = oxygen content.

The O_2 delivery equation demonstrates that DO_2 is directly proportional to cardiac output and O_2 content within the blood. As cardiac output or O_2 content of the blood increases, O_2 delivery will also increase. Decreased cardiac output or O_2 content will lead to subsequent decreased O_2 delivery.

Altitude Effects on Gas Exchange

Altitude is defined as height in relation to sea or ground level, and with increases, there is a decrease in atmospheric pressure. Atmospheric pressure refers to the total pressure of the total components of air at a specific height. While changes in atmospheric pressure with altitude have no direct effect on O_2 concentration within inspired air, it reduces the overall partial pressure of O_2 which is the main driver of gas exchange as discussed earlier. With this decreased partial pressure of inspired O_2, the partial pressure of O_2 in the alveoli and subsequently the artery is decreased compared to sea level. Interestingly, the alveolar-arterial gradient is actually increased compared to sea level due to gas exchange and diffusion not being limited to ventilation-perfusion matching. This is because blood traveling through the lung capillaries is inadequately oxygenated as a result of reduced drive pressure which in turn causes hypoxic vasoconstriction and thus longer time for gas exchange to occur. Exercise at high altitudes can lead to hypoxia due to the larger role of V/Q matching with inability to maintain slow transit time due to higher cardiac output. Over time, the body can acclimate to the changes in gas exchange at higher altitudes. However, if the rise in altitude is too rapid, then the hypoxia and resulting pulmonary hypertension can lead to pulmonary edema and altitude sickness [33].

Normal Physiologic Parameters

In this chapter, the authors have introduced fundamental topics in lung anatomy and physiology. The subsequent tables are intended to serve as a reference of normal physiologic parameters for arterial blood gas (Table 2.1), PaO_2 (Table 2.2), arterial pH and $PaCO_2$ in men (Table 2.3), arterial pH and $PaCO_2$ in women (Table 2.4), respiratory parameters for adults (Table 2.5), and venous blood gas values (Table 2.6).

Table 2.1 Normal arterial blood gas values [34]

Parameter	Normal range
pH	7.36–7.44
$PaCO_2$	35–45 mmHg
PaO_2	80–100 mmHg
SaO_2	95–97%
HCO_3	22–26 mEq/L
Base excess	±3 mmol/L

Table 2.2 PaO_2: Altitude- and age-adjusted normal values [35]

Age	0 m	1000 m	2000 m
	PaO_2	PaO_2	PaO_2
19–24	102.1–103.5	86.7–88.2	74.2–75.6
25–34	99.6–101.8	84.3–86.5	71.7–73.9
35–44	97.1–99.4	81.8–84.0	69.3–71.5
45–54	94.7–96.9	79.4–81.6	66.8–69.0
55–64	92.2–94.5	76.9–79.1	64.4–66.6
65–74	92.0–89.8	74.5–76.7	61.9–64.1
75–84	87.3–89.5	72.0–74.2	59.5–61.7

Table 2.3 Arterial pH and $PaCO_2$ in men [35]

Altitude	pH	$PaCO_2$
0 m	7.42 (7.38–7.46)	38.3 (33.0–43.7)
1000 m	7.43 (7.39–7.47)	35.1 (29.8–40.5)
2000 m	7.44 (7.40–7.48)	32.5 (27.1–37.8)

Table 2.4 Arterial pH and $PaCO_2$ in women [35]

Altitude	pH	$PaCO_2$
0 m	7.43 (7.39–7.46)	37.2 (31.8–42.5)
1000 m	7.44 (7.40–7.47)	34.0 (28.6–39.3)
2000 m	7.45 (7.41–7.48)	31.3 (26.0–36.7)

Table 2.5 Normal values for respiratory parameters for average adult [36–38]

Parameter	Normal value
End tidal CO_2	30–35 mmHg
Dead space (Vd)	150 mL
Tidal volume (Vt)	500 mL
Vd/Vt	28–33%
Minute ventilation (VE)	5–8 L/min
Arterial oxygen content (CaO_2)	19–20 ml O_2/dl blood
Oxygen delivery (DO_2)	900–1100 mL/min
Oxygen consumption (VO_2)	200–250 mL/min
Mixed venous oxygen saturation (SvO_2)	65%

Table 2.6 Normal venous blood gas values

Parameter	Normal value
pH	7.31–7.41
pCO_2	40–50 mmHg
pO_2	36–42 mmHg
SO_2	60–80%
Bicarbonate	22–26 mEq/L
Base excess	±3 mmol/L

Conflicts of Interest   None

Financial Disclosures   None

References

1. Gilroy AM, MacPherson BR, Wikenheiser J. Atlas of anatomy. 4th ed. New York, NY: Thieme Medical Publishers, Inc.; 2020.
2. Wikenheiser J. Clinical anatomy, histology, embryology, and neuroanatomy: an integrated textbook. New York, NY: Thieme Medical Publishers, Inc.; 2021.
3. Costanzo LS. Physiology. 6th ed. Amsterdam: Elsevier, Inc.; 2018.
4. Desai JP. Pulmonary compliance. Treasure Island, FL: StatPearls; 2020. NCBI Bookshelf. NCBI. https://www.ncbi.nlm.nih.gov/books/NBK538324/
5. Edwards Z, Annamaraju P. Physiology, lung compliance. Treasure Island, FL: StatPearls; 2020. NCBI Bookshelf. NCBI. https://www.ncbi.nlm.nih.gov/books/NBK554517/
6. Hurley JJ, Hensley JL. Physiology, airway resistance. Treasure Island, FL: StatPearls; 2020. NCBI Bookshelf. NCBI. https://www.ncbi.nlm.nih.gov/books/NBK542183/
7. Williams EC, Motta-Ribeiro GC, Vidal Melo MF. Driving pressure and transpulmonary pressure: how do we guide safe mechanical ventilation? Anesthesiology. 2019;131(1):155–63. https://doi.org/10.1097/ALN.000000000000273.
8. Dekerlegand RL, Cahalin LP, Perme C. Respiratory failure. Phys Rehabil. 2007:689–717. https://doi.org/10.1016/b978-072160361-2.50029-6.
9. Buchan TA, Wright SP, Esfandiari S, et al. Pulmonary hemodynamic and right ventricular responses to brief and prolonged exercise in middle-aged endurance athletes. Am J Physiol Heart Circ Physiol. 2019;316(2):H326–34. https://doi.org/10.1152/ajpheart.00413.2018.
10. Bidani A, Flumerfelt RW, Crandall ED. Analysis of the effects of pulsatile capillary blood flow and volume on gas exchange. Respir Physiol. 1978;35(1):27–42. https://doi.org/10.1016/0034-5687(78)90038-5.
11. Dawson A. Regional pulmonary blood flow in sitting and supine man during and after acute hypoxia. J Clin Invest. 1969;48(2):301–10. https://doi.org/10.1172/JCI105986.
12. Carlsson AJ, Bindslev L, Santesson J, Gottlieb I, Hedenstierna G. Hypoxic pulmonary vasoconstriction in the human lung: the effect of prolonged unilateral hypoxic challenge during anaesthesia. Acta Anaesthesiol Scand. 1985;29(3):346–51. https://doi.org/10.1111/j.1399-6576.1985.tb02212.x.
13. Singleton GJ, Olsen CR, Smith RL. Correction for mechanical dead space in the calculation of physiological dead space. J Clin Invest. 1972;51(10):2768–72. https://doi.org/10.1172/JCI107097.
14. Nunn JF, Campbell EJ, Peckett BW. Anatomical subdivisions of the volume of respiratory dead space and effect of position of the jaw. J Appl Physiol. 1959;14(2):174–6. https://doi.org/10.1152/jappl.1959.14.2.174.
15. Marsh MJ, Ingram D, Milner AD. The effect of instrumental dead space on measurement of breathing pattern and pulmonary mechanics in the newborn. Pediatr Pulmonol. 1993;16(5):316–22. https://doi.org/10.1002/ppul.1950160508.
16. Sackner JD, Nixon AJ, Davis B, Atkins N, Sackner MA. Effects of breathing through external dead space on ventilation at rest and during exercise. II. Am Rev Respir Dis. 1980;122(6):933–40. https://doi.org/10.1164/arrd.1980.122.6.933.
17. Tobin CE, Zariquiey MO. Arteriovenous shunts in the human lung. Proc Soc Exp Biol Med. 1950;75(3):827–9. https://doi.org/10.3181/00379727-75-18360.
18. Rowe GG, Castillo CA, Maxwell GM, Clifford JF, Crumpton CW. Atrial septal defect and the mechanism of shunt. Am Heart J. 1961;61(3):369–74. https://doi.org/10.1016/0002-8703(61)90608-1.
19. Forster RE. Exchange of gases between alveolar air and pulmonary capillary blood: pulmonary diffusing capacity. Physiol Rev. 1957;37(4):391–452. https://doi.org/10.1152/physrev.1957.37.4.391.
20. Harris EA, Kenyon AM, Nisbet HD, Seelye ER, Whitlock RM. The normal alveolar-arterial oxygen-tension gradient in man. Clin Sci Mol Med. 1974;46(1):89–104. https://doi.org/10.1042/cs0460089.

21. Ploysongsang Y, Wiltse DW. Effects of breathing pattern and oxygen upon the alveolar arterial oxygen pressure difference in lung disease. Respiration. 1985;47(1):39–47. https://doi.org/10.1159/000194747.

22. Austrian R, McClement JH, Renzetti AD, Donald KW, Riley RL, Cournand A. Clinical and physiologic features of some types of pulmonary diseases with impairment of alveolar-capillary diffusion. Am J Med. 1951;11(6):667–85. https://doi.org/10.1016/0002-9343(51)90019-8.

23. Peris LV, Boix JH, Salom JV, Valentin V, Garcia D, Arnau A. Clinical use of the arterial/alveolar oxygen tension ratio. Crit Care Med. 1983;11(11):888–91. https://doi.org/10.1097/00003246-198311000-00010.

24. Kramer EL, Sanger JJ. 81mKr gas and 99mTc-MAA V/Q ratio images for detection of V/Q mismatches. Eur J Nucl Med. 1984;9(8):345–50. https://doi.org/10.1007/BF00252867.

25. Rhodes CG, Valind SO, Brudin LH, et al. Quantification of regional V/Q ratios in humans by use of PET. II. Procedure and normal values. J Appl Physiol. 1989;66(4):1905–13. https://doi.org/10.1152/jappl.1989.66.4.1905.

26. Meignan M, Simonneau G, Oliveira L, et al. Computation of ventilation-perfusion ratio with Kr-81m in pulmonary embolism. J Nucl Med. 1984;25(2):149–55.

27. Austin WH, Lacombe E, Rand PW, Chatterjee M. Solubility of carbon dioxide in serum from 15 to 38 C. J Appl Physiol. 1963;18:301–4. https://doi.org/10.1152/jappl.1963.18.2.301.

28. Chittamma A, Vanavanan S. Comparative study of calculated and measured total carbon dioxide. Clin Chem Lab Med. 2008;46(1):15–7. https://doi.org/10.1515/CCLM.2008.005.

29. Andrews JL, Copeland BE, Salah RM, Morrissey B, Enos EJ, Spilios A. Arterial blood gas standards for healthy young nonsmoking subjects. Am J Clin Pathol. 1981;75(6):773–80. https://doi.org/10.1093/ajcp/75.6.773.

30. Caiozzo VJ, Davis JA, Berriman DJ, Vandagriff RB, Prietto CA. Effect of high-intensity exercise on the VE-VCO2 relationship. J Appl Physiol. 1987;62(4):1460–4. https://doi.org/10.1152/jappl.1987.62.4.1460.

31. Allen CJ, Jones NL. Rate of change of alveolar carbon dioxide and the control of ventilation during exercise. J Physiol (Lond). 1984;355:1–9. https://doi.org/10.1113/jphysiol.1984.sp015401.

32. Malte H, Lykkeboe G. The Bohr/Haldane effect: a model-based uncovering of the full extent of its impact on O2 delivery to and CO2 removal from tissues. J Appl Physiol. 2018;125(3):916–22. https://doi.org/10.1152/japplphysiol.00140.2018.

33. Peacock AJ. ABC of oxygen: oxygen at high altitude. BMJ (Clin Res ed). 1998;317(7165):1063–6. https://doi.org/10.1136/bmj.317.7165.1063.

34. Miaskiewicz JJ. Pulmonary function testing. In: McKean SC, Ross JJ, Dressler DD, Scheurer DB, editors. Principles and practice of hospital medicine, 2e. New York: McGraw-Hill. Accessed 03 June 2021. https://accessmedicine.mhmedical.com/content.aspx?bookid=1872&sectionid=146978117.

35. Crapo RO, Jensen RL, Hegewald M, Tashkin DP. Arterial blood gas reference values for sea level and an altitude of 1,400 meters. Am J Respir Crit Care Med. 1999;160(5 Pt 1):1525–31. https://doi.org/10.1164/ajrccm.160.5.9806006.

36. Respiratory physiology & anesthesia. In: Butterworth IV JF, Mackey DC, Wasnick JD. eds. Morgan & Mikhail's clinical anesthesiology, 6e. New York: McGraw-Hill. Accessed 03 June 2021. https://accessmedicine.mhmedical.com/content.aspx?bookid=2444&sectionid=193560150

37. Alveolar ventilation. In: Levitzky MG. ed. Pulmonary physiology, 9e. New York: McGraw-Hill. Accessed 03 June 2021. https://accessmedicine.mhmedical.com/content.aspx?bookid=2288&sectionid=178856748

38. Alba Yunen R, Oropello JM. Pulmonary artery catheterization. In: Oropello JM, Pastores SM, Kvetan V, editors. Critical care. New York: McGraw-Hill. Accessed June 03, 2021. https://accessmedicine.mhmedical.com/content.aspx?bookid=1944&sectionid=143523126.

Chapter 3
Respiratory Mechanics and Ventilation

Sonali Rao, Meleeka Akbarpour, and Jessica J. Tang

History of Mechanical Ventilation

The story of mechanical ventilators parallels the broader story of developments in medicine and engineering.

References to artificial ventilation can be found in passages as early as from the Bible. However, some of the earliest attempts to mechanically ventilate patients can be traced back to the late eighteenth century. The Royal Humane Society of England began supporting the use of bellows as a means of artificial respiration. Although the force and volume of air could not be well controlled through this method, it mimicked one of the fundamental processes of breathing: forcing air directly into the lungs. This system is known as positive-pressure ventilation (PPV).

Another early attempt at ventilation was developed in the 1830s by Dr. John Dalziel. Dr. Dalziel's device consisted of an airtight box that was used to rhythmically pump air to rescue drowning sailors. This technique would later be known as negative-pressure ventilation (NPV) [1]. Rather than pushing air into the respiratory system like positive-pressure ventilation, this process changes the external air pressure, indirectly forcing air into and out of the lungs as the body equalizes the pressure between the atmosphere and respiratory system. Many early ventilators were modeled on this negative-pressure principle, including one of the most commonly recognized ventilation devices from the early twentieth century, the iron lung.

NPV works by exposing the surface of the thorax to pressures below that of atmospheric pressure during inspiration, thereby indirectly facilitating the movement of air into the lungs. In a NPV such as the iron lung, the patient lies on a bed

S. Rao (✉) · M. Akbarpour
Irvine School of Medicine, University of California, Irvine, CA, USA
e-mail: sonaliar@hs.uci.edu; akbarpom@hs.uci.edu

J. J. Tang
Kaiser Permanente Santa Clara, Santa Clara, CA, USA

© The Author(s), under exclusive license to Springer Nature Switzerland AG 2022
A. A. Hakimi et al. (eds.), *Mechanical Ventilation Amid the COVID-19 Pandemic*,
https://doi.org/10.1007/978-3-030-87978-5_3

with their body covered by a sealed tank from the neck down. The tank mimics the movement of the human diaphragm such that as the diaphragm in the tank expands, it creates a negative pressure within the tank and the patient's body. This pressure gradient between the atmosphere and the lungs ultimately draws air into the lungs during inhalation [1]. When the pressure surrounding the thorax increases and reaches atmospheric pressure, expiration occurs passively. Ultimately, the inspiratory changes with NPV, in pleural and alveolar pressures, replicate those during spontaneous breathing.

In 1904, Dr. Ferdinand Sauerbruch created a negative-pressure operating chamber which enclosed the patient's entire body except for the head [1]. This chamber was large enough for surgeries to be performed inside it. Later in 1928, the Drinker-Shaw iron lung was developed, which became the first widely used negative-pressure ventilator. Inspired by Dr. Drinker's iron lung, John Emerson, an engineer of medical equipment, sought to improve his predecessor's model [1]. Emerson built and successfully tested his first model in 1931. It was a quieter, lighter, and less expensive version of Dr. Drinker's device, and by the 1940s was widely adopted as the ventilator of preference during the polio epidemic (Fig. 3.1).

In the 1960s, the use of NPV began to decline as these ventilators were heavy and would frequently leak, making it difficult to maintain effective ventilation and high airway pressure. By the end of World War II, focus was instead shifted towards developing volume-targeted ventilators and small intermittent positive-pressure breathing (IPPB) devices [1].

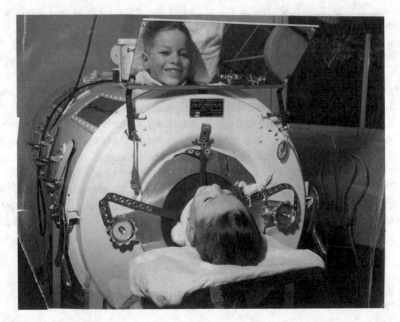

Fig. 3.1 The Emerson respirator, more commonly known as an "iron lung." Photo credit: "NCP4145" by otisarchives4 is licensed under CC BY 2.0

Noninvasive Positive-Pressure Ventilation

Noninvasive positive-pressure ventilation (NPPV) provides ventilatory support without the use of artificial airways, such as an endotracheal or tracheostomy tube. NPPV was first used in 1780, and was described as a bellows-type device [1]. In 1910, Green and Janeway introduced a novel approach to providing NPPV, in which a patient's head was placed into a sealed chamber filled with positive pressure. By the twentieth century, the Bennett TV and PR ventilators along with the Bird Mask series of ventilators became commonly used for life support [1]. The use of noninvasive ventilation has increased over the past two decades in the management of both acute and chronic respiratory failure, both in the home and critical care settings.

Positive-Pressure Invasive Ventilators

By the 1940s and 1950s, a new form of ventilation began to emerge. This new method required more invasive interventions, requiring endotracheal tubes, but provided volume-control ventilation. The most basic ventilator was the Morch ventilator, a single-circuit piston ventilator without monitors, alarms, or specific settings [1]. Operators would count the respiratory rate and measure tidal volume on another device. The most advanced ventilator was the Engstrom ventilator, which had a double circuit, allowing for anesthesia delivery or ventilation, and included airway pressure and tidal volume monitoring. This allowed for a more exact control of respiratory rate. The Emerson postoperative ventilator was a hybrid of the Morch and Engstrom ventilators. It was a single-circuit volume-controlled ventilator that provided machine-triggered inspiration, but had pressure and volume monitoring.

The second generation of mechanical ventilators incorporated simple patient monitors which monitored tidal volume and respiratory rate. However, the most distinguishing feature of this generation of ventilators was patient-triggered inspiration. After the introduction of intermittent mandatory ventilation (IMV), pressure-support and pressure-control ventilation shortly followed with the introduction of Servo 900C in 1981 [1].

Third-generation mechanical ventilators included the Puritan Bennett 7200, the Bear 1000, the Servo 300, and the Hamilton Veolar [1]. These ventilators incorporated microprocessor control, allowing for multiple approaches to gas delivery and monitoring. Almost every third-generation mechanical ventilator included pressure support, pressure control, volume control, and synchronized intermittent mandatory ventilation. Additionally, waveforms of pressure, flow, and volume, as well as pressure-volume and flow-volume loops, were first introduced with these ventilators. The present-day mechanical ventilators are fourth-generation machines which are the most complex and versatile.

Today's mechanical ventilators include a myriad of ventilation modes that are based on closed-loop control and a pressure-targeted approach. These new ventilators are customizable and can display and monitor up to 40 unique variables. SmartCare is a form of closed-loop control of pressure support for weaning. The ventilator automatically adjusts the pressure support level every few minutes to maintain a predefined respiratory rate, tidal volume, and end-tidal partial pressure of CO_2 (P_{CO2}). When the pressure support level is reduced to a predetermined level, the ventilator automatically performs a spontaneous breathing trial (SBT). If the patient fails the SBT, the ventilator automatically resumes ventilation. If the patient passes the SBT, the ventilator notifies the user that the patient should be considered for extubation.

Proportional assist ventilation and neurally adjusted ventilatory assist are available among the fourth-generation ventilators, but will likely be more commonly used in the future. With these, the mode, pressure, flow, volume, and time are not set. Instead, the proportion of a patient's ventilatory effort that is unloaded without forcing a ventilatory pattern is set. Proportional assist ventilation functions by responding to the mechanical output of the diaphragm and accessory muscles of inspiration. The neurally adjusted ventilatory assist functions by responding to the neural input to the diaphragm.

Basics of Mechanical Ventilation

Breaths delivered by a mechanical ventilator are defined by four phases: the trigger phase (how the breath is initiated), the inspiratory phase (how the breath gets delivered), the cycle phase (how inspiration ends and expiration begins), and the expiratory phase (the baseline pressure during the period between breaths). Each of these four phases can be manipulated on the ventilator to achieve optimal oxygenation.

The trigger phase is activated by the patient's inspiratory (negative) pressure or inspiration reaching a set point. Alternatively, a third trigger is time based on the setting for the respiratory rate. If the patient does not trigger any breaths, the ventilator will deliver breaths based on time. For example: with a rate or frequency set at 10 breaths per minute (BPM) in a patient who is not making any efforts to breathe, a breath will be given every six seconds to achieve 10 BPM.

Inspiratory flow delivered by the ventilator is most often a set rate, known as a square flow pattern or a decelerating (also known as ramp) flow pattern where flow starts at a high level and then tapers down with no preset value for peak flow. Newer generations of ventilators can provide a combination of fixed and variable flows in the use of dual modes such as volume-assured pressure support and pressure augmentation. The cycle phase is a function of the preset inspiratory time and preset tidal volume (or flow over time to deliver a targeted tidal volume). The baseline pressure may be zero, where pressure is not elevated between breaths, or elevated above zero to a positive pressure that is held in the lungs by the action of the exhalation valve in the ventilator.

Ventilator Settings

Ventilator settings are the controls on a mechanical ventilator that can be set or adjusted in order to determine the amount of support that is delivered to the patient. Support is provided in the form of ventilation and oxygenation. These two factors can be adjusted by manipulating settings such as mode, tidal volume, FiO_2, positive end-expiratory pressure (PEEP), and respiratory rate.

Examples of the basic ventilator settings:

- Mode
- Tidal volume
- Frequency (rate)
- FiO_2
- Flow rate
- I:E ratio
- Sensitivity
- PEEP
- Alarms

Each of these topics is discussed in more detail in subsequent chapters.

Conflicts of Interest The authors have no relevant conflicts of interest to disclose.

Funding This work was not funded.

Reference

1. Kacmarek RM. The mechanical ventilator: past, present, and future. Respir Care. 2011;56(8):1170–80. https://doi.org/10.4187/respcare.01420.

Chapter 4
Mechanical Ventilators and Monitors: An Abridged Guide for Engineers

Jay Shen, Luke Hoffmann, and Linsey Wilson

Who Uses a Ventilator? What Level of Training Is Needed?

Since their invention, ventilators have mainly been used in hospitals to assist patients with different forms of respiratory failure. During the nineteenth and first half of the twentieth centuries, negative-pressure ventilators were large cumbersome devices that were mostly stationary and filled large hospital wards [1]. As positive-pressure ventilators began to take hold in the second half of the twentieth century, these devices have become smaller and more portable, which expanded their footprint from hospitals to the field, and even to patient homes. Modern-day ventilators are no bigger than a purse, can be battery powered, and simply require an oxygen tank for fresh gas flow.

In the hospital and nursing home settings, physicians or mid-level providers (physician assistants and nurse practitioners) typically write the ventilator setting orders, which are then carried out by the respiratory therapist (RT). Because ventilator settings can be changed multiple times a day, this pathway ensures that ventilator settings are not updated by multiple parties, which can lead to confusion for care teams. Bedside nurses are also usually quite familiar with using the ventilator, but are generally encouraged to follow the above pathway, unless there is no RT or physician present.

J. Shen (✉)
Department of Anesthesiology & Perioperative Care, Irvine Medical Center,
University of California, Orange, CA, USA
e-mail: jayys@hs.uci.edu

L. Hoffmann · L. Wilson
Irvine School of Medicine, University of California, Irvine, CA, USA

© The Author(s), under exclusive license to Springer Nature Switzerland AG 2022
A. A. Hakimi et al. (eds.), *Mechanical Ventilation Amid the COVID-19 Pandemic*,
https://doi.org/10.1007/978-3-030-87978-5_4

RTs are certified medical professionals who create and carry out treatment plans for patients with respiratory issues. They must have a minimum of an associate degree from an accredited respiratory therapy education program, but many go on to earn further credentialing [2]. The responsibility of an RT can drastically vary at different institutions, but in general they work alongside physicians by carrying out physician orders, documenting aspects of respiratory care, administering respiratory therapy, and creating treatment plans for improving a patient's respiratory function. Although most physicians are at some point trained on how to use ventilators, physicians with specified training in critical care are usually titrating the ventilator on a daily basis. Anesthesiologists are also daily users of ventilators, as patients are often on mechanical ventilation during surgery.

In the field, paramedics often are the first to initiate mechanical ventilation for patients in respiratory failure or distress. Paramedic training requires between 1200 and 1800 hours and may last for 6–12 months. They then need to pass certification exams for both skills and knowledge [3].

When used at home, ventilator settings are usually non-titratable as patients that need variable settings are generally kept at nursing home facilities or hospitals. Home caregivers, however, must be able to provide supportive care, such as pulmonary hygiene, and recognize signs of ventilatory dysfunction.

Which Patients Benefit from This Device?

Patients that benefit from mechanical ventilation include the following: Those who (1) require high oxygen concentrations in the lungs, (2) need help clearing carbon dioxide, (3) require respiratory support so their body can concentrate on fighting other processes, (4) no longer have the ability to breathe by themselves, and (5) require help with breathing because they are unconscious [4]. All of these processes describe patients in respiratory failure. Ventilators, in general, are used to support patients in various forms of respiratory failure.

Interestingly, respiratory failure can be caused by problems with the lungs themselves (e.g., pneumonia), but oftentimes has an etiology unrelated to the pulmonary system. For example, common causes of respiratory failure include sepsis (bloodstream infections) or heart failure. During times of physiologic stress, the demand on the respiratory system to bring in oxygen or clear carbon dioxide is increased. Patients can develop respiratory failure simply from this inability to keep up with the increased demand. Respiratory failure is usually split into hypoxemic (problems with low oxygen in the blood), hypercapnic (problems with clearing carbon dioxide in the blood), or mixed (both) etiologies. Ultimately, ventilators assist patients with one or both problems. In most cases, ventilators buy the patient time by providing support until the underlying problem is addressed. A subset of patients may never be able to come off the ventilator. These patients are termed ventilator dependent.

Monitoring Physiologic Parameters

Oxygenation and Pulse Oximetry

Oxygen is an essential element utilized by our cells to produce energy through aerobic cellular respiration. It is brought into the lungs through inhalation, diffuses across the respiratory membrane into the bloodstream, and is attached to hemoglobin molecules as it is transported to various organs and bodily tissues. Because oxygen is vital to cellular function, measuring how much oxygen is in the blood provides important data regarding how well the lungs are functioning [5]. The measurement of quantifying how much hemoglobin in the blood is bound by oxygen is called oxygen saturation. Oxygen saturation is obtained non-invasively through pulse oximetry, which is an electronic device that is usually taped or clipped to the patient's finger. It emits light that travels through the patient's finger to a sensor located on the opposite side which will then measure how much light was not absorbed as it passes through the patient [5]. That measurement is then used to calculate the ratio of oxygenated to deoxygenated hemoglobin and reports the oxygen saturation as a percentage [5]. For a healthy person, a normal oxygen saturation is 95–100%. Pulse oximetry offers a rapid, continuous method of detecting oxygen saturation in patients and is particularly useful in hospital settings to monitor patients undergoing surgery and those whose lung function or breathing may be compromised [6].

Carbon Dioxide and Capnography

Carbon dioxide (CO_2) is a by-product of our cells and is transported through the bloodstream to be eliminated by the body through exhalation. The amount of CO_2 released in one exhaled breath is termed end-tidal CO_2 ($ETCO_2$). This measurement provides information on how well CO_2 is being transported to and expired from the lungs, but also is indicative of cardiac function and blood flow through the lungs. $ETCO_2$ can be measured with noninvasive capnography devices and is generally reported in mmHg with normal values between 35 and 45 mmHg [7]. Capnography allows monitoring of the patient's ventilation status in real time and is a valuable tool to inform the provider of any physiological or equipment complications that need to be quickly addressed. There are two main types of capnography devices: mainstream and sidestream. Each has its advantages and disadvantages in how $ETCO_2$ is measured and in what patient situations it is indicated [7, 8].

Mainstream capnography is designed with the capnograph's CO_2 sensor attached to an airway adapter that is located between the patient's endotracheal tube and the breathing circuit (Fig. 4.1). The airway adapter has an infrared sensor that emits light toward a photodetector on the opposite side of the adapter, which allows for measurement of $ETCO_2$ [8]. Mainstream capnography is used in intubated patients and

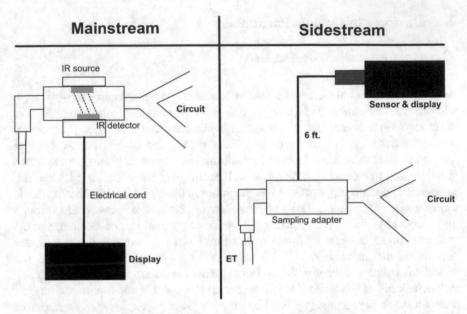

Fig. 4.1 Diagrams illustrating the equipment design of mainstream capnography vs. sidestream capnography

can be used for neonates and children [8]. Many of the advantages of this device type are due to the absence of a sampling tube in the apparatus. Because the $ETCO_2$ is being measured along the same pathway as the endotracheal tube and breathing circuit, there are no obstructions, pressure drops, or recording delay and there is minimal dispersion of gases [8]. Disadvantages of mainstream capnography include the sensor windows being more easily affected by secretions and the device design being less practical for patients in positions where they are not lying on their back [8].

Sidestream capnography is configured with the CO_2-sensing device located separately from the patient's endotracheal tube rather than directly along the airway (Fig. 4.1) [8]. CO_2 exhaled from the patient is pumped from the airway through a six- to eight-foot sampling tube to reach the CO_2-sensing unit. Additionally, any anesthetic gases that are exhaled with the CO_2 can be diverted to a gas scavenger or back to the patient via the breathing circuit [8]. One main advantage of sidestream capnography is that it can be used in patients who are not intubated. The apparatus can be fitted with nasal adapters that allow $ETCO_2$ measurements to be taken from patients receiving oxygen through nasal cannula [8]. Another advantage is the ability to use the device in patients who are not supine given the sampling tube's length. However, because the sampling tube is separate from the patient's airway, recording delays are expected as the gases must travel farther distances to the sensor and obstructions within the sampling tube can occur [8]. Furthermore, $ETCO_2$ measurements may be altered due to water vapor pressure changes or pressure drops within the sampling tube [8]. A particular issue that has been noted regarding sidestream capnography within the pediatric population is capnogram alteration due to increased gas dispersion within the sampling tube [8].

Volume Capnography

Volume capnography provides a continuous visual representation of the partial pressure of CO_2 (PCO_2) compared to the volume exhaled by the patient [9]. It offers many advantages for patient care such as real-time monitoring of ventilation quality, ventilation/perfusion (V/Q) ratio, CO_2 production, and early detection of pathological respiratory conditions that may compromise patient safety. An example of a volume capnogram is shown in Fig. 4.2. The volume capnogram is divided into three phases characterized by different expired gas components from distinct locations within the respiratory tract [9]. Phase I is composed of the gas from the end of the previous inspiration that is located within areas that do not undergo gas exchange such as anatomical dead space (e.g., conducting airways) and artificial dead space (e.g., the breathing circuit) [9, 10]. Thus, no CO_2 from the body is exchanged here and the PCO_2 (measured along the y-axis) remains zero. Increases in dead space will cause phase I prolongation [10]. If the PCO_2 is greater than zero during this phase, it suggests that the patient is breathing in previously expired CO_2 or that there is sensor malfunction [10]. Phase II consists of gas that travels to the sensor from the distal airway as well as from the first alveoli that empty upon expiration [9]. The slope is equal to the transition velocity between these two areas of the respiratory tract. Increased airway resistance or V/Q mismatch may extend this phase [10]. Phase III is made up of gas exclusively from the alveoli [10]. The positive slope during this phase represents real-time diffusion of CO_2 into the alveoli and out of the respiratory tract [9].

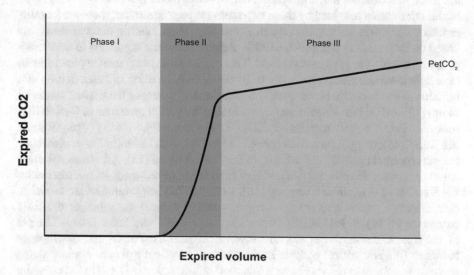

Fig. 4.2 Volume capnogram showing the relationship between expired volume of air and expired PCO_2 (measured in mmHg) during phases I, II, and III

Transcutaneous CO_2 Monitoring

Transcutaneous CO_2 monitoring is another continuous noninvasive method to measure a patient's CO_2 levels and evaluate the quality of ventilation. A transcutaneous monitor is placed on the patient's skin where it measures the partial pressures of oxygen and carbon dioxide, which can be used to estimate the arterial oxygen and carbon dioxide partial pressures [11]. The device works by increasing the skin's temperature at the device's attachment site, leading to increased blood flow to the local area. This increased heat changes the solubility of CO_2 in the blood [11]. It also causes the skin's metabolic rate to increase by 4–5% for each additional degree Celsius gained and thus increases CO_2 production at the site [11]. The sensor, commonly a Severinghaus electrode, measures pH changes to calculate the PCO_2 [12]. An algorithm is then applied that corrects for the additional CO_2 produced locally by the skin as a result of increased temperature and estimates the arterial PO_2 and PCO_2. Transcutaneous CO_2 monitoring can prove to be useful in mechanical ventilation to detect hypoventilation, hypoperfusion, revascularization status, ventilation adequacy, and therapeutic responses to medical interventions [11]. It is especially helpful for monitoring patients who do not have arterial access or cannot have frequent blood draws [11, 12].

Arterial Blood Gas vs. Venous Blood Gas

Two additional ways to monitor gases such as O_2 and CO_2 in a patient's bloodstream are through an arterial blood gas (ABG) or a venous blood gas (VBG). While some of the information provided by these two methods may be similar, there are key differences that must be acknowledged, especially when making clinical decisions based on their measurements. An ABG is performed by gaining access to a patient's artery to sample the oxygenated blood. This can be done using needle punctures to take individual samples periodically or by using an indwelling catheter (a tube that remains in the patient's blood vessel) to continuously sample the patient's arterial blood [13]. ABGs provide information including the partial pressures of O_2 and CO_2 (normal PaO_2 >~80 mmHg, $PaCO_2$ 35–45 mmHg), acidity (physiologic pH 7.35–7.45), oxygen saturation (generally >95%), and concentration of bicarbonate ions (normal range 21–27 mEq/L) in the arterial blood [13]. All values are measured except for the bicarbonate levels, which are obtained through calculation by the Henderson-Hasselbalch formula [13]. PaO_2 and oxygen saturation are useful in determining a patient's oxygen status and whether there is too much or too little oxygen in the blood. $PaCO_2$ helps to evaluate a patient's ventilation status. The pH of the sample demonstrates the relationship between the $PaCO_2$ and bicarbonate balance. This is a critical number in determining a patient's overall clinical status since disturbances in pH are not well tolerated physiologically [13]. However, while ABGs provide a wealth of information, they can be technically challenging to obtain and may not be a feasible option in all patients [13].

A VBG is obtained by sampling blood from the veins through intermittent needle punctures or through a patient's indwelling venous catheter. Similar to an ABG, a VBG also measures the partial pressures of O_2 and CO_2 (now PvO_2 and $PvCO_2$, respectively), oxygen saturation, pH, and bicarbonate concentration [14]. Because blood is being sampled from the veins and has previously released some of its oxygen into the body, a patient's true oxygenation status cannot be determined with a VBG. Additionally, VBG measurements differ from those of ABGs to varying degrees depending on the site collection and the patient's clinical status, and historically have been perceived as less accurate [14]. Therefore, while VBGs can provide helpful information and may be easier to perform, they should be correlated with ABG values when making critical clinical decisions.

Airway Pressures

During normal physiologic inspiration, the contraction of the diaphragm and external intercostal muscles allows the thoracic cavity to expand. Using Boyle's law (pressure is inversely proportional to volume with temperature constant), as the thoracic cavity expands, the volume increase causes a decrease in pressure. This is referred to as negative pressure. The lungs expand in synchrony with the thoracic cavity as they are held to the thoracic cage by the visceral and parietal membranes. The negative pressure within the lungs causes a pressure gradient with the external environment, allowing air from the outside environment to flow into the lungs down the pressure gradient (from high to low pressure). This is called negative-pressure ventilation [15].

For patients on mechanical ventilation, the process is changed. Inspiration on a mechanical ventilator occurs as positive pressure is injected through a breathing tube into the trachea to the lungs. Breathing tubes usually have a balloon, or cuff, that prevents the leakage of the positive airway pressure from going forward. Assuming no blockages in the breathing circuit, the positive pressure from the ventilator needs to overcome the patient's chest wall, airway, and lung resistances in order to generate a breath.

Peak Inspiratory Pressure vs. Plateau Pressure

Peak inspiratory pressure (PIP) is the total pressure generated by the ventilator to overcome airway and alveolar resistance. This is necessary to allow inspiratory flow and designated tidal volume. A simplified equation of *PIP* is

$$\text{Peak airway pressure} = \text{Resistive pressure} + \text{Elastic pressure} + \text{Positive end} - \text{expiratory pressure}$$

Resistive pressure is the summation of resistance within the ventilator circuit, the endotracheal tube, and the patient's airways. Elastic pressure is defined as the product of chest wall and lung recoil. Positive end-expiratory pressure (PEEP) refers to the pressure in the lungs at the end of expiration greater than atmospheric pressure.

Peak inspiratory pressure measures the highest pressure applied to the lungs during inhalation whereas plateau pressure, P_{plat}, also known as transpulmonary pressure, is the pressure the alveoli and small airways of the lung are exposed to at peak inspiration when there is no air movement. PIP is the sum of the P_{plat} and the pressure needed to overcome airway resistance. As a result, P_{plat} must be smaller than PIP and is only a direct measurement of the pressure within the airways when there is no airflow [16]. The P_{plat} is measured through the inspiratory pause maneuver as shown in Fig. 4.3.

This maneuver pauses airflow through the lungs, thereby eliminating the pressure contribution from airway resistance, and thus revealing the pressure contribution solely from the alveoli and airways. Peak pressures are considered elevated when there is a 5 mmHg or greater difference between peak pressure and plateau pressure. This occurs when there is a lung pathology causing elevated airway resistance within the respiratory system. Lung pathologies associated with an increased airway resistance include bronchospasms, bronchiectasis, retained secretions, and endotracheal tube tip occlusions. An elevated peak pressure and plateau pressure occur when the difference between peak pressure and plateau pressure is small, suggesting a lung pathology with poor alveolar compliance. Lung pathologies associated with an elevated plateau and peak pressure include pneumothorax, pulmonary edema, acute respiratory distress syndrome, and pneumonia [17].

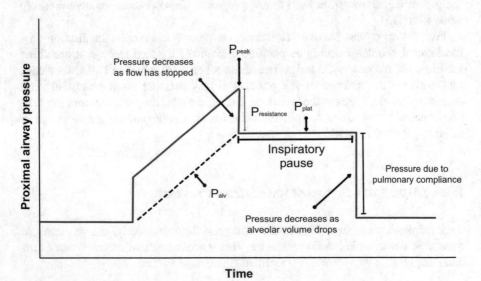

Fig. 4.3 P_{peak} is the maximum pressure applied to the lungs at full expiration whereas P_{plat} is the pressure of the alveoli and small airways during an inspiratory pause maneuver, when there is no flow circulating through the lungs. As indicated in the figure, the primary difference between P_{peak} and P_{plat} is that P_{peak} accounts for the resistance that needs to be overcome to allow airflow into the terminal airways and alveoli

Auto-PEEP vs. Extrinsic PEEP

In healthy lungs, the end-expiratory pressure is in equilibrium with the environmental pressure. However, in patients with lung pathology where there is an airflow limitation or obstruction, the end-expiratory pressure can be positive. This is referred to as intrinsic PEEP or auto-PEEP. Intrinsic PEEP occurs when the expiratory time is shorter than the time needed to fully deflate the lungs, preventing the lung and chest wall from reaching an elastic equilibrium. This leads to air trapping within the distal alveoli. Intrinsic PEEP can be measured by the expiratory hold maneuver as indicated in Fig. 4.4. This measurement can be performed on the ventilator by pausing the breath in expiration, preventing the delivery of more breaths, and allowing the alveolar pressure to equilibrate with the ventilator circuit. The circuit pressure at the end of the expiratory hold can be measured as the intrinsic PEEP, a rough approximation of the alveolar pressure at the end of expiration [18].

Extrinsic PEEP is the pressure applied by the ventilator throughout the respiratory cycle to maintain alveolar patency and prevent the alveoli from collapsing. Allowing the alveoli to stay open improves oxygenation by increasing the surface area for gas exchange and by decreasing air shunting [19]. Along with improving oxygenation to the distal alveoli, extrinsic PEEP can be used to improve ventilation/perfusion (V/Q) mismatches. A V/Q mismatch occurs (1) when one or more areas of the lung are well oxygenated but have poor blood flow or (2) when the lungs receive adequate blood flow but have poor airflow. The application of a positive pressure through a patient's lungs can open airways that were previously collapsed, improving alveolar oxygenation and thus decreasing V/Q mismatch [20].

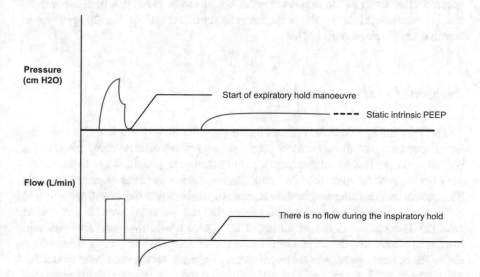

Fig. 4.4 The expiratory hold maneuver pauses the ventilator during expiration, allowing the alveolar pressure to equilibrate with the ventilator circuit. The alveolar pressure at the end of the expiratory hold is known as intrinsic PEEP or auto-PEEP

Extrinsic PEEP decreases the work of breathing for patients that have stiff lungs with low compliance because the positive pressure delivered to alveoli improves oxygenation and compensates for the decreased lung compliance [20]. Patients with stiff lungs will have to increase the number of breaths and total inhaled air volume into their lungs to compensate for their decreased lung compliance. This leads to an overall increase in energy expenditure and lactic acid production that can be counteracted by the ventilator providing an extrinsic PEEP.

A major concern with extrinsic PEEP is that it can decrease blood return to the heart, causing an overall decreased cardiac output. In normal respiratory physiology, the negative pressure created in the airways during inspiration decreases the pressure within the right atrium, generating a suction effect to increase venous return to the heart. Extrinsic PEEP applied from the ventilator generates a more positive pressure in the airways than the typical negative pressure created in normal respiratory physiology. This altered respiratory physiology increases right atrial pressure and decreases venous return to the heart, leading to an overall decrease in cardiac output. This is an important concern for intubated patients who have distributive shock or low blood pressure, as extrinsic PEEP can exacerbate the already decreased cardiac output in these patients [20].

Respiratory Rate

Respiratory rate (RR) is defined as the number of breaths a patient takes in 1 min, known as breaths per minute (bpm). The mechanical ventilator sets the RR to a specific value to allow the same number of breaths to be given to a patient per minute. For example, if the set RR is 20, then the ventilator will deliver 20 bpm or one breath every three seconds [21].

Respiratory Set vs. Actual Rate

The set respiratory rate is the bpm set by the provider on the ventilator. The ventilator will ensure that the set rate is delivered regardless of how many breaths the patient initiates. The actual rate is how many breaths the patient wants to take without intervention. As such, there are multiple combinations of set vs. actual rate. (1) The patient is breathing below the set rate: In these cases, the ventilator will add breaths to the patient's actual rate to ensure that the patient is breathing at the set rate. (2) The patient is not breathing at all: Once again, the ventilator will add breaths to ensure that the patient breathes at the set rate. (3) The patient is breathing above the set rate: Here, what happens largely depends on the ventilator mode. For assist control modes, the ventilator will deliver a fixed tidal volume or drive pressure (depending on the setting of volume control or pressure control) during every inspiration, regardless of whether the breath is initiated by the patient or the ventilator.

During synchronized intermittent mandatory ventilation (SIMV), the ventilator will deliver a fixed tidal volume or drive during every inspiration up until the set rate. Anything above the set rate, the ventilator will deliver pressure support breaths [22].

Ventilator Sensed Rate

Ventilators can deliver flow- vs. time-cycled breaths. Flow-cycled breaths occur when the ventilator senses changes in flow, usually initiated by the patient, and a breath is delivered. Time-cycled breaths occur when enough time has elapsed based on the set rate, leading to a breath delivery.

In order for the ventilator to recognize a patient's breath, it must be able to sense changes in pressure within the patient's respiratory system. The ventilator has sensors within its tubing that detect the increase in negative pressure within the thoracic cavity that occurs with inspiration. If the change in pressure surpasses the ventilator's trigger-sensitivity threshold, the ventilator will deliver a breath at the fixed tidal volume. However, if the patient fails to make a new inspiratory effort, the ventilator is programmed to initiate a breath in a time-dependent manner, known as time-triggered breaths. Time-triggered breaths will always follow the set rate of bpm established by the ventilator unless the patient attempts to inspire [23].

Humidity (Heat and Moister Exchangers vs. Heated Humidifier vs. Heated-Wire Circuits)

When a person breathes normally, the upper respiratory tract acts to filter, warm, and humidify the inspired air before it reaches the alveolar air sacs in the lungs. However, mechanical ventilation bypasses much of the anatomy that carries out these important bodily functions and places the burden of accomplishing them on the lower respiratory tract [24]. This can lead to lower respiratory tract damage that can negatively affect the patient's ventilation and cause complications. To avoid this, mechanical ventilators are equipped with devices that can optimize the humidity of the ventilated air. Humidifiers can be divided into two general categories: passive and active.

Passive humidifiers use a heat and moisture exchanger (HME) or artificial nose which contains a condenser that captures the water vapor and heat from the patient's exhaled air and adds it to the air that will be subsequently inhaled [24]. The device is located between the patient and the Y-piece, where the inspiratory and expiratory limbs separate to connect to the ventilator [24]. HMEs can further be characterized by their design elements as hygroscopic, hydrophobic, combined hydrophobic hygroscopic, and filtered [24, 25]. Hygroscopic HMEs contain hygroscopic salts such as lithium chloride or calcium chloride that have a high capacity to absorb moisture from exhaled air and release it back into inhaled air [24]. Hydrophobic

HMEs have condensers that repel water and maintain the temperature gradient, allowing water vapor droplets to accumulate on the filter's surface to humidify the next inhaled breath [24]. Combined hydrophobic hygroscopic HMEs contain both a water-repelling and hygroscopic salt element. Additionally, pleated filters with dense fibers or electrostatic filters can be applied to each of these HME types to create barriers to viral and bacterial pathogens [24]. Passive humidifiers are advantageous because they remove condensation that may accumulate in other problematic portions of the breathing circuit. However, they are associated with increased airway resistance and dead space, are more prone to occlusion, and are contraindicated in certain patient populations [24, 25].

Active humidifiers function by utilizing a heated water reservoir that warms the air. The device is located in the inspiratory limb of the ventilator circuit between the patient and ventilator [24]. Heated humidifiers (HH) can be further designated as bubble, passover, inline vaporizer, and counterflow [24]. Bubble humidifiers push gas into a tube that opens at the bottom of the water reservoir. As the gas forms bubbles that rise to the top of the reservoir, the amount of water vapor the gas contains increases. Additional ways to increase water vapor content using a bubble humidifier include slowing the flow rate, using a longer water column, and having a diffuser that creates smaller bubbles [24]. For passover humidifiers, air travels over the heated water reservoir which supplies it with increased water vapor. Passover humidifiers can further be modified with wicks or membranes which increase the gas-water interface and thus the water vapor content of the gas being inhaled by the patient [24]. Inline vaporizers consist of a plastic capsule in the circuit's inspiratory limb that adds water vapor to the gas and heats it via a disk heater. Because the capsule is located closer to the patient, this system does not use heated wires or additional temperature monitoring [24]. Lastly, counterflow humidifiers work by using externally heated water that travels through a humidifier and down a surface while gas travels across that surface in the opposite direction. Both inline vaporizers and counterflow humidifiers are newer technologies that are still being researched [24]. Compared to passive humidifiers, active humidifiers can be used more broadly and can attain a greater breadth of humidity and temperature. However, active humidifiers have a greater risk of contamination due to possible condensation of water vapor within the breathing circuit [24].

Heated humidifiers can be designed with water traps or heated wires to mitigate the risk of water vapor condensing along the inspiratory limb as a result of temperature differences along its length [24]. Specifically in regard to heated-wire circuits, these are located within the inspiratory limb of the breathing circuit and help regulate the temperature at the Y-piece [24]. Temperature probes are located at the humidifier and at the Y-piece and provide feedback to the system to achieve the desired temperature [24]. Heated-wire circuits can be divided into single-heated-wire (SHW) and double-heated-wire (DHW) circuits. While both have a heated wire within the inspiratory limb, DHW circuits contain a second wire in the expiratory limb to decrease condensation of water vapor within that portion as well [24]. The decrease in condensation with the use of heated-wire circuits makes these versions of active heated humidifiers advantageous compared to those without heated wires [24, 26].

Tidal Volume

Tidal volume (Vt) is defined as the amount of air that is moved into or out of the lungs during normal inhalation or exhalation and is typically about 500 mL in a healthy adult [27]. Vt is an important value to monitor and set in mechanical ventilation particularly in volume control modes. Too small of a Vt may cause inadequate oxygenation/ventilation and too large of a Vt may cause barotrauma to the lungs. Therefore, the set Vt must be titrated to the patient's physiological status and oxygen needs [27]. For a patient with healthy lungs, providers commonly start with a Vt of 6–8 mL/kg of predicted body weight [28]. For patients whose lung function is compromised such as in acute respiratory distress syndrome, the Vt may be set lower at 4–6 mL/kg [28]. Generally, Vt is not set above 10 mL/kg as research has shown increases in morbidity with similar or greater values [28].

Set Vt may be the same as or different than actual inhaled Vt depending on the ventilator setting being used. In continuous mandatory ventilation (CMV), the ventilator will provide breaths at a set Vt and RR despite the patient's own breathing efforts. CMV is commonly used in patients who are paralyzed and therefore the set Vt should match the actual inhaled Vt [29]. However, there are other volume control modes that allow for spontaneous breaths by the patient in addition to those initiated by the ventilator. In assist-control ventilation (ACV), the ventilator also has a set Vt and RR [29]. Unlike CMV, ACV also responds to the patient's spontaneous breaths by providing the set Vt when triggered and resetting the time it will deliver the next set breath. Because the ventilator is still providing the set Vt to each mechanically or patient-induced breath, set Vt should equal actual inhaled Vt [29]. Intermittent mandatory ventilation (IMV) is another mode that allows for spontaneous breathing by the patient while it continues to deliver set Vt at the set rate. For patients with this setting, there is no assistance by the ventilator during these spontaneous breaths [29]. This can lead to a discrepancy between the set Vt and actual inhaled Vt depending on the patient's spontaneous breathing against the airway circuit resistance. Finally, synchronous intermittent mandatory ventilation (SIMV) combines preset breaths with the patient's spontaneous breathing and synchronizes the timing of the mechanical breaths to avoid stacked breathing (delivering a mechanical breath while the patient has already initiated a spontaneous breath) [29]. If the patient's spontaneous breathing does not match the ventilator's settings, it is possible for set Vt to differ from actual inhaled Vt [29].

Exhaled Vt is another parameter that is important to monitor as it can provide information on both mechanical and spontaneous ventilation. Generally, the exhaled Vt should be approximately the same as the set Vt. If the exhaled Vt is lower than the set Vt, there may be air leakage within the ventilatory circuit [29]. Common causes of air leakage occur around the endotracheal (ET) tube if the inflatable cuff does not create a leakproof seal or if a cuffless ET tube is too small to prevent air leakage around it [29]. Lower exhaled Vt compared to set Vt can also suggest insufficient exhalation time which could be due to the patient's lung health or due to mismatched timing of the ventilator-assisted breathing and the patient's spontaneous breathing rates [29].

Patient-Ventilator Synchrony Monitoring

Patient-Ventilator Synchrony/Dyssynchrony Introduction

Patient-ventilator synchrony refers to the mechanical ventilator functioning in synchrony with the patient's own respiratory drive. The respiratory system is dynamic and is constantly being influenced by the body's own mechanical, chemical, behavioral, and reflex mechanisms to create subtle changes in breath-to-breath adjustments. This multitude of factors affecting each patient's breathing pattern can present a major challenge for the ventilator to respond appropriately to the patient's expiratory and inspiratory signals [30].

Respiratory drive is dependent on both voluntary and autonomic control. These control centers act in synchrony to determine whether inspiration or expiration should be inhibited or stimulated, sending outgoing neuronal information to the phrenic and intercostal nerves to adjust the various aspects of ventilation. The ventilator must respond to these adjustments to maintain patient-ventilator synchrony. Patient-ventilator dyssynchrony (PVD) occurs when the ventilator is unable to recognize or adjust to a patient's breathing pattern [30].

Ineffective Triggering

Ineffective triggering is a form of PVD where the ventilator fails to trigger a breath when the patient attempts inhalation. Ventilators respond by initiating a breath when the flow or pressure within a patient's respiratory drive changes. A pressure-triggered breath occurs when the inspiratory effort by the patient creates a large enough negative pressure within the airways that it surpasses the pressure threshold on the ventilator. With a flow-triggered breath, the patient's inspiration must draw a continuous flow greater than the flow threshold on the ventilator. In either case, if the flow or pressure generated by a patient's inspiratory effort is unable to surpass the ventilator's threshold value, then the ventilator will not initiate a breath when the patient attempts inhalation, leading to ineffective triggering. Ineffective triggering occurs in patients with severe respiratory weakness and can even exacerbate their weakness by forcing them to increase their inspiratory efforts in an attempt to produce a triggered breath. Ways to prevent ineffective triggering include lowering the flow or pressure threshold on the ventilator and addressing the underlying cause of the patient's respiratory weakness [30].

Double Triggering and Reverse Triggering

As respiratory drive increases, the duration of a patient's inspiration, also known as neural inspiratory time (neural T_i), can outlast the ventilator's programmed inflation time (ventilator T_i), causing the ventilator to trigger an additional breath in response to the patient's continued inhalation, known as double triggering. Double triggering occurs when the patient's diaphragm continues to contract as the ventilator begins the expiratory phase. When the diaphragm continues to contract, the pressure sensor on the ventilator will recognize the increased negative pressure in the patient's proximal airways and immediately initiate a new breath. As a result, the ventilator will deliver two breaths without exhalation in between, thereby essentially doubling the patient's fixed Vt. The elevated Vt can lead to overdistention of the alveoli and small airways and cause clinical manifestations such as pneumothorax, pneumomediastinum, and other pathologies associated with volutrauma or barotrauma. Figure 4.5 represents double triggering with neural T_i being longer than ventilator T_i, forcing the ventilator to respond to the lengthened neural T_i time by initiating a new breath. In order to correct double triggering, the ventilator can be turned off to allow the episode causing the double triggering to resolve. The ventilator's flow or volume settings should be adjusted to meet the patient's respiratory demands in order to correct the double triggering when the cause of double triggering does not resolve on its own [30, 31].

Reverse triggering, also known as entrainment, is another type of patient-ventilator dyssynchrony that occurs when a patient's respiratory center is activated by the ventilator passively inflating the lungs. Reverse triggering that occurs during pressure-controlled ventilation shows detectable flow changes during the inspiratory phases and continued patient effort during expiratory flow. During volume-controlled ventilation, reverse triggering is identified by pressure changes during the inspiratory phases or continued patient effort during the expiratory flow waveform. Reverse triggering originates in the patient's diaphragm as it contracts in response to the ventilator triggering a breath. If the diaphragm continues to contract during the ventilator exhalation, the patient will be inhaling while the ventilator is in the expiratory phase, forcing the ventilator to initiate another breath, known as

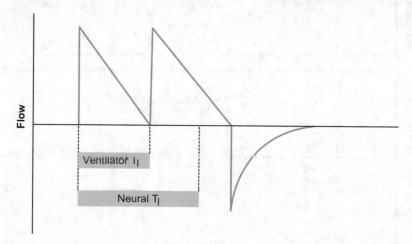

Fig. 4.5 The patient's inspiration time, neural T_i, is greater than the ventilator's inspiration time, ventilator T_i, prompting the ventilator to initiate a new breath. This phenomenon is known as double triggering

breath stacking. Similar to double triggering, breath stacking can cause excessive regional lung stress as the tidal volume can dramatically increase due to excessive inspiratory volume delivery [30, 31].

Flow Dyssynchrony and Auto-Triggering

An increased respiratory drive oftentimes necessitates an increased flow from the ventilator. Flow dyssynchrony occurs when the ventilator is unable to meet the patient's increased flow demand. For example, this occurs when the flow rate set by the ventilator is too low to meet the patient's own inspiratory demand. During volume ventilation while the flow is fixed, flow dyssynchrony can be identified on pressure-time waveforms as a "scooped" appearance on the pressure wave during inhalation, as demonstrated in Fig. 4.6. Improving flow dyssynchrony necessitates a reduction in a patient's inspiratory demand or an increase in flow through the ventilator. Increasing ventilator flow delivery can be accomplished by directly increasing the flow or by adjusting the inspiratory flow patterns [30].

Inappropriate ventilator sensitivity levels can cause auto-triggering, a process by which the ventilator misinterprets the initiation of a patient's breath and triggers a breath spontaneously. Signals that can induce auto-triggering include condensation in the circuit, ET cuff leaks, circuit leaks, cardiogenic oscillations, increased cardiac output, or elevated ventricular filling pressure. The management of auto-triggering is to minimize both ET and circuit leaks, remove condensation from the circuit, and decrease the sensitivity of the trigger threshold [30].

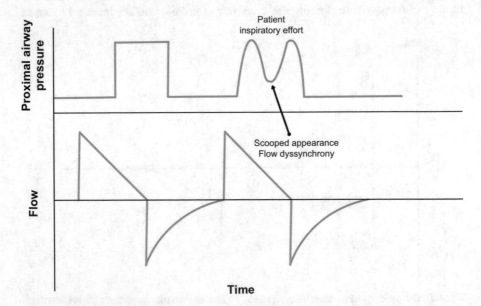

Fig. 4.6 The scooped appearance in the figure showcases flow dyssynchrony as the flow rate set by the ventilator is insufficient to meet the patient's elevated inspiration flow rate

Setup and Form Factor of Contemporary Ventilators

Modern mechanical ventilators come in an array of shapes and sizes and have gone through many generations of modifications. In the ICU, the ventilator is usually positioned at the head of the patient's bed to be closer to the patient's airway. It can be either to the left or the right of the patient, but is commonly positioned closer to the entrance of the room for ease of access. A standard intensive care unit (ICU) ventilator typically has wheels so that it can be moved from room to room. However, once it is set up for a patient, it is usually not moved around the room. It also requires an AC plug for power and wall gas hookups, unless it is a portable transport ventilator.

The current generation of ICU ventilators (fourth generation) are mainly distinguished from older ventilators by their plethora of features and ventilation modes available to the user. With the advent of microprocessor chips, ventilators have become extremely advanced in their ability to control oxygen percentage, pressures/volumes, flows, and respiratory cycle times [1]. As seen in Fig. 4.7, modern ventilators have a computer screen with dials and buttons that allow the user to make

Fig. 4.7 Avea™ CVS Ventilation System by Vyaire Medical with touch screen

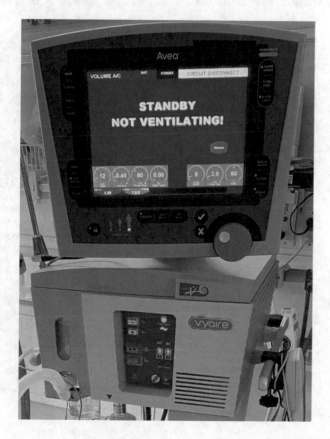

setting changes to the ventilator. Many modern-day ventilators are even touch screen with high-resolution monitors. Each setting on the ventilator is dialed in through the buttons, screen, and dials, allowing the medical professional intricate control.

Since ventilators can deliver anywhere from 21% oxygen (room air) to 100% oxygen, each ventilator also requires gas connections of air and oxygen. In the United States, room air is indicated with the color yellow, and oxygen with the color green. Specialty-specific ventilators may have connections for other forms of gas (e.g., anesthesia ventilators usually have a nitrous oxide line which is indicated with the color blue). Gas connections can come directly from the hospital's central supply, which directly hook into the wall (Fig. 4.8), or can come in the form of cannisters. Special pegs and keys on the cannisters and wall hookups are used to ensure that the different gases are not interchanged, which would cause the ventilator to deliver the wrong gas. This could cause significant harm to the patient by delivering hypoxic gas mixtures.

Modern-day ventilators are usually circle-system circuits. They have an inspiratory and expiratory limb controlled by one-way valves that regulate the direction of airflow. One end of the circuit is hooked up to the ventilator (Fig. 4.9) and the other end converges at the "Y" connector, which is then hooked to the patient's

Fig. 4.8 Oxygen (green) and Air (yellow) wall hookup. BeaconMedæs™

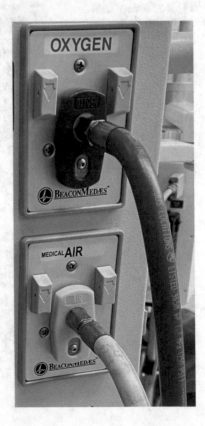

Fig. 4.9 Inspiratory and expiratory limbs of the ventilator circuit with accordion tubing

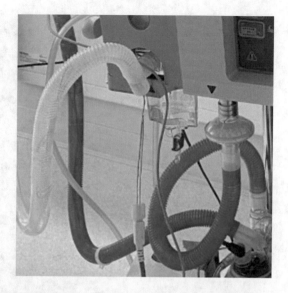

Fig. 4.10 "Y" connector that hooks up to the endotracheal tube

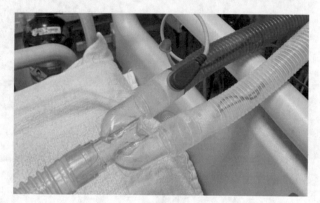

endotracheal tube or noninvasive ventilator mask (Fig. 4.10). The circuit tubing is usually configured in an accordion shape, which allows it to stretch and reach the patient, but also works to trap water droplets in the warm and humidified air.

Transport ventilators (Fig. 4.11) are smaller battery-operated ventilators that can appear in ambulances, helicopters, and aircrafts to transport patients between hospital settings. Transport ventilators are also used in the hospital to transport patients between different areas in the hospital, such as between the ICU and operating room. Many mishaps can occur when patients are transported with ventilators [32]. Thus transport ventilators are built for their ease of maneuverability, compact size and form factor, and simplistic operating functions. Transport ventilators usually use air and oxygen cannisters as their source of fresh gas flow. Studies have shown that these ventilators are effective and safe for short periods of time, despite their simplistic design [33].

Fig. 4.11 LTV™1200 by
Vyaire Medical transport
ventilator with oxygen
cannister

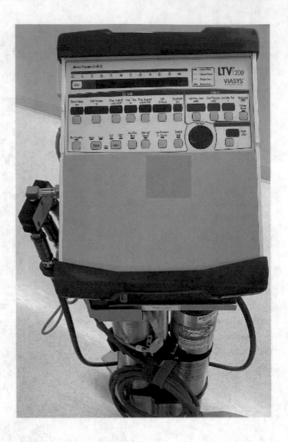

Financial Disclosures The authors have no relevant conflicts of interest to disclose.

Funding This work was not funded.

References

1. Kacmarek RM. The mechanical ventilator: past, present, and future. Respir Care. 2011;56(8):1170–80.
2. Your Complete Guide to Becoming a Respiratory Therapist | University of Cincinnati. University of Cincinnati. Published May 2019. Accessed 3 July 2021.
3. What's the Difference Between an EMT and a Paramedic? UCLA CPC. Published September 18, 2014. Accessed 3 July 2021.
4. American Thoracic Society Patient Educations Information Series: Mechanical Ventilation. Am J Respir Crit Care Med. 196, P3–4, 201. https://www.thoracic.org/patients/patient-resources/resources/mechanical-ventilation.pdf. Accessed July 2021.
5. Hafen BB, Sharma S. Oxygen Saturation. Nih.gov. Published May 7, 2021. Accessed 3 July 2021.
6. Pulse Oximetry. Yale Medicine. Published March 2, 2021. Accessed 3 July 2021.

7. Richardson M, Moulton K, Rabb D, et al. Introduction. Nih.gov. Published March 2016. Accessed 3 July 2021.
8. Bhavani Shankar Kodali MD. Types of Capnographs - Capnography. Capnography. Published 2021. Accessed 3 July 2021.
9. Kreit JW. Volume capnography in the intensive care unit: potential clinical applications. Ann Am Thorac Soc. 2019;16(4):409–20. https://doi.org/10.1513/annalsats.201807-502cme.
10. Munir K, Himmelstoss M. Volumetric capnography. Bonaduz: Hamilton Medical; 2016.
11. Transcutaneous CO_2 Monitoring, October 2018. American Association of Sleep Technologists.
12. Restrepo RD, Hirst KR, Wittnebel L, Wettstein R. AARC Clinical Practice Guideline: Transcutaneous Monitoring of Carbon Dioxide and Oxygen: 2012. Respir Care. 2012;57(11):1955–62. https://doi.org/10.4187/respcare.02011.
13. Theodore AC. Arterial Blood Gases. UpToDate. Published 2021. Accessed 3 July 2021.
14. Theodore AC. Venous Blood Gases and Alternatives to Arterial Blood Gases. UpToDate. Published 2021. Accessed 3 July 2021.
15. Mechanics of Breathing | Boundless Anatomy and Physiology. Lumenlearning.com. Published 2021. Accessed 3 July 2021.
16. Jade H. Peak airway pressure in mechanical ventilation definition & interpretation. Health Jade. Published December 18, 2019. Accessed 4 July 2021.
17. Cassone M, Cocciolone A, Melnychuk E. Your First Shift in the Unit: Demystifying Ventilator Alarms. Emra.org. Published December 16, 2019. Accessed 4 July 2021.
18. Yartsev A. Intrinsic PEEP and the expiratory hold manoeuvre | Deranged Physiology. Derangedphysiology.com. Published 2015. Accessed 4 July 2021.
19. Merck Manuals. Noninvasive positive pressure ventilation (NIPPV) using bilevel positive airway pressure. Merck Manuals Professional Edition. Published 2021. Accessed 4 July 2021.
20. Mora AL, Mora JI. Positive End-Expiratory Pressure. Nih.gov. Published August 29, 2020. Accessed 4 July 2021.
21. Mora AL, Mora JI. Ventilation Assist Control. Nih.gov. Published April 28, 2021. Accessed 4 July 2021.
22. Modes of Mechanical Ventilation. Openanesthesia.org. Published 2021. Accessed 4 July 2021.
23. Mancebo J. Chapter 6. Assist-control ventilation. In: Principles and practice of mechanical ventilation, 3e. New York: AccessMedicine, McGraw Hill Medical; 2021. Mhmedical.com. Accessed 4 July 2021.
24. Al Ashry HS, Modrykamien AM. Humidification during mechanical ventilation in the adult patient. Biomed Res Int. 2014;2014:1–12. https://doi.org/10.1155/2014/715434.
25. Cerpa F, Cáceres D, Romero-Dapueto C, et al. Humidification on ventilated patients: heated humidifications or heat and moisture exchangers? Open Respir Med J. 2015;9(1):104–11. https://doi.org/10.2174/1874306401509010104.
26. Restrepo RD, Walsh BK. Humidification during invasive and noninvasive mechanical ventilation: 2012. Respiratory Care. 2012;57(5):782–8. https://doi.org/10.4187/respcare.01766.
27. Hallett S, Toro F, Ashurst JV. Physiology, tidal volume. Nih.gov. Published May 9, 2021. Accessed 4 July 2021.
28. Hyzy RC, Mcsparron JI. UpToDate. Published 2021. Accessed 4 July 2021.
29. Staff RT. Ventilation modes and monitoring. RT: For decision makers in respiratory care. Published February 7, 2007. Accessed 4 July 2021.
30. Mellott KG, Grap MJ, Munro CL, Sessler CN, Wetzel PA. Patient-ventilator dyssynchrony: clinical significance and implications for practice. Crit Care Nurse. 2009;29(6).41–55. https://doi.org/10.4037/ccn2009612.
31. Poor H. Patient-ventilator dyssynchrony. Basics of Mechanical Ventilation. Published online 2018:75–93. https://doi.org/10.1007/978-3-319-89981-7_7.
32. Waydhas C. Intrahospital transport of critically ill patients. Crit Care. 1999;3(5):R83–9. https://doi.org/10.1186/cc362. Epub 1999 Sep 24. PMID: 11094486; PMCID: PMC137237
33. Hurst JM, Davis K Jr, Branson RD, Johannigman JA. Comparison of blood gases during transport using two methods of ventilatory support. J Trauma. 1989;29(12):1637–40.

Chapter 5
An Overview of Mechanical Ventilation and Development of the UC San Diego MADVent

Lonnie Petersen, Sidney Merritt, and James Friend

Introduction

Mechanical ventilation is a lifesaving intervention for a broad group of patients when spontaneous respiration ceases from trauma, cardiac arrest, or sedation, or when it becomes insufficient in pneumonia, allergic reaction, or fatigue. The term *mechanical ventilation* covers anything from short-term manual bag ventilation potentially applied outside the hospital or during transportation to in-hospital urgent or intensive care, or chronic life-sustaining treatment lasting months or years. Over the years, ventilators have been adapted to support these diverse settings. During emergencies, such as natural disasters or the current COVID-19 pandemic, ventilator resources can quickly become depleted and lives are lost. As with previous pandemics, such as the influenza pandemics [1] and the polio outbreaks [2] of the early twentieth century, the current COVID-19 pandemic inspired a large number of

L. Petersen
Department of Mechanical and Aerospace Engineering, Jacobs School of Engineering, University of California San Diego, La Jolla, CA, USA
e-mail: l8petersen@health.ucsd.edu

S. Merritt
Department of Anesthesiology, School of Medicine, University of California San Diego, La Jolla, CA, USA
e-mail: skmerritt@health.ucsd.edu

J. Friend (✉)
Department of Mechanical and Aerospace Engineering, Jacobs School of Engineering, University of California San Diego, La Jolla, CA, USA

Department of Surgery, School of Medicine, University of California San Diego, La Jolla, CA, USA
e-mail: jfriend@ucsd.edu

© The Author(s), under exclusive license to Springer Nature Switzerland AG 2022
A. A. Hakimi et al. (eds.), *Mechanical Ventilation Amid the COVID-19 Pandemic*,
https://doi.org/10.1007/978-3-030-87978-5_5

novel technologies and strategies to ensure ventilation despite the repeated surges of critically ill patients. Many of these innovations borne out of sheer desperation hold valuable lessons that must be learned so that we are better able to overcome the next healthcare emergency.

Spontaneous Respiration

The primary function of the pulmonary system is to facilitate gas exchange between the air and pulmonary vasculature [3]. The respiratory system is located in the thoracic cavity and consists of the upper airways; nasal and oral cavities; and the pharynx and larynx which allow for the conduction (*see* later sections regarding *dead space*) and heating of inspired air. The lower structures consist of the tracheobronchial tree, which successively differentiates from the trachea into bronchi, bronchioles, and alveoli, the location where gas exchange occurs [3]. A normal spontaneous inspiration is accomplished by synchronized downward movement of the diaphragm and upward movement of the external intercostals, thereby increasing the thoracic cavity and lowering the pressure of the pulmonary system below ambient pressure. This passively draws in air [4]. This drop in intrathoracic pressure simultaneously facilitates venous blood return to the heart and filling of the lungs. Due to evolutionary pressure, over time this process has optimized the perfusion-to-ventilation ratio to best facilitate gas exchange. Exchange of oxygen and carbon dioxide takes place across the thin alveolar walls to the pulmonary capillaries and vice versa. Perfusion is driven primarily by the concentration gradients of oxygen and carbon dioxide across this barrier. The rate of gas perfusion across the walls is closely tied to the rate of ventilation of air into and out of the alveoli. Expiration is accomplished by the passive, elastic recoil of the diaphragm and pulmonary tissue, and may include the additional contraction of the internal intercostals and abdominal muscles in case of a forced expiration.

The Purpose and Basic Functions of a Ventilator

Failure of spontaneous ventilation or impaired gas exchange on the level of the alveoli necessitates mechanical ventilation. Modern ventilators used for life support offer numerous feedback loops, alarms, and features to increase patient safety and simplify usage over a wide range of ventilation modes and settings. Highly trained staff—*respiratory therapists*—are necessary to set them up and operate them in the clinical setting [5]. Regulations in advanced nations are numerous and complex, all in an attempt to reduce the risk of patient morbidity and mortality during intervention for nearly any possible medical condition. A categorized illustration of the variety of ventilator types is provided in Fig. 5.1.

					Constant Flow CPAP	Conventional CPAP
Mechanical Ventilators	Positive Pressure Ventilators	Non-invasive PPV (NIPPCV)	Constant Airway Pressure	Continuous Positive Airway Pressure (CPAP)		Bubble CPAP
					Auto. / Variable Flow CPAP	
				Nasal Cannula	High Frequency Nasal Cannula (HFNC)	
					Low Frequency Nasal Cannula (LFNC)	
			Variable Airway Pressure	Nasal High Frequency Ventilator (n-HFV)		
				Nasal Biphasic Positive Airway Pressure (n-BPAP)		
				Nasal Synchronized Intermittent PPV (n-SIPPV)		
		Invasive PPV (IPPV)	Pt. triggered	Synchronized Intermittent Mandatory Ventilator (SIMV)		
				Pressure Support Ventilator (PSV)		
			Continuous	Pressure control		
				Volume control		
	Negative Pressure Ventilator			Iron Lung		

Fig. 5.1 Types of ventilators. A categorized list of ventilator types, indicating the broad variety of devices devised over the years that are still in current use to support respiration

The core purpose of a ventilator is to pass oxygen into and draw carbon dioxide out of the lungs of a patient unable to do so on their own. It must do so at a sufficient rate, flow, and capacity to ensure that the patient's blood remains oxygenated (defined as P_{O2}) at greater than 88–90% and sufficiently free of carbon dioxide ($Pa_{CO2} < 40$ mmHg) to maintain life. It must also do so without injuring the patient and while accommodating the patient's dynamic condition and treatment needs. All ventilators have similar, essential features [6] and monitor specific parameters as provided in Table 5.1. Under normal circumstances, the lungs of an adult human are exquisitely capable of respiration, providing an area of approximately 140 m^2 in contact with the blood, about the size of a tennis court, to exchange gases.

A ventilator typically delivers a gas into the patient's lungs by producing a differential pressure between the lungs and the external environment sufficient to inflate them. Crucially, oxygen is a part of that gas in ventilation. The magnitude of

Table 5.1 Common parameters monitored with ventilators

Parameter	Acronym	Default	Range	Purpose
Positive end expiratory pressure	PEEP	3–5 cm H_2O	0–30 cm H_2O	Oxygenation; prevent lung collapse [6]
Fraction inhaled oxygen	FiO_2	21% (air)	21–100%	Oxygenation
Minute ventilation	MV or $\dot{V}_T$; MV = RR$\cdot V_T$	5–6 L/min	5–8 L/min	Ventilation
Tidal or inspiratory volume	$V_T = V_I$	600 mL or 6 mL/kg patient body weight	50–2000 mL	Ventilation
Respiratory rate	RR	20 breaths/min	1–80 cm H_2O	Ventilation
Peak inspiratory pressure	PIP	3–5 cm H_2O	10–80 cm H_2O	Gas flow resistance
Plateau pressure	P_{plat}	30 cm H_2O	–	Pulmonary compliance
Maximum inspiratory airflow	$\dot{V}_{max}$	60 L/min	–	Prevent lung injury due to excess $\dot{V}$

this pressure is an important factor in patient safety and the effectiveness of the ventilation, usually ranging between 5 and 40 cm_{H_2O}. Excessive pressure is an important contributor to barotrauma [7], though the relationship is complex as it also depends upon the patient's lung capacity, lung compliance, and volume of gas delivered by the ventilator per cycle. Regardless, barotrauma is devastating to patients in critical care, and is most prevalent in patients with compromised lungs. It has been an important issue during the COVID-19 pandemic with the disease's particularly pernicious effects upon the lungs [8] from pneumonia to acute respiratory distress syndrome (ARDS). It is more broadly a risk in patients with chronic obstructive pulmonary disease (COPD), interstitial lung disease, and asthma. Barotrauma appears more often in younger patients and in the first 3 days of ventilation.

The volume of gas delivered into the patient's lungs is the *tidal volume* at a rate defined as the *inspiratory airflow*. This may be either directly controlled between 50 and 2000 mL (typically) or indirectly defined from the set peak pressure or *peak inspiratory pressure* (PIP), depending on how the ventilator is operated as discussed later. While the gas is being delivered, the positive end-expiratory pressure (PEEP) is typically monitored via a separate safety valve, preventing excess pressure regardless of how the ventilator is otherwise operating. The *baseline airway pressure* (BAP) is the *actual* pressure present in the airway of the patient, and is otherwise a synonym for PEEP. There are other pressures that are typically monitored in modern ventilation, including the PIP and the *plateau pressure* (P_{plat}). These are associated with the condition of the lungs and, in some cases, the ventilation system.

Upon release of the differential pressure, the natural recoil of the lung tissue accomplishes the exhalation, completing the respiration cycle. The exhaled gases are passed along another path to avoid re-inhaling (rebreathing) the exhaled gases. There is always some volume of air left in both the patient's pulmonary system [9] and a portion of the ventilator that is rebreathed from respiration to respiration; the latter part is the *dead space* [10] of the ventilator that cannot be large in comparison to the lung capacity of the patient.

The cycling of the ventilation and exhalation occurs at the *respiratory rate*, usually independently adjustable between 1 and 40 breaths/min, and sometimes to much higher rates, to 80 bpm or more. The rate is typically adjusted alongside the tidal volume to prevent blood acidosis (pH <7.35) or alkylosis (pH >7.45). Depending on the operating mode, the ventilator can produce a respiration cycle independent of the patient's behavior, as (continuous) *mandatory ventilation* or *controlled ventilation*, or upon detection of a patient's desire to inhale as (continuous) *spontaneous ventilation*, usually with a patient-driven increase in the inhaled flow or a drop in the pressure within the vent tubing connected to the patient. The latter tends to be less sensitive to the patient, but the former is more difficult to sense. To avoid upsetting a patient during mandatory ventilation, they are usually sedated. If the respiratory rate is too high, it can lead to *breath stacking*, a condition where a new lung inspiration is driven by the ventilator before the previous breath has been fully expired.

The flow rate of the gas into the patient's lungs—the *inspiratory flow rate*, $\dot{V}$ —is also controlled, and tends to default to 60 L/min. The flow rate is particularly important in spontaneous ventilation, where the work done by the patient to maintain a desired breathing rate and volume may become a significant burden if there is a mismatch with the ventilator settings such that the product of the flow rate and volume per breath is insufficient. More generally, unassisted breathing by mammals evolves to minimize the work necessary to obtain adequate alveolar respiration [11]. A discrepancy between this state and the settings of the ventilator is uncomfortable for the patient and can be a confounding factor in adverse patient outcomes.

Some ventilators provide a controllable method to introduce more oxygen than available in standard air, up to 100% at the risk of oxygen toxicity or poisoning [12]. The parameter defined for this purpose, the *fraction inhaled oxygen* (FiO_2), is the percentage of oxygen in the gas; values greater than 60% for prolonged periods greatly increase the risk of toxicity. Increasing the oxygen concentration above the standard 21% of air reduces the amount of gas that needs to be ventilated and therefore eases life support, especially for patients with compromised lung function. In almost every case, the additional oxygen is provided from an external source, whether from compressed bottles or oxygen generator plants. Whatever the case, medical oxygen is an urgent unmet need [13] in developing regions during the COVID-19 pandemic.

The interface between patient and ventilator depends upon the patient condition. Other than tracheostomy, an unusual procedure for critical care of infected patients, endotracheal intubation is the most invasive and carries the most risk. It prevents the patient from speaking, and typically in conjunction with mandatory continuous ventilation it requires the patient to be sedated, leaving them completely in the care of the medical staff and dependent upon the ventilator for survival. From hypoxemia (<88% in the COVID-19 pandemic [14]) to cardiac arrhythmia and arrest, the serious complications of intubation in the critical care setting [15] are prevalent, with reports of over 25% of patients encountering them. Critical care is the standard in a pandemic, with patients coming in extremely ill and in need of immediate attention. Beyond the direct risks of intubation, the removal of the intubation and weaning of the patient from ventilation also carry risks [16]. Weaning in the modern context follows a carefully defined protocol including a spontaneous breathing trial and a spontaneous awakening trial.

In the context of the COVID-19 pandemic, these risks were judged to be sufficiently adverse that there were strong public pleas [14] for doctors to avoid intubating COVID-19 patients wherever possible, instead suggesting alternative methods for treating these patients and delaying or entirely avoiding a transition to mandatory intubated ventilation during the course of the disease. The decision to place a patient on a ventilator is based on clinical assessment and prediction of the disease evolution along a trajectory perceived in the doctor's mind as informed from knowledge of past patient outcomes. Decreasing oxygen saturation and concerning changes in the patient's respiration frequency may lead to a doctor's rapid decision to intubate and ventilate. In some cases the need is acute and ventilatory treatment is initiated immediately, while other cases develop gradually, based on developing fatigue and a growing need to support the respiratory work of the patient. Some of the non-intubation alternatives will be briefly discussed later, but here it is important to note that noninvasive ventilation also carries patient risks that should be considered [17].

As a life support device, the ventilator is one of the few instruments that accompany the patient wherever they go. In transition, manual bag-based respirators (or manual ventilators or bag-valve masks [18]) are used to maintain respiration, but only for a short time. These same respirators form the core of most inexpensive ventilator designs, not only because they facilitate a translation of simple compressive motion into appropriate gas flow for respiration, but also because they have been vetted and approved by key regulatory authorities like the U.S. Food and Drug Administration (FDA), reducing the burden of regulatory approval for some aspects of the inexpensive ventilator. Modern ventilators tend to fall into two groups: portable ventilators with integrated pressure generation or regulation of pressurized gas provided from another source, and facility ventilators that tend to be larger, more complex, and capable of a greater range of ventilation modes.

Whatever the case, the standard of care is to provide each patient with their own ventilator. In patient surges, including well-publicized events in Italy, the United States, India, and other nations during the COVID-19 pandemic, but also prior to that in several events including the 2017 Las Vegas mass shooting [19], there were attempts to support several patients on a single ventilator due to shortages. Several medical associations teamed together to discourage the concept due to safety concerns [20]. The problem is the inability to guarantee the matching of patients that share a ventilator over time. For example, the lungs of patients suffering from

COVID-19 exhibit rapidly changing lung capacities and compliances. An initially successful attempt to match ventilation peak pressures, tidal volumes, and PEEP can rapidly devolve to a mismatched set of patients, leaving one or more with inadequate ventilation and risk of hypoxia or death with no warning from the ventilator. Some strategies to avoid this outcome have been produced [21], though they require careful and continual monitoring beyond the standard ventilation protocol, a problem when facing a patient surge.

Finally, modern ventilators incorporate numerous alarms and indicators to inform the respiratory technician, nurse, or doctor of life support problems. Most of the complexity in ventilators is due to their use as a critical life support instrument for unresponsive patients. Beyond the potential problems that an otherwise ill or injured patient may exhibit, the ventilator tubing can become pinched or come loose, the power can be cut, or the ventilator's settings can be inadvertently changed or set to automatically change by the operator that later are not appropriate for the patient. Obvious and easily understood alarms are necessary to ensure that a harried staff member can comprehend and quickly fix problems in ventilation as they arise.

The Evolution of Assisted Ventilation

From Aelius Galenus, Ibn al-Nafis, and Vesalius' furtive descriptions of respiration in the second, thirteenth, and sixteenth centuries, respectively, to the first reports of resuscitation in 1472 for an infant and 1744 for an adult [22], the Industrial Revolution was well underway when the first effective ventilators appeared in the nineteenth century, operating with a negative pressure around the patient's torso while their head was exposed to ambient air pressure to form a pressure difference sufficient to drive inhalation [23]. These came into wide use in the 1920s–1950s mainly due to poliomyelitis outbreaks, with the iron lung (Drinker and Shaw tank) emblematic of that era. Unfortunately, the ventilators enclosed the entire lower body and weighed nearly 750 kg, and strained healthcare budgets with the expenses of procuring and operating them. Lighter and less expensive, the negative pressure-based Both respirator was devised in Australia and became popular as well for a brief period before positive-pressure ventilators were devised.

Newer ventilators generally employ positive-pressure ventilation instead, after the convincing results by Bjørn Ibsen in treating a poliomyelitis outbreak in Denmark, using it in conjunction with tracheostomy on 27 August 1952, drastically improving mortality outcomes overnight. Positive-pressure ventilation began appearing from the 1940s as a much lighter, less expensive, portable, and effective method [23], though with a downside: the perfusion of blood in the lungs is reduced with positive-pressure ventilation during the inspiration phase, while it (and filling of the ventricles) is increased with negative ventilation in this phase. Even today, there remain conditions in which negative-pressure ventilation is preferred [24]. Notably, there are physiological advantages to positive-pressure ventilation, including alveolar recruitment in respiration, improved lung compliance, and functional residual capacity of the lungs. Altogether, there appear to be no clear advantages of one method over the other for the majority of patients. Due to the greater complexity, cost, and size of negative-pressure ventilation, positive-pressure ventilation became and remains predominant.

Sadly, the rapid surge of patients in the COVID-19 pandemic in late 2019 to 2021 as of this writing caused many to be concerned about the lack of ventilation equipment and technicians to manage them [25]. Beyond the desperate measures taken in some cases to split the ventilators as previously described, many of the same lessons learned during the last major respiratory infectious pandemic only to be forgotten [26] were learned all over again in this one. Coming at the end of the World War I, the mortality rate of the 1917–1918 influenza pandemic was nearly the same as that of COVID-19 [27]. Largely thought to arise from an outbreak in Leavenworth, Kansas, in the United States, it came to be known as the Spanish flu.

Spain was one of the few countries willing to publically acknowledge a serious infectious disease during wartime. Furthermore, most countries wanted to return to a sense of normalcy after years of death and destruction that marked the first of many large wars in the twentieth century. The pandemic was mostly forgotten along with the war. Ironic in a retrospective sense, Warren Harding won in a landslide on a policy of "America First" and a withdrawal from international obligations towards populist interests on parallel with the Trump administration [28]. Many of the same measures eventually taken to slow COVID-19 were adopted with greater zeal to overcome the influenza pandemic, including mandatory masks (with fines in many locales), outdoor-only venues [29], and quarantines. Moreover, the 1917–1918 pandemic led to public health reforms in data aggregation, employer-provided health insurance, and founding of epidemiology as a discipline.

Unfortunately, progress on these matters did not continue onward to nationalized healthcare or medical insurance that is the standard in all advanced nations of the world except for the United States [30]. Before the devastating COVID-19 pandemic, which has claimed the lives of over 900,000 Americans and 3.3 million people worldwide as of this writing, coronavirus, Zika, and other infectious diseases were known to potentially be capable of sustaining a serious pandemic. There was sufficient concern in the United States to cause the Obama administration to find the Directorate for Global Health Security and Biodefense in the National Security Council of the United States in 2014, making it responsible for advance detection of global health threats. Unfortunately, the Trump administration dissolved the group in May 2018 [31].

A positive consequence of the COVID-19 pandemic has been the reinvention of inexpensive ventilator technologies, adopting microcontrollers and motors devised for 3D printing and robotics. These components, combined together with Internet-based, need-driven, and crowdsourced solutions, very rapidly responded to the well-founded concern of being overwhelmed by very sick patients and being unable to keep them alive with ventilators [32]. In the remainder of this chapter, we aim to provide the reader with information on ventilator design and production standards necessary to consider for their clinical use in the United States, in hopes that the efforts the reader undertake may indeed be translated to clinical use to save lives.

Types of Modern Ventilation

Ventilators deliver three basic forms of breathing sequences—continuous mandatory (CMV), intermittent mandatory (IMV), and continuous spontaneous (CSV) ventilation—in five basic patterns: pressure-control (PC)-CMV, PC-IMV, PC-CSV, volume-control (VC)-CMV, and VC-IMV [33], with the difference in flow and pressure illustrated in Fig. 5.2 for PC and VC operation. Moreover, there are several schemes to control the parameters (Table 5.1) and automatically adjust them to the patient's needs. The complexity of the situation is not helped by medical device manufacturer's penchant for uniquely naming some of these schemes as features to improve their market position or sales. In an attempt to overcome the cacophony of "over 100 different names for in excess of 30 mutually exclusive *ventilation modes*," the 140-page standard (International Standards Organization ISO/TC 210 2019) ISO 19223 was defined and published by the International Standards Organization (ISO) in 2019. Within, it aims to define standard terms for positive-pressure ventilation; we use these terms in this chapter. The standard provides 35 figures of airway pressure versus time for different forms of ventilation support alone. The reader would benefit from consulting the standard in considering how best to define a ventilator's operation or features. We summarize the main forms of ventilation as follows.

CMV: Continuous Mandatory Ventilation

Ventilation is delivered at a set interval without any accommodation for patient initiation.

A/C: Assist/Control Ventilation

Ventilation is delivered at a set interval unless the patient initiates a cycle before an interval elapses.

IMV: Intermittent Mandatory Ventilation

Ventilation is delivered at a set interval. Between these intervals, the patient may breathe without restriction or initiate another form of ventilation.

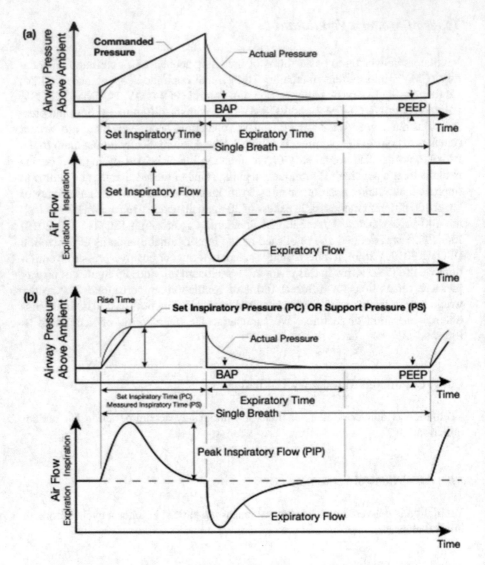

Fig. 5.2 Ventilator operation. A ventilator delivers gas into the lungs of a patient by either (**a**) volume (flow) control (VC) or (**b**) pressure control (PC). Some of the other parameters are monitored by most modern ventilators to ensure patient safety

SIMV: Synchronized Intermittent Mandatory Ventilation

Ventilation is delivered at a set interval, but this interval synchronizes with spontaneous breathing, if any. Between these intervals, the patient may breathe without restriction or initiate another form of ventilation.

S/T: Spontaneous/Timed Ventilation

Ventilation is triggered by a patient action, usually an inhalation. If the patient fails to initiate the ventilator after a set time elapses, the ventilator provides ventilation.

CSV: Continuous Spontaneous Ventilation

Ventilation is triggered by a patient action, usually an inhalation. No support ventilation is provided if the patient fails to trigger the ventilation.

APRV: Airway Pressure Release Ventilation

Almost ubiquitously termed *BiPAP, bilevel positive airway pressure* provides two set pressures for the patient to breathe above ambient pressure, one during inhalation and another during exhalation.

CPAP: Continuous Positive Airway Pressure

The device provides a set pressure for the patient to breathe above ambient pressure.

These ventilation modes are coded with a specific control variable, either volume (VC) or pressure control (PC) and any secondary intentions, listed below, to define a complete ventilation scheme. For example, CMV-VC provides continuous mandatory ventilation with volume control, ensuring that the delivered gas volume in a cycle is as commanded, adjusting the time, flow rate, or pressure of the delivery in order to achieve the desired outcome.

Pressure Support (PS)

The ventilator offers a fixed pressure above ambient to the patient upon the patient's inhalation and it is terminated by patient's respiratory action.

Patient-Triggered

The ventilator provides breathing by sensing the patient's inhalation, either via a drop in airway pressure or gas flow into the patient.

Ventilator-Initiated

The breath is triggered by the ventilator without sensing patient activity.

Time-Terminated

A breathing cycle is terminated at a fixed time, regardless of other factors.

Volume-Targeted

The ventilator is set to operate so that it delivers a desired inspiratory volume for each breath.

It is likely that in the coming years additional ventilation modes will be defined and added to the ISO standard. Recently, artificial intelligence and machine learning have become popular monikers to define the adaptability algorithms written into control systems for myriad applications, from robotics to medical devices [34]. Moreover, this technique is being creatively used to identify patients at risk of further morbidity and mortality [35], a fascinating extension of existing medical equipment in patient care. However, the reader should keep in mind that improvements in life support equipment are considered *changes* by the FDA and similar regulatory authorities, leading to a lengthy and expensive effort to prove the safety, efficacy, and ease of use of these new technologies. Most successful efforts of this sort appear after years of effort and only via the support of large medical device manufacturers.

Other forms of ventilation include continuous positive airway pressure (CPAP), a closely related variant, bilevel continuous positive airway pressure (Bi-PAP), and nasal high flow (NHF), the latter especially useful with increased oxygen [36, 37]. These aid respiration without cycling, and are mainly used to maintain airway patency or to provide greater oxygen partial pressures than standard air, improving blood oxygen concentration without sedation. They, however, incur a risk of spreading disease as the exhaled gas—along with viral particles and aerosols—is passed into the patient room unless precautions are taken [38]. Because negative-pressure patient care rooms are rare, even in developed nations, there were several attempts to devise patient care containment devices to protect healthcare workers and retain non-intubated ventilation as an option for COVID-19 treatment [39].

Extracorporeal membrane oxygenation (ECMO) is a last-ditch device that basically functions as a heart-lung bypass machine or an external heart and lung unit. It can be used when the lungs—even if mechanically ventilated—cannot support gas exchange. The most severe cases of ARDS-like pulmonary distress that arose from COVID-driven pneumonia lead to such significant inflammation of the lung tissue that oxygen and carbon dioxide exchange becomes impossible. This increased the need for ECMO beyond capacity in many hospital systems, in turn causing difficult triage decisions to be made on saving only a subset of patients. Not broadly available, ECMO is typically concentrated in specialist centers, and ECMO for COVID-19 patients who present a risk of infecting others including medical staff is even more selective. Patients that are young, have no comorbidities, and have not been on mechanical ventilation for a long period (with a recommendation of a week or less) were typically considered for ECMO. Because ECMO provides complete support, if the patient does not improve while on ECMO, the medical staff must consider ending ECMO support after some time (with 21 days usually cited) [40]. Even with excellent care, COVID-19 patient prognosis after ECMO is modest [40].

Designing Ventilators for Clinical Use

Regulations and Standards

A medical device designer is not free to create a ventilator according to any notional plan, as there are many regulatory bodies with detailed requirements that must be followed in a demonstrated way from the initial concept to receive permission to use the ventilator in a clinical setting. For example, besides the FDA in the United States, the United Kingdom (Medicines and Healthcare products Regulatory Agency, MHRA), the European Union (Council Directive 93/42/EEC on Medical Devices), Australia (Therapeutic Goods Administration, TGA), Japan (Pharmaceuticals and Medical Devices Agency, PMDA), and China (National Medical Products Administration, NMPA) have their own medical device regulatory authorities with unique requirements. Other nations also have unique requirements, but many will accept FDA or EU approval as sufficient.

Within the regulations promulgated by these organizations, there is a necessity to follow certain basic standards for medical device design, construction, and support during their use in the clinical setting. The most common among these are maintained by the International Standards Organization (ISO) and the International Electrotechnical Commission (IEC). With ventilators, the standards are surprisingly detailed, even for an *Emergency Use Authorization* (EUA) as was issued by the Chief Scientist of the FDA on 24 March 2020. This EUA was in response to the COVID-19 pandemic for accelerated approval of ventilators based upon a perceived shortage of them and related equipment. The framework of the EUA was the standard approval process, and documentation was provided in the EUA on how to later or simultaneously proceed with a *de novo*/510(k) clearance or *pre-market approval* (PMA) after the EUA was rescinded. Essentially, all of the standard approval requirements were still present, but some were relaxed based upon reasoned judgement that the urgent need was not compatible with the lengthy testing required to satisfy them.

The overarching standards for a life-support ventilator are ISO 80601-2-80 (International Standards Organization ISO/TC 121/SC 3 2018) and ISO 80601-2-12 (Organization 2020), the latter important in a healthcare facility setting. These standards define myriad aspects of a ventilator, from gas leakage limits to sterilization, shock robustness to displays, and oxygen handling to control placement. Moreover, these standards reference numerous other standards that a device designer must be aware of and conform to. The most notable among these include the following standards[1]:

IEC 60601-1:2005+AMD1:2012+AMD2:2020 CSV

This defines electrical and electromagnetic interference requirements for equipment used in medical practice.

IEC 60601-1-11

It tests for the integrity of the enclosure against water, dust, and patient or user's fingers, and cleaning and disinfection.

ISO 18652

It offers biocompatibility requirements for medical devices, and a key reason why many low-cost ventilators employ previously approved resuscitation bags for their past approval of the gas flow path to and from the patient [31].

ISO 5356-1

This provides dimensions and other requirements for ventilators and other breathing equipment to safely and reliably interface with each other.

21 CFR Part 820 or ISO 13485

The medical device manufacturer must operate with a validated quality management system as defined by these two standards. This, importantly, also includes feedback on device failure and patient or operator injury after the ventilator has

---

[1] Note that all of these standards have subparts and are frequently updated. The reader should carefully review the latest requirements with their regulatory authority.

been provided to the end user. Records of these events must be maintained and reported to the FDA.

ISO 14971

The medical device manufacturer must demonstrate that the design was produced with risk management principles, identifying and documenting potential failure modes in components and processes used in the device. Any mitigation strategies, changes, and controls to avoid failure are to be documented.

IEC 62304:2015

Design and development of medical device software. The process of writing life-support software demands a level of documentation and oversight well beyond standard software encapsulated in a life cycle for the software and a quality management system to supervise its development.

AAMI TIR69:2017 and ANSI/IEEE C63.27:2017

These are wireless equipment coexistence and compatibility standards, with the former dedicated specifically to medical equipment.

ISO 7010

The source of many of the "stick man" figures and iconic labels on equipment. This standard defines the shape, color, content, and size of warning and informational labels that must be attached to the equipment.

An important effect of these regulations and standards is that the process of documenting the design, production, sales, and clinical use of the device is what matters, not merely the end result. The net result of these regulations and standards is very limited flexibility in medical device design, consequence of adverse patient outcomes over decades of clinical experience, and an aim to avoid these and potential future problems by standardizing the technology. In other words, these rules were "written in blood" over many years.

What appears to be a creative and useful new idea in technology may instead risk a patient's life due to the operator not understanding the implications of the new idea. Progress is slow as safety remains paramount. In the context of a pandemic, however, the urgent need may outweigh the risk, and the EUA is the means to waive some or all of the regulations that maintain patient safety.

Example Design: Inexpensive Bag-Based Ventilator

Based upon the perceived urgent need of ventilators for the COVID-19 pandemic, we quickly set upon a program of designing and producing prototype ventilators in March–May of 2020 [31]. We made use of the EUA issued by the FDA, and sought to satisfy as many of the standards and regulations as possible, knowing that while the urgency would alleviate some of the requirements, most would remain enforced to protect patients. Notably, our approach attempted to address the patient segment most likely requiring intubation and ventilation, those suffering from ARDS.

From the clinical experience of our team, the standards, and published literature, we judged the following aspects to be vital for ventilators during COVID-19: operation using the pressure-control (PC) mode of ventilation, control of the respiratory rate and the inspiratory time, and (ISO 5356-1) compatibility with external components typically used in ventilation, including, in particular, adjustable positive end-expiratory pressure (PEEP) valves [41]. At the time, the vast majority of low-cost ventilators were designed as (VC) volume-control ventilators, delivering a requisite amount of air into the lungs, whether or not it was to an excess pressure. This can cause barotrauma, especially in patients with ARDS, one of the most common symptoms of COVID-19 in hospitalized cases [42].

Because the device supports life, basic alarms were required to indicate out-of-range operation, specifically high- and low-pressure conditions, and, likewise, high and low volumes delivered. Unlike most low-cost ventilators, and in adherence to FDA/ISO standards, we fully alarmed our ventilator to include faults in the motor and circuits, kinked or disconnected ventilation tubing, or failure of the backup battery. The battery was included to satisfy the requirement for at least 30 min of operation without power.

Because most COVID-19 patients at that time that were subjected to ventilation were intubated and sedated [43, 44], we decided to adopt a mandatory ventilation scheme to avoid the extremely expensive flow sensors required for accurate spontaneous inhalation detection. This also helped us avoid writing and validating software that would be needed to ensure that the ventilator sensed and operated properly upon a patient's inhalation. This simplified the settings of the ventilator and its troubleshooting as a mandatory closed-loop pressure-controlled (PC) time-terminated (tt) ventilator. It provided predictable breath delivery, and streamlined device production with only the requirement of pressure sensors and an algorithm for predicting the volume of gas delivered based upon the compression of the respiration bag, itself predicted by the angle of the arm used to compress it.

We also sought to minimize the number of parts used to produce the device, particularly hardware, and to make it possible to hang or mount the ventilator in an arbitrary direction. With the parts we selected, we sought to use parts that were not compromised by supply-chain constraints that were prevalent at the outset of 2020 due to COVID-19-driven lockdowns in China and elsewhere. Notably, we avoided gas flow sensors, ventilator-only pressure sensors, or specialized stepper motors—instead choosing identical motors used for 3D printing, and selecting simple laser-machined parts for the structure that could be manufactured nearly anywhere. The process produced a list of parts that cost about $300. The compression mechanism did have a pinch point, a problem according to ISO 60601-1-11, but our mitigation included a guard and automatic sensing to stop any detected pinch and an alarm to announce the problem.

An important part of the process is validation of the design. Validation of any novel medical device is a lengthy process that usually starts on the benchtop and only after extensive testing and having passed regulatory control finds its way to patient service in the form of clinical trials. In our case, there is fortunately an explicitly defined gold standard, the mechanical lung, for example the Dual Adult Test Lung by Michigan Instruments (4717 Talon Court SE, Grand Rapids, MI 49512 USA) paired with a ventilation data acquisition system (MP160, BioPac, 42 Aero Camino Goleta, CA 93117 USA). Clinical ventilators are routinely validated and calibrated using mechanical lung simulators according to FDA standards. We validated our new ventilator using these same procedures, first testing the adverse condition alarms that would inform the healthcare provider of problems, then testing ventilation under normal to extreme conditions, and finally continuously testing the ventilator for 24 h.

High- and low-volume ventilation problems were simulated by altering the PEEP values to trigger the ventilator's respective alarms. High pressure perhaps from a coughing patient or a ventilator tube kink that may block airflow likewise produced an alarm, but only after repeated coughing as desired. Causing an alarm after transient coughing or movement of the patient can become annoying enough to cause the healthcare provider to shut the alarm off permanently, making events that risk the patient's health undiscovered. Once our anesthesiologists were satisfied with the alarms and controls, our ventilator was then taken through the validation steps defined by ISO 80601-2-80:2018: a 24-h ventilation test and 12 cases of adverse ventilation, defined to explore the edge cases and limits of the ventilator's operation with different lung compliances and capacities on a mechanical lung. Our particular system showed little to no deviation from the defined values for these tests while being supervised by independent anesthesiologists, and this helped to confirm that our system would be safe for use. In normal conditions, testing would include many other aspects as defined by the standards, but with an EUA during a pandemic, these are the most important considerations to validate. The reader is cautioned, however, to remember that even with an EUA the vast majority of standards and regulations continue to be enforced, and so partnership with companies skilled in advancing technology from this stage to clinical use and beyond is vital.

Conclusions

In this chapter we have sought to provide a basic foundation for understanding human respiration, supporting it via mechanical ventilation, how mechanical ventilation is applied to treating patients, and the process to design a ventilator that may be appropriate for clinical use according to the regulations in place—even during desperate conditions that may rise during a global infectious pandemic. Unfortunately, the combination of continued growth in the human population, facile mobility, and widespread displacement due to climate change and conflict virtually guarantees new and serious infectious pandemics in our future. Our response to these events can save lives by providing innovative healthcare solutions drawn from new technologies and achievements in the interim. Mechanical ventilation is a key part of supporting life despite illness and disease, and devising low-cost, effective, and safe ventilators is crucial to our collective future. More responsive ventilators able to support life despite poor lung compliance or capacity, ventilators that are available and work in even the most disadvantaged areas of the world, and better ventilation options to help avoid sedation and intubation are but a few of the most important improvements that need to be made in the years to come. By making best use of the combination of physiological knowledge and regulations written to define a safe route to clinically useful medical devices, along with a brief example drawn from our own experience during COVID-19, we hope that the reader of this chapter can help define a better future in healthcare ventilation.

Conflicts of Interest The authors declare no relevant conflicts of interest.

Funding This work was funded by the Office of Naval Research (USA) through grant 1300847376 and a matching gift grant from Kratos Defense to L.P. and J.F.

References

1. Kilbourne ED. Influenza pandemics of the 20th Century. Emerg Infect Dis. 2006;12(1):9.
2. Tebbens D, Radboud J, Pallansch MA, Kew OM, Cáceres VM, Sutter RW, Thompson KM. A dynamic model of poliomyelitis outbreaks: learning from the past to help inform the future. Am J Epidemiol. 2005;162(4):358–72.
3. Chaudhry R, Bordoni B. Anatomy, thorax, lungs. Treasure Island, FL: StatPearls; 2021.
4. West JB, Luks A. West's respiratory physiology: the essentials. Alphen aan den Rjin: Wolters Kluwer; 2016. https://books.google.com/books?id=Wtj_oQEACAAJ
5. Morrison S. Ford and GM are making tens of thousands of ventilators. It may already be too late. Vox Media, LLC; 2020. https://www.vox.com/recode/2020/4/10/21209709/tesla-gm-ford-ventilators-coronavirus.
6. Silva PL, Rocco PRM. The basics of respiratory mechanics: ventilator-derived parameters. Ann Transl Med. 2018;6(19):376. https://doi.org/10.21037/atm.2018.06.06.
7. Anzueto A, Frutos–Vivar F, Esteban A, Alía I, Brochard L, Stewart T, Benito S, et al. Incidence, risk factors and outcome of barotrauma in mechanically ventilated patients. Intensive Care Med. 2004;30(4):612–9.
8. Udi J, Lang CN, Zotzmann V, Krueger K, Fluegler A, Bamberg F, Bode C, Duerschmied D, Wengenmayer T, Staudacher DL. Incidence of barotrauma in patients with Covid-19 pneumonia during prolonged invasive mechanical ventilation – a case-control study. J Intensive Care Med. 2021;36(4):477–83. https://doi.org/10.1177/0885066620954364.
9. Gray JS, Grodins FS, Carter ET. Alveolar and Total Ventilation and the Dead Space Problem. J Appl Physiol. 1956;9(3):307–20. https://doi.org/10.1152/jappl.1956.9.3.307.

10. Lucangelo U, Blanch L. Dead space. Intensive Care Med. 2004;30(4):576–9.
11. Mortola JP. How to breathe? Respiratory mechanics and breathing pattern. Respir Physiol Neurobiol. 2019;261:48–54.
12. Cooper JS, Phuyal P, Shah N. Oxygen toxicity. Treasure Island, FL: StatPearls; 2020. [Internet Only, Accessed 12 May 2021]. https://www.ncbi.nlm.nih.gov/books/NBK430743/
13. Usher AD. Medical oxygen crisis: a belated Covid-19 response. Lancet. 2021;397(10277):868–9.
14. Villarreal-Fernandez E, Patel R, Golamari R, Khalid M, DeWaters A, Haouzi P. A plea for avoiding systematic intubation in severely hypoxemic patients with Covid-19-associated respiratory failure. Crit Care. 2020;24(1):337.
15. Jaber S, Amraoui J, Lefrant J-Y, Arich C, Cohendy R, Landreau L, Calvet Y, Capdevila X, Mahamat A, Eledjam J-J. Clinical practice and risk factors for immediate complications of endotracheal intubation in the intensive care unit: a prospective, multiple-center study. Crit Care Med. 2006;34(9):2355–61.
16. McConville JF, Kress JP. Weaning patients from the ventilator. N Engl J Med. 2012;367(23):2233–9.
17. Gay PC. Complications of noninvasive ventilation in acute care. Respir Care. 2009;54(2):246–58.
18. Bucher JT, Vashisht R, Ladd M, Cooper JS. Bag mask ventilation (Bag Valve Mask, BVM). Treasure Island, FL: StatPearls; 2020.
19. Neyman G, Irvin CB. A single ventilator for multiple simulated patients to meet disaster surge. Acad Emerg Med. 2006;13(11):1246–9.
20. Petersen LG, Friend J, Merritt S. Single ventilator for multiple patients during Covid-19 surge: matching and balancing patients. Crit Care. 2020;24(1):1–3.
21. Young JD, Sykes MK. Assisted ventilation. 1. Artificial ventilation: history, equipment and techniques. Thorax. 1990;45(10):753–8.
22. Slutsky AS. History of mechanical ventilation. From Vesalius to ventilator-induced lung injury. Am J Respir Crit Care Med. 2015;191(10):1106–15.
23. Shneerson JM. Assisted ventilation. 5. Non-invasive and domiciliary ventilation: negative pressure techniques. Thorax. 1991;46(2):131–5.
24. Rothfield M, Sengupta S, Goldstein J, Rosenthal BM. 13 Deaths in a Day: an 'Apocalyptic' Coronavirus Surge at an N.Y.C. Hospital. New York: The New York Times; n.d.
25. Pal S. Forgotten: the Spanish influenza pandemic of 1918. In: Historians without borders. Milton Park: Routledge; 2019. p. 185–200.
26. Barry JM. The great influenza: the epic story of the deadliest plague in history. In: The great influenza: the story of the deadliest pandemic in history. London: Penguin Books; 2005.
27. Wilson DL, Coolidge C. The Presidency of Warren G. Harding. Lawrence: Regents Press of Kansas; 1977.
28. Hobday RA, Cason JW. The open-air treatment of pandemic influenza. Am J Public Health. 2009;99 Suppl 2(Suppl 2):S236–42.
29. Spinney L. "How the 1918 Flu Pandemic Revolutionized Public Health." n.d.. url: https://www.smithsonianmag.com/history/how 1918-flu-pandemic-revolutionized-public-health-180965025/; Smithsonian Magazine.
30. Sun LH. Top white house official in charge of pandemic response exits abruptly. Washington: The Washington Post; n.d.
31. Vasan A, Weekes R, Connacher W, Sieker J, Stambaugh M, Suresh P, Daniel E. Lee, et al. MADVent; a low-cost ventilator for patients with COVID-19. Med Dev Sens. 2020;3(e10106):1–14.
32. Dellaca' Raffaele L, Veneroni C, Farre' R. Trends in mechanical ventilation: are we ventilating our patients in the best possible way? Breathe. 2017;13(2):84–98. https://doi.org/10.1183/20734735.007817.
33. Gholami B, Phan TS, Haddad WM, Cason A, Mullis J, Price L, Bailey JM. Replicating human expertise of mechanical ventilation waveform analysis in detecting patient-ventilator cycling asynchrony using machine learning. Comput Biol Med. 2018;97:137–44.

34. Mamandipoor B, Frutos-Vivar F, Peñuelas O, Rezar R, Raymondos K, Muriel A, Bin D, et al. Machine learning predicts mortality based on analysis of ventilation parameters of critically ill patients: multi-centre validation. BMC Med Inform Decis Mak. 2021;21(1):1–12.

35. Pinto VL, Sharma S. Continuous positive airway pressure. Treasure Island, FL: StatPearls; 2020. [Internet only, accessed 12 May 2021]. https://www.ncbi.nlm.nih.gov/books/NBK482178/

36. Frat J-P, Thille AW, Mercat A, Girault C, Ragot S, Perbet S, Prat G, et al. High-flow oxygen through nasal cannula in acute hypoxemic respiratory failure. N Engl J Med. 2015;372(23):2185–96.

37. Tran K, Cimon K, Severn M, Pessoa-Silva CL, Conly J. Aerosol generating procedures and risk of transmission of acute respiratory infections to healthcare workers: a systematic review. PLoS One. 2012;7(4):e35797.

38. Tilvawala G, Grant A, Wen JH, Wen TH, Criado-Hidalgo E, Connacher WJ, Friend JR, Morris T. Vacuum exhausted isolation locker (VEIL) to reduce inpatient droplet/aerosol transmission during COVID-19 pandemic. Infect Control Hosp Epidemiol. 2021:1–10. https://doi.org/10.1017/ice.2020.1414.

39. Bartlett RH, Ogino MT, Brodie D, McMullan DM, Lorusso R, MacLaren G, Stead CM, et al. Initial ELSO guidance document: ECMO for COVID-19 patients with severe cardiopulmonary failure. ASAIO J. 2020;66(5):472.

40. The Society of Critical Care Medicine (SCCM), American Association for Respiratory Care (AARC), American Society of Anesthesiologists (ASA), Anesthesia Patient Safety Foundation (APSF), American Association of Critical-Care Nurses (AACN), and American College of Chest Physicians (CHEST). n.d. "Joint Statement on Multiple Patients Per Ventilator." https://www.asahq.org/about-asa/newsroom/news-releases/2020/03/joint-statement-on-multiple-patients-per-ventilator.

41. Barbaro RP, MacLaren G, Boonstra PS, Iwashyna TJ, Slutsky AS, Fan E, Bartlett RH, et al. Extracorporeal membrane oxygenation support in Covid-19: an international cohort study of the extracorporeal life support organization registry. Lancet. 2020;396(10257):1071–8.

42. Brower RG, Matthay MA, Morris A, David S, Taylor Thompson B, Wheeler A, Acute Respiratory Distress Syndrome (ARDS) Network. Ventilation with lower tidal volumes as compared with traditional tidal volumes for acute lung injury and the acute respiratory distress syndrome. N Engl J Med. 2000;342(May):1301–8.

43. Meng L, Qiu H, Wan L, Ai Y, Xue Z, Guo Q, Deshpande R, et al. Intubation and ventilation amid the Covid-19 outbreak Wuhan's experience. Anesthesiology. 2020;132(6):1317–32.

44. Bourenne J, Hraiech S, Roch A, Gainnier M, Papazian L, Forel J-M. Sedation and neuromuscular blocking agents in acute respiratory distress syndrome. Ann Transl Med. 2017;5:291–303. https://doi.org/10.21037/atm.2017.07.19.

Chapter 6
An Introduction to Noninvasive Ventilation

Melissa Huang, Karen Katrivesis, and Trung Q. Vu

Introduction

Noninvasive ventilation (NIV) offers an alternative treatment for respiratory insufficiency compared to invasive ventilation. Some of the benefits of NIV versus invasive ventilation include patient's comfort, avoidance of directly manipulating the patient's airway, minimized use of sedation, avoidance of ventilator-induced lung injury (VILI), ease of use outside of the intensive care unit, and an option for patients with "do not intubate" orders. The drawbacks of NIV versus invasive ventilation are that it does not offer airway protection from aspiration, it may feel claustrophobic for the patient, and it may cause facial pressure ulcers with the use of certain masks, especially if used for prolonged periods. Additionally, NIV has been found to have significant failure rates, shown to be up to 52% in one study [1], and these patients may experience complications from delayed intubation. NIV may be insufficient if the patient remains hypoxic or hypercapnic despite NIV, is at risk of aspiration, or has impaired consciousness. Another concern for the use of NIV in a patient with an infectious disease such as COVID-19 is aerosolization, which puts healthcare workers at risk.

High-Flow Nasal Cannula

High-flow nasal cannula (HFNC), or high-flow nasal oxygen (HFNO), is a form of noninvasive ventilation that delivers heated and humidified oxygen through a nasal cannula. It can heat gas up to 37 °C with 100% relative humidity and deliver

M. Huang · K. Katrivesis · T. Q. Vu (✉)
Department of Anesthesiology & Perioperative Care, Division of Anesthesiology
Critical Care Medicine, University of California, Irvine, CA, USA
e-mail: vut@hs.uci.edu

© The Author(s), under exclusive license to Springer Nature Switzerland AG 2022
A. A. Hakimi et al. (eds.), *Mechanical Ventilation Amid the COVID-19 Pandemic*,
https://doi.org/10.1007/978-3-030-87978-5_6

21–100% FiO$_2$ at flow rates up to 70 liters/minute (L/min). Normal nasal cannula delivers cold and dry air, which can decrease moisture to the nasopharynx and decrease secretion clearance. The warmed humidified gas promotes secretion clearance and provides more comfort to the patients. Furthermore, the high flow rate allows for greater rates of oxygen delivery, whereas other methods, such as the non-rebreather mask and simple face mask, deliver flow rates of up to 15 L/min and 12 L/min, respectively. HFNC also generates low levels of positive end-expiratory pressure (PEEP), which improves oxygenation by recruiting alveoli to increase surface area for gas exchange.

HFNC in COVID-19 Patients

HFNC is often the first-line intervention for respiratory support in patients with COVID-19 who are no longer tolerating supplemental oxygen, as it is easy to use and typically better tolerated and more comfortable than continuous positive airway pressure (CPAP) and bilevel positive airway pressure (BiPAP) therapies. At the height of the pandemic, experiences from other institutions around the world have shown that COVID-19 patients who required endotracheal intubation have a higher mortality. Rather, therapy that seems to have a positive clinical outcome is proning and avoidance of endotracheal intubation. Thus, HFNC served as a beneficial alternative for COVID-19 patients due to its ease of application, its ability to deliver high-flow-rate oxygen to match patients' increased respiratory rate, and its increased comfort for patients while being proned for an extended amount of time. Simulated studies have shown that bioaerosol dispersion using HFNC is similar to that of a standard oxygen mask which raises concern for healthcare providers [3]. Nevertheless, a study of HFNC use for COVID-19 patients has found that there is no evidence of increased COVID-19 infection among healthcare workers treating patients using HFNC as long as personal protective equipment are used [4].

CPAP

CPAP delivers constant pressure to the lungs throughout the respiratory cycle. The continuous positive pressure is achieved via an airtight face mask. The maintenance of constant airway pressure leads to improved oxygenation by decreasing atelectasis, recruitment of alveoli, and improvement of respiratory compliance and ventilation-perfusion mismatch. CPAP can be useful in patients with hypoxemic or hypercarbic respiratory failure, congestive heart failure, and obstructive sleep apnea and in the pediatric and neonatal intensive care unit.

CPAP in COVID-19 Patients

Early studies of CPAP use in the treatment of respiratory failure in patients with COVID-19 showed that the use of CPAP led to avoidance of mechanical ventilation in 58% of patients with a survival rate of 79% in one cohort of 24 patients [5]. Concerns of CPAP use in COVID-19 patients include pressure ulcers, barotrauma, and increased SARS-CoV-2 aerosolization. Aerosolization refers to small droplets and particles that remain suspended in air and may transmit viruses such as SARS-CoV-2. The particles are generated with procedures such as intubation, extubation, bronchoscopy, nebulization, suctioning, and delivery of high-flow oxygen. Other variables that contribute to aerosolization include flow velocity, leak, and coughing.

Aerosolization with CPAP devices has been studied with different methods to reduce aerosol exposure. Physical barriers such as intubation shields have been developed. One study looked at attaching filters to remove viral particles in the air from the expiratory limb of CPAP devices, which was observed with a minor increase in imposed work of breathing [6]. Another technology that was developed to reduce infection of healthcare workers is the constant-flow canopy, which is a plastic canopy that fits over the upper bed and contains a fan, filtering system, and a negative-pressure exhaust system that exchanges the filtered air [7]. Follow-up studies on flow canopies in a simulated setting confirm a significant reduction in aerosol count during intubation [8].

CPAP delivered via helmet has the benefit of decreased aerosolization compared to the face mask, greater comfort to the wearer, and reduction in pressure ulcers. A study of 157 patients with moderate-to-severe hypoxemic respiratory failure from COVID-19 treated with helmet CPAP found a failure rate of 44.6% [9]. The HEMIVOT trial compared the use of HFNC versus helmet ventilation in patients with moderate-to-severe hypoxemic respiratory failure and found that helmet ventilation had improved oxygenation and dyspnea. This trial also found a reduced rate of intubation compared to HFNC, although the duration of respiratory support was not significantly different [10].

BiPAP

BiPAP has two levels of continuous airway pressure, inspiratory airway pressure (IPAP) and expiratory positive airway pressure (EPAP). Unlike CPAP where the continuous airway pressure provides no direct ventilation, the difference in pressure between IPAP and EPAP provides the pressure support to assist with ventilation. BiPAP is useful for those with hypercapnic (elevated CO_2 levels) respiratory failure or a combination of hypercapnic and hypoxemic respiratory failure. Some patients may also find BiPAP to be more comfortable than CPAP as it reduces airway pressure when a patient is exhaling. It has been used for this purpose in patients with acute chronic obstructive pulmonary disease exacerbations and cardiogenic pulmonary edema. It is also used to transition patients off mechanical ventilation. Basic BiPAP ventilator settings include IPAP, EPAP, and FiO_2 with the addition of minimum respiratory rate and inspiratory time.

BiPAP in COVID-19 Patients

In COVID-19 patients who have risk factors for hypercapnia such as obstructive sleep apnea and obesity hypoventilation syndrome, BiPAP may be preferred to CPAP as the addition of inspiratory pressure should further reduce the work of breathing. However, studies on BiPAP use in COVID-19 patients are limited as CPAP is more commonly used. One study of COVID-19 patients found an association between BiPAP use and lower baseline P_aO_2/FiO_2 ratio compared to those using CPAP, although all-cause mortality was the same between these two groups [11].

Survival Mode with Noninvasive Ventilation in a Resource-Limited Setting

In a resource-limited setting, the capacity for invasive ventilation may be limited due to lack of intensive care unit beds, hospital staff, ventilators, or other infrastructure. Noninvasive ventilation and other alternative methods of delivering oxygen are crucial for respiratory support when invasive ventilation is not a widely available option. Supplemental oxygenation delivered through nasal cannula, non-rebreathing mask, or facial mask is the first option for oxygen delivery, as well as prone position. NIV adds the benefit of adding respiratory support and decreasing the work of breathing for patients, which will reduce fatigue and exhaustion [12].

Conflicts of Interest   None

Financial Disclosures   None

References

1. Pierson DJ. History and epidemiology of noninvasive ventilation in the acute-care setting. Respir Care. 2009;54(1):40.
2. Menzella F, Barbieri C, Fontana M, et al. Effectiveness of noninvasive ventilation in COVID-19 related-acute respiratory distress syndrome. Clin Respir J. 2021;15:779–87.
3. Li J, Fink JB, Ehrmann S. High-flow nasal cannula for COVID-19 patients: low risk of bio-aerosol dispersion. Eur Respir J. 2020;55(5):2000892.
4. Westafer LM, Soares WE 3rd, Salvador D, Medarametla V, Schoenfeld EM. No evidence of increasing COVID-19 in health care workers after implementation of high flow nasal cannula: a safety evaluation. Am J Emerg Med. 2021;39:158–61.

5. Nightingale R, Nwosu N, Kutubudin F, et al. Is continuous positive airway pressure (CPAP) a new standard of care for type 1 respiratory failure in COVID-19 patients? A retrospective observational study of a dedicated COVID-19 CPAP service. BMJ Open Respir Res. 2020;7(1):e000639.
6. Donaldsson S, Naver L, Jonsson B, Drevhammar T. COVID-19: minimising contaminated aerosol spreading during CPAP treatment. Arch Dis Child Fetal Neonatal Ed. 2020;105(6):669–71.
7. Misra S. Ketamine-associated bladder dysfunction—a review of the literature. Curr Bladder Dysfunct Rep. 2018;13(3):145–52.
8. Derrick J, Thatcher J, Wong JCP. Efficacy of an enclosure for reducing aerosol exposure during patient intubation. Med J Aust. 2020;213(8):372–3.
9. Aliberti S, Radovanovic D, Billi F, et al. Helmet CPAP treatment in patients with COVID-19 pneumonia: a multicentre cohort study. Eur Respir J. 2020;56(4):2001935.
10. Grieco DL, Menga LS, Cesarano M, et al. Effect of helmet noninvasive ventilation vs high-flow nasal oxygen on days free of respiratory support in patients with COVID-19 and moderate to severe hypoxemic respiratory failure: the HENIVOT randomized clinical trial. JAMA. 2021;325(17):1731–43.
11. Carpagnano GE, Buonamico E, Migliore G, et al. Bilevel and continuous positive airway pressure and factors linked to all-cause mortality in COVID-19 patients in an intermediate respiratory intensive care unit in Italy. Expert Rev Respir Med. 2021;15(6):853–857.
12. Dondorp AM, Hayat M, Aryal D, Beane A, Schultz MJ. Respiratory support in COVID-19 patients, with a focus on resource-limited settings. Am J Trop Med Hyg. 2020;102(6):1191–7.

Chapter 7
Noninvasive Ventilation and Mechanical Ventilation to Treat COVID-19-Induced Respiratory Failure

Timmy Cheng, Richard Anthony Lee, and Walter B. Gribben

Introduction

Severe COVID-19 frequently results in respiratory complications, especially hypoxic respiratory failure. While the true incidence of hypoxic respiratory failure in patients with COVID-19 is not clear, a report of 72,314 cases from the Chinese Center for Disease Control and Prevention revealed that 81% of cases were reported to be mild (defined in this study as no pneumonia or mild pneumonia), 14% were severe (defined as dyspnea, respiratory frequency ≥ 30 breaths/min, oxygen saturation [SpO_2] $\leq 93\%$, a ratio of arterial partial pressure of oxygen to fraction of inspired oxygen [$PaO2/FiO_2$] <300 mm Hg, and/or lung infiltrates >50% within 24–48 h), and 5% were critical (defined as respiratory failure, septic shock, and/or multiorgan dysfunction or failure) [1].

The optimal oxygen saturation (SpO_2) in adults with COVID-19 remains uncertain; however, indirect evidence from experience in patients without COVID-19 suggests that an SpO_2 <92% or >96% may be harmful. Retrospective analyses of two electronic medical record databases including the e-ICU Collaborative Research Database and the Medical Information Mart for Intensive Care III database reported that an optimal range of SpO_2 was 94–98%, and the percentage of time patients were within the optimal range of SpO_2 was associated with decreased hospital mortality [2]. A systematic review and meta-analysis of 25 randomized controlled trials (16,037 patients with sepsis, critical illness, stroke, trauma, myocardial infarction,

T. Cheng (✉)
Department of Internal Medicine, Division of Pulmonary and Critical Care,
Irvine Medical Center, University of California, Irvine, CA, USA
e-mail: timmy@chs.uci.edu

R. A. Lee · W. B. Gribben
Irvine Medical Center, University of California, Irvine, CA, USA
e-mail: richaral@hs.uci.edu; wgribben@hs.uci.edu

© The Author(s), under exclusive license to Springer Nature Switzerland AG 2022
A. A. Hakimi et al. (eds.), *Mechanical Ventilation Amid the COVID-19 Pandemic*,
https://doi.org/10.1007/978-3-030-87978-5_7

or cardiac arrest, and patients who had emergency surgery) suggested that a liberal oxygen strategy (with median SpO_2 of 96%), compared with a conservative oxygen strategy, is associated with increased risk of hospital mortality in acutely ill patients [3]. The recent LOCO2 trial randomized patients with acute respiratory distress syndrome (ARDS) to a conservative oxygen arm (target SpO_2 88–92%) or a liberal oxygen arm (target $SpO_2 \geq$96%). The trial was stopped early for futility and possible increased 28-day mortality after 61 deaths had occurred in 205 included patients, and the conservative oxygen arm had a higher risk of death at 90 days [4]. Considering the associated patient harm at the extremes of SpO_2 targets and the increased cost of liberal oxygen use, as well as the potential to reduce equity if oxygen resources are depleted, a reasonable SpO_2 range for patients receiving oxygen is 92–96%. Surviving Sepsis Campaign: guidelines on the management of critically ill adults with Coronavirus Disease 2019 (COVID-19) issued a strong recommendation against using oxygen to target SpO_2 >96%, and a strong recommendation to avoid lower values (SpO_2 <90%) [5].

In adults with COVID-19 and acute hypoxemic respiratory failure, conventional oxygen therapy may be insufficient to meet the oxygen needs of the patient necessitating enhanced respiratory support with options including high-flow nasal cannula, noninvasive positive-pressure ventilation, intubation and invasive mechanical ventilation, or extracorporeal membrane oxygenation (ECMO).

Before discussing these respiratory support strategies for treating COVID-19 pneumonia, it is important to introduce important terms and concepts frequently used. The following concepts are important to understand when discussing different modalities of respiratory support.

Oxygenation—It is the process of delivering oxygen into the lungs to be picked up by the circulating blood. This is mainly affected by positive end-expiratory pressure (PEEP) and fraction of inspired oxygen (FiO_2).

Ventilation—It is the processing of removing carbon dioxide from the bloodstream through the lungs. The term "minute ventilation" is the amount of ventilation performed in 1 min and is calculated by multiplying the respiratory rate by the tidal volume (RR × TV).

PEEP—It is the positive end-expiratory pressure. This is the amount of air pressure placed on the lungs at the end of the expiration. This pressure is thought to keep the lungs expanded at the end of a breath to prevent collapse of portions of the lungs. Keeping more portions of the lungs expanded will improve oxygenation.

FiO_2—It is the concentration of oxygen being delivered to the patient. Air at sea level usually carries 21% oxygen (21% FiO_2). Depending on a patient's needs, up to 100% FiO_2 can be delivered to improve oxygenation.

Respiratory rate—It is the number of breaths per minute. Increasing the respiratory rate increases the minute ventilation, thus increasing carbon dioxide excretion.

Tidal volume—It is the volume of each breath. Increasing the tidal volume increases the minute ventilation, thus increasing carbon dioxide excretion.

Plateau pressure—It is the air pressure measured in the lungs at the end of an inspiration when there is no movement of air in or out of the lungs. The plateau pressure can also be calculated with the formula PEEP plus driving pressure. The plateau pressure is often used as a measure of likelihood of barotrauma, or damage to the lungs due to high pressures in the lungs. In general, the plateau pressure should be kept under 30 cmH$_2$O to prevent barotrauma.

Driving pressure—It is the amount of pressure either delivered or required for each breath. The driving pressure is sometimes called "inspiratory pressure" or "pressure support."

Noninvasive Ventilation (NIV)

High-flow nasal cannula is an oxygen delivery system similar to simple or "low-flow" nasal cannula oxygen support systems. In both high-flow and low-flow nasal cannula systems, oxygen is delivered through a cannula to the nostrils for the patient to inhale. In a low-flow nasal cannula system, 100% oxygen is delivered at a flow rate of up to 6 L/min. The flow rate of a low-flow nasal cannula is limited by nasal mucosal irritation and drying of the nasal passages that may lead to bleeding. A normal human breath generates a peak inspiratory flow rate of around 30–60 L/min at rest, and up to 120 L/min in a patient who is short of breath. Therefore, in a low-flow nasal cannula system, the flow of delivered oxygen is not sufficient to meet the patient's peak inspiratory flow. Therefore, ambient air (FiO$_2$ 21%) is concurrently inhaled and mixed with the delivered oxygen. The final inspired concentration of oxygen depends on the flow rate of the delivered oxygen and the patient's inspiratory flow rate.

High-flow nasal cannula differs from low-flow nasal cannula in a number of ways. First is the ability to deliver flow rates up to 60 L/min. By meeting the patient's respiratory flow rate needs, the patient's breath does not need to mix with the surrounding air. This allows for the ability to control the FiO$_2$ delivered to the patient. To help the patient tolerate such a fast flow rate and prevent mucosal bleeding, the air that is delivered is heated and humidified to prevent drying of the nasal passages. There are several benefits of the high flow rate. One benefit is the theoretical positive pressure placed on the respiratory system throughout the respiratory breath. Positive pressure during the inspiratory phase augments the patient's tidal volumes, theoretically increasing patient's ventilation. At the end of the expiratory cycle, positive pressure results in a small amount of PEEP to keep alveoli open, thus improving the patient's oxygenation. The high flow rate has also been postulated to help with washing out carbon dioxide from the areas of the lung that do not usually receive significant airflow (also known as the physiologic dead space). Together, these mechanisms allow for increased oxygenation support, increased ventilatory support, and finer control of the delivered FiO$_2$ when compared to traditional low-flow nasal cannula systems.

Although high-flow nasal cannula provides many benefits over conventional low-flow nasal cannulas, high-flow nasal cannulas also have their limitations. Since the system is still open to the outside environment, there is a chance for a poor seal with the patient's nostrils and leakage from the system. In the dyspneic patient, the high-flow nasal cannula system may not be able to provide adequate flow to meet the patient's needs, so mixing with the surrounding air is still possible. The amount of pressure delivered to the patient cannot be controlled. Finally, the amount of pressure is likely relatively low when compared to the pressures that can be delivered through other noninvasive or invasive ventilatory support systems.

High-flow nasal cannula is preferred over noninvasive positive-pressure ventilation in patients with acute hypoxemic respiratory failure based on data from an unblinded clinical trial in patients without COVID-19 without hypercapnia who had acute hypoxemic respiratory failure with a ratio of arterial partial pressure of oxygen to fraction of inspired oxygen [PaO_2/FiO_2] $\leq$300 mm Hg, in which study participants were randomized to high-flow nasal cannula, conventional oxygen therapy, or noninvasive positive-pressure ventilation. The patients in the high-flow nasal cannula group had significantly more ventilator-free days (24 days) than those in the conventional oxygen therapy group (22 days) or noninvasive positive-pressure ventilation group (19 days) and 90-day mortality was lower in the high-flow nasal cannula group than in either the conventional oxygen therapy group or the noninvasive positive-pressure ventilation group [6]. In the subgroup of more severe hypoxemic patients (PaO_2/FiO_2 $\leq$200 mm Hg), the intubation rate was lower for high-flow nasal cannula than that for conventional oxygen therapy or noninvasive positive-pressure ventilation [6]. In a meta-analysis of eight trials with 1084 patients conducted to assess the effectiveness of oxygenation strategies prior to intubation, compared to noninvasive positive-pressure ventilation, high-flow nasal cannula reduced the rate of intubation and mortality in the intensive care unit (ICU) [7].

Noninvasive positive-pressure ventilation is an aerosol-generating procedure and may generate aerosol spread of SARS-CoV-2 and thus increase nosocomial transmission of the infection. In a systematic review of five case-control and five retrospective cohort studies which evaluated transmission of SARS to healthcare workers, noninvasive positive-pressure ventilation was among the procedures reported to present an increased risk of transmission [8]. It remains unknown whether high-flow nasal cannula presents a lower risk of nosocomial SARS-CoV-2 transmission than noninvasive positive-pressure ventilation.

Prone Positioning

Prone positioning may provide a more uniform distribution of transpulmonary pressures during mechanical ventilation by recruiting nonaerated tissue and by reducing the vertical pleural pressure gradient [9]. Factors that could contribute to this differential ability of the prone position to alter dorsal lung transpulmonary pressures include, among others, the compressive effects of consolidated lung, direct transmission of the weight of abdominal contents to caudal regions of the dorsal lung, and direct transmission of the weight of the heart to the regions of the lung located beneath it [10]. In a study of anesthetized and mechanically ventilated healthy volunteers, regional lung ventilation did not differ with position, whereas perfusion was more uniform in the prone position [11].

Prone positioning has been shown to improve oxygenation and outcomes in patients with moderate-to-severe ARDS receiving mechanical ventilation [12, 13]. There is less evidence regarding the benefit of prone positioning in awake patients who require supplemental oxygen without mechanical ventilation. In a retrospective study of 15 COVID-19 patients treated with noninvasive ventilation and pronation, all patients had an improvement in SpO_2 and $PaO_2:FIO_2$ during pronation; 12 patients (80%) had an improvement in SpO_2 and $PaO_2:FIO_2$ after pronation while the remainder had either the same value or worsened value [14]. In a prospective study of 24 awake, non-intubated, spontaneously breathing COVID-19 patients with hypoxemic respiratory failure managed outside of the ICU, 15 patients (63%) could tolerate prone positioning for more than 3 h, and oxygenation increased during prone positioning in only 25% and was not sustained in half of those after resupination [15]. In another prospective cohort study of awake prone positioning of 56 patients with COVID-19 receiving high-flow nasal cannula of noninvasive positive-pressure ventilation, prone positioning was maintained for at least 3 h in 84% of the patients [16]. Oxygenation substantially improved during prone positioning; however improvement in oxygenation was not sustained 1 h after resupination and there was no difference in intubation rate between patients who maintained improved oxygenation (responders) and those for whom improved oxygenation was not maintained (nonresponders) [16].

It remains unknown which hypoxemic, non-intubated patients with COVID-19 pneumonia benefit from prone positioning, how long prone positioning should be continued, or whether prone positioning prevents the need for intubation or improves survival. Awake prone positioning is contraindicated in patients with respiratory distress who require immediate intubation. It is essential to monitor hypoxemic patients with COVID-19 closely for signs of respiratory decompensation requiring an invasive mechanical ventilation.

Mechanical Ventilation

If noninvasive ventilation starts to fail, then the physician must consider the use of invasive mechanical ventilation. In most patients, this will require the placement of an endotracheal tube through the vocal cords in order to provide oxygen directly into the patient's lungs. Signs of worsening respiratory failure include worsened level of consciousness, worsened work of breathing (heavy accessory muscle use), and worsening hemodynamics and vital signs (as provided by pulse oximetry, telemetry, and arterial blood gas data).

The insertion of an endotracheal tube into an ICU patient usually requires that the patient be sedated. Paralysis is also often used to ensure the smooth passage of the endotracheal tube through the vocal cords into the trachea. Following the successful insertion of the endotracheal tube, the tube is then connected to a mechanical ventilator. Using mechanical ventilation, the physician can set parameters for tidal volume, respiratory rate, positive end-expiratory pressure, and fraction of inhaled oxygen. In contrast to traditional volume-control ventilation, a pressure-control ventilation strategy can be used. In this strategy, the physician sets a certain inspiratory and expiratory pressure, and then the physician observes the resulting tidal volumes.

No studies have shown any significant mortality benefit to one type of mechanical ventilation over another (such as volume control versus pressure control). The administration of mechanical ventilation can, unfortunately, cause damage to the lung, through administration of too much pressure (barotrauma) or too much volume (volutrauma). In patients with ARDS, an approach using a low tidal volume of 4–6 mL per kilogram of ideal body weight was shown to reduce mortality when compared to a traditionally used higher tidal volume of 8–10 mL per kilogram ideal body weight [17]. A French study showed that a strategy of allowing the patients to be turned on their stomach in a prone position for a significant part of the day could improve alveolar recruitment. This was the second study to show any potential benefit to reducing mortality in ARDS [12]. The third strategy in mechanical ventilation involves the use of continuous paralysis. Paralysis is typically employed in patients experiencing ventilator dyssynchrony, in which the patient's own initiated breaths clashed with the mechanical ventilator-delivered mandatory breaths. Administering neuromuscular blockade takes away the patient's ability to breathe on their own. As a result, the patient only receives the mandatory breaths set by the physician via the mechanical ventilator. A 2010 study seemed to show a slight mortality benefit for patients treated with neuromuscular blockade for 48 h [18]. However, a follow-up study in 2019 cast doubt on these findings [19]. Physicians still tend to use neuromuscular blockade in cases of individual ventilator dyssynchrony.

Mechanical ventilation provides several benefits to the patient. For one, it removes all of the patients' work of breathing, and displaces it onto the mechanical ventilator. This can be especially helpful in patients who are also experiencing shock. Second, it allows the physician to increase patients' PEEP to levels above what could be delivered via noninvasive ventilation. Without the leak allowed by a face mask, the endotracheal tube easily allows delivery of very high levels of PEEP, up to 20 cmH_2O or more. This can help improve oxygenation in patients who remain hypoxic even with an FiO_2 level of 100%. Third, the physician is able to set a respiratory rate higher than what the patient could be able to breathe on their own. Respiratory rates of 30 or even 35 breaths/min can be set and maintained for hours or even days on end. This would not be possible for the patient to do on his or her own, as it would cause an eventual tiring of the patient's respiratory muscles.

There are also disadvantages that are associated with mechanical ventilation. One disadvantage is that the presence of an endotracheal tube is typically uncomfortable for ICU patients. The tube must be wedged between the patient's vocal cords, and this often causes significant discomfort for the patients. As a result, patients must be treated continuously to provide pain relief, as well as to provide sedation. In most ICUs today, a continuous infusion of fentanyl, and synthetic opioid, is used to provide continuous pain relief. However, older, longer acting opiates such as morphine or hydromorphone can also be used. Patients who are receiving mechanical ventilation also often require a sedative to keep them calm while mechanical ventilation is being delivered. Several medications have been tried to provide this. Traditionally, benzodiazepines were used for sedation. However, these can cause a resulting delirium, which can prolong mechanical ventilation, as well as the patient's length of ICU stay. Other agents that have been tried include ketamine, propofol, and, most recently, dexmedetomidine. All of these agents provide some benefits above benzodiazepines. However, all of them also carry their own side effects.

The insertion of an endotracheal tube through the patient's vocal cords bypasses the nasopharynx and oropharynx. These are populated by cilia which normally help to filter out bacteria that can be present in the air. This artificial breathing system leaves the patient at increased risk of developing nosocomial infections, such as ventilator-acquired pneumonia (VAP). Several strategies, such as regular oral care, keeping the head of the bed elevated, and providing acid suppression therapy, have shown to reduce the risk of VAP. However, so far, nothing has been found to eliminate this risk. Another disadvantage of mechanical ventilation via endotracheal tube is that the patient is not able to eat by mouth (due to the presence of the tube) or to communicate by talking (because the tube passes through the vocal cords). The endotracheal tube can be maintained in place indefinitely. However, certain complications start to develop after prolonged medical mechanical ventilation, especially over more than 2–3 weeks. These complications include the development of tracheal stenosis, as well as possible mechanical erosion through the vocal cords or the trachea. Also, patients typically continue to require continuous infusions of opiates and sedatives to keep them comfortable while the endotracheal tube remains in place.

Once the endotracheal tube is inserted, the patient is started on mechanical ventilation and remains on mechanical ventilation. However, once the patient's respiratory status starts to improve, the physician will start working towards the eventual removal of the endotracheal tube, a procedure that is called extubation. Once patients are able to be weaned down on their sedation, a procedure called a spontaneous breathing trial (SBT) can be attempted. During this procedure, the ventilator is switched to a mode which allows the patient to breathe on their own. The patient is still provided a continuous positive expiratory pressure of at least 5 cmH$_2$O to overcome the resistance of the endotracheal tube. Often, the patient is also given some additional assistance in the form of pressure support to allow the patient to breathe more easily while connected to the ventilator. This SBT is ordered by the physician, and initiated by the respiratory therapist. The therapist will start the patient on a spontaneous breathing mode, and then observe the patient for signs of respiratory distress. These include tachypnea, low tidal volumes, and significant agitation. If these are observed, and persist, then the trial is considered to have been failed, and the patient is put back onto a mandatory mechanical ventilation mode. If, however, the patient does show that they are able to breathe on their own, as seen by good tidal volumes, a normal respiratory rate, and absence of agitation, then the patient is allowed to breathe spontaneously for about 30–120 min. Successful completion of one of these spontaneous breathing trials is often referred to as "passing" a SBT. This is one of the criteria used by the physician in determining whether the patient can be successfully extubated. However, extubation, just like intubation, is ultimately a clinical decision. Certain tools, such as the rapid shallow breathing index, have been devised to help calculate the probability of extubation success. However, per large review trials, about 10–15% of patients who are extubated will eventually require re-intubation for recurrent respiratory failure.

Tracheostomy

In patients who are not able to be weaned from the ventilator after about 2 weeks, tracheostomy should be considered. The tracheostomy procedure involves the insertion of a plastic tube through the cartilage of the anterior trachea, allowing it to sit below the vocal cords in the trachea. This procedure can be performed by a surgeon, pulmonologist, intensivist, or certain other specially trained physicians. This procedure can be done either in the operating room or at the bedside in the ICU. The advantage of performing a tracheostomy is that it allows for long-term mechanical ventilation. Indeed, some patients with spinal cord injuries, who have irreversible and permanent respiratory failure, are able to be maintained on continuous mechanical ventilation for years or even decades with this strategy. After the tracheostomy tube is inserted, the endotracheal tube is removed from the patient's vocal cords. Since the tracheostomy tube does not pass through the vocal cords, it typically results in the patients feeling a lot less pain and anxiety than with an endotracheal tube. Typically, within a day or two, opiate and sedation drips can be weaned down, or even off. The removal of these chemical agents can facilitate the process of ventilator weaning. At this point, patients can be started on increasingly longer trials of spontaneous breathing. The goal, eventually, is that they are able to breathe on their own completely for more than 24 h/day. At this point, the patient can be changed over to an uncuffed tracheostomy, or even be completely decannulated (the complete removal of the tracheostomy tube). After the tracheostomy tube is removed, the stoma closes quickly over the subsequent days, and the scar will eventually heal over. The primary long-term complication of tracheostomy is the development of scar tissue that can result in tracheal stenosis. Rarely, the tracheostomy site can also erode into adjacent blood vessels and result in significant bleeding.

One other advantage of the tracheostomy tube is that it allows patients to talk again on their own, with the use of special assistive devices that can be placed over the tracheostomy tube. Older devices, such as the Passy Muir valve, required the patient to be able to be temporarily off the ventilator in order to use them. However, new devices can be inserted in line with the ventilator circuit, to allow the patient to communicate even while connected to the mechanical ventilator.

Conflicts of Interest No relevant conflicts of interest to disclose.

Funding This work was not funded.

References

1. Wu Z, McGoogan JM. Characteristics of and important lessons from the coronavirus disease 2019 (COVID-19) outbreak in China: summary of a report of 72314 cases from the Chinese Center for Disease Control and Prevention. JAMA. 2020;323(13):1239–42.
2. van den Boom W, Hoy M, Sankaran J, et al. The search for optimal oxygen saturation targets in critically ill patients: observational data from large ICU databases. Chest. 2020;157(3):566–73.
3. Chu DK, Kim LH, Young PJ, et al. Mortality and morbidity in acutely ill adults treated with liberal versus conservative oxygen therapy (IOTA): a systematic review and meta-analysis. Lancet. 2018;391(10131):1693–705.
4. Barrot L, Asfar P, Mauny F, et al. Liberal or conservative oxygen therapy for acute respiratory distress syndrome. N Engl J Med. 2020;382(11):999–1008.
5. Alhazzani W, Moller MH, Arabi YM, et al. Surviving sepsis campaign: guidelines on the management of critically ill adults with coronavirus disease 2019 (COVID-19). Crit Care Med. 2020;48(6):e440–e69.
6. Frat JP, Thille AW, Mercat A, et al. High-flow oxygen through nasal cannula in acute hypoxemic respiratory failure. N Engl J Med. 2015;372(23):2185–96.
7. Ni YN, Luo J, Yu H, Liu D, Liang BM, Liang ZA. The effect of high-flow nasal cannula in reducing the mortality and the rate of endotracheal intubation when used before mechanical ventilation compared with conventional oxygen therapy and noninvasive positive pressure ventilation. A systematic review and meta-analysis. Am J Emerg Med. 2018;36(2):226–33.
8. Tran K, Cimon K, Severn M, Pessoa-Silva CL, Conly J. Aerosol generating procedures and risk of transmission of acute respiratory infections to healthcare workers: a systematic review. PLoS One. 2012;7(4):e35797.
9. Cornejo RA, Diaz JC, Tobar EA, et al. Effects of prone positioning on lung protection in patients with acute respiratory distress syndrome. Am J Respir Crit Care Med. 2013;188(4):440–8.
10. Albert RK, Hubmayr RD. The prone position eliminates compression of the lungs by the heart. Am J Respir Crit Care Med. 2000;161(5):1660–5.
11. Nyren S, Radell P, Lindahl SG, et al. Lung ventilation and perfusion in prone and supine postures with reference to anesthetized and mechanically ventilated healthy volunteers. Anesthesiology. 2010;112(3):682–7.
12. Guerin C, Reignier J, Richard JC, et al. Prone positioning in severe acute respiratory distress syndrome. N Engl J Med. 2013;368(23):2159–68.
13. Fan E, Del Sorbo L, Goligher EC, et al. An Official American Thoracic Society/European Society of Intensive Care Medicine/Society of Critical Care Medicine Clinical Practice Guideline: Mechanical Ventilation in Adult Patients with Acute Respiratory Distress Syndrome. Am J Respir Crit Care Med. 2017;195(9):1253–63.
14. Sartini C, Tresoldi M, Scarpellini P, et al. Respiratory parameters in patients with COVID-19 after using noninvasive ventilation in the prone position outside the intensive care unit. JAMA. 2020;323(22):2338–40.
15. Elharrar X, Trigui Y, Dols AM, et al. Use of prone positioning in nonintubated patients with COVID-19 and hypoxemic acute respiratory failure. JAMA. 2020;323(22):2336–8.
16. Coppo A, Bellani G, Winterton D, et al. Feasibility and physiological effects of prone positioning in non-intubated patients with acute respiratory failure due to COVID-19 (PRON-COVID): a prospective cohort study. Lancet Respir Med. 2020;8(8):765–74.
17. Acute Respiratory Distress Syndrome N, Brower RG, Matthay MA, et al. Ventilation with lower tidal volumes as compared with traditional tidal volumes for acute lung injury and the acute respiratory distress syndrome. N Engl J Med. 2000;342(18):1301–8.
18. Papazian L, Forel JM, Gacouin A, et al. Neuromuscular blockers in early acute respiratory distress syndrome. N Engl J Med. 2010;363(12):1107–16.
19. National Heart L, Blood Institute PCTN, Moss M, et al. Early neuromuscular blockade in the acute respiratory distress syndrome. N Engl J Med. 2019;380(21):1997–2008.

Part II
SARS CoV-2 Transmission and Innovative Protective Barriers

Chapter 8
COVID-19 Pathophysiology and COVID-19-Induced Respiratory Failure

Nikhil A. Crain, Ario D. Ramezani, and Taizoon Dhoon

Pathophysiology of COVID-19

With the rapidly emergent COVID-19 pandemic, infectious disease experts across the world have worked to understand the viral mechanisms of SARS-CoV-2 and the underlying reasons for multi-organ pathophysiology observed in affected patients. There is evidence that SARS-CoV-2 has the ability to evade a human's antiviral defenses and thus render a delayed immune response, with reports indicating incubation periods from 2 to 14 days with a median of roughly 5.1 days [1–3]. Primarily, it has been shown that SARS-CoV-2 targets the angiotensin-converting enzyme 2 (ACE2) receptor to invade host cells found in organs including the lungs, liver, heart, kidney, blood, and nervous system [4–6]. The binding to ACE2 receptors in the lungs has been shown as the primary mechanism to facilitate the transfer of COVID-19 between humans regardless of the symptomatic state [7].

The subsequent cascade of effects following ACE2 receptor binding include direct cell damage, breakdown of renin-angiotensin-aldosterone system (RAAS), massive cytokine release, oxidative stress, thrombosis, and systemic inflammation [5, 8, 9]. Symptoms have been shown to last from 2 to 4 weeks, which can vary between individuals of different risk factors and unique immune responses [5]. As described by Loganathan et al., the pathophysiology of SARS-CoV-2 can be categorized into three major stages: (1) invasion of type II pneumocytes via ACE2 receptors and replication with transmembrane protease, serine 2 (TMPRSS2) assistance; (2) viral replication in respiratory tract and prompt elevation of CXCL10 and epithelial β INF and γ-INF; and (3) sustained viral loads leading to acute respiratory distress syndrome (ARDS) [5].

N. A. Crain · A. D. Ramezani · T. Dhoon (✉)
Irvine Medical Center, University of California, Orange, CA, USA
e-mail: ario.ramezani@westernu.edu; tdhoon@hs.uci.edu

© The Author(s), under exclusive license to Springer Nature Switzerland AG 2022
A. A. Hakimi et al. (eds.), *Mechanical Ventilation Amid the COVID-19 Pandemic*,
https://doi.org/10.1007/978-3-030-87978-5_8

Severe acute respiratory syndrome coronavirus 2 (SARS-CoV-2) is a positive-sense RNA virus of the *Coronaviridae* family that has a non-segmented genome and viral envelope [10]. Coronaviruses are spherical, or "crown-like," in shape, and contain over 30,000 nucleotides, rendering it a large positive-sense RNA virus [5]. There are four major proteins that are translated by the viral genome: matrix (M), nucleocapsid (N), envelope (E), and most importantly spike (S) glycoprotein which binds to the ACE2 receptor [11, 12]. Specifically, the S protein has two subunits: while S1 attaches to the host's cell membrane via the ACE2 receptor, S2 enables cell-to-cell fusion called syncytium [13–15]. The enzyme TMPRSS2, a special type of protease, is essential to cleave the S proteins and allows S1 binding to the ACE2 receptor [6, 14]. It is the N- and O-linked glycans of SARS-CoV-2 that enable the virus to avoid innate immune system defenses [15]. E proteins serve an arguably novel role in regulating ion conduction and altering the cell environment. N proteins serve the pivotal task to aid in replication and transcription [5].

The transmembrane protein ACE2 produces angiotensin 2, which is a peptide hormone that serves a critical role in the RAAS [16]. Understanding the location of where SARS-CoV-2 can gain entry to the host cells via ACE2 receptors is important in determining the sites of originating infection and possible distribution [17]. Goblet and ciliated cells of the nasal cavity and pharyngeal epithelium of the upper airway contain high levels of ACE2 and TMPRSS2 co-expression, which indicate likely sites of initial infection [18–23]. The lower airway, including the bronchial epithelium and type II pneumocytes, also highly expresses ACE2 and TMPRSS2, thereby enabling entry to the lungs and subsequent respiratory disease from COVID-19 [18–21]. Along with the additional expression of CD147 and CD26, the respiratory barrier epithelium is a key target for viral attack and spread, rendering a loss of barrier function with the eventual recruitment of macrophages and lymphocytes which cause inflammation and cell lysis [24].

It has been demonstrated that SARS-CoV-2 can increase the levels of both pro-inflammatory mediators, such as interferon-gamma and interleukins β, 6, and 12, as well as chemokines, like CXCL10 and CCL2 [25, 26]. As a result of the massively elevated release of these molecules, two well-documented manifestations, called *cytokine storm* and *hyper-inflammatory syndrome*, can be provoked by COVID-19 infections and result in severe symptomatic states [25–29]. Importantly, it has been shown that nuclear factor kappa-light-chain-enhancer of activated B cells, or simply NF-κB, along with signal transducer and activator of transcription 3 (STAT3) creates an important cytokine feedback loop [30]. Of note, IL-6 in particular serves an important role in generating the viral inflammatory response from SARS-CoV-2, with studies showing increased levels in patients with pulmonary inflammation, lung damage, and severe COVID-19 infection [30–36].

While COVID-19 has received great attention for its ability to cause characteristic fever, fatigue, dry cough, and dyspnea among infectious individuals [26, 37], many organs can become affected through viral spread and immune and inflammatory responses [38]. Nevertheless, it is primarily a pulmonary illness which causes a pneumonia-like syndrome that is often indistinguishable in radiological imaging from other viral respiratory diseases [39–41]. Bilateral interstitial diffusion and ground-glass opacities with "crazy-paving" patterns have been reported, as well as progressive pleural effusions in advanced cases [42, 43]. Generally, the manifestation of pneumonia results from the high presence of ACE2 in lungs [44, 45]. Moreover, inflammation and injury of alveolar cells can result in acute respiratory distress syndrome (ARDS), which activates RAAS pathways and disrupts adaptive immunity mechanisms [46]. In the case of COVID-19, endotheliitis within the lungs has emerged as a distinct characteristic, which results in a complex cascade of endothelial injury, vascular "microthrombosis" within capillaries, and intussusceptive angiogenesis [47–55].

Nevertheless, endotheliitis is not exclusive to the lungs, and has been reported in the heart, kidney, and small intestine [49]. In the most critically severe COVID-19 cases, it has been shown that deaths resulted from ARDS, acute kidney injury (AKI), and myocardial injury, with a history of cardiovascular disease as a significant complicating factor [56, 57]. The ACE2 receptor is postulated to also be a primary reason for direct inflammation of the myocardium in progressive cases [58–61]. Histopathologic cardiac changes observed in patients with SARS-CoV-2 have been fibrosis and myocyte hypertrophy [62]. Two myocardial biomarkers, creatine-kinase-MB (CK-MB) and high-sensitivity cardiac troponin I (hs-cTnI), were shown to be increased in critical patients with myocardial injury [37]. Similarly, the resulting cytokine storm, which may lead to infiltrating inflammatory cells and eventual necrosis, has been cited to be another mechanism that can result in heart injury [63–65]. While cardiac involvement has been widely reported, it is important to note that COVID-19 autopsies may prove difficult to distinguish between direct viral involvement and preexisting conditions, especially if samples are coupled with unclear, overlapping, and nonspecific findings [48, 52, 66]. Nevertheless, cardiac injury is a critical feature of COVID-19 progression associated with increased risk of fatality [67].

Other systemic implications have been cited in recent SARS-CoV-2 research. Along with atrophy of the spleen and lymph nodes, and thus possible reduced turnover of lymphocytes, lymphocytopenia has been reported as another complication of COVID-19 [68–70]. Under histopathological evaluation, the spleen of COVID-19 patients has shown congested pulps, evidence of hemorrhagic spots, and paucity of lymphoid follicles and CD8+ cells [55, 68]. Neural involvement has been proposed to be related to either direct peripheral nerve attachment, and subsequent transfer to the central nervous system (CNS), or indirect harm from cytokine release and sepsis [71]. Specifically, the olfactory nerve may heighten CNS infection to the medulla oblongata, which may further complicate cardiorespiratory drive [4]. While gastrointestinal involvement, including nausea, vomiting, diarrhea, and anorexia, has been reported as a symptom of COVID-19, a recent meta-analysis showed that abdominal pain was the only significant factor associated with severe cases compared to mild-to-moderate illnesses [72]. Signs of skin complications have manifested in either viral exanthems (e.g., rashes, macules, urticaria, and vesicles) or vasculopathies (e.g., cyanosis, livedo, papules) [73, 74]. Microscopically, examinations have shown a range of findings, from perivascular dermatitis and keratinocyte necrosis to erythrocyte extravasation [73–75].

Given the multisystem progression which can be seen in individuals afflicted with COVID-19, there have been several risk factors which are associated with severe illness. Chronic obstructive pulmonary disease (COPD), cerebrovascular disease, diabetes mellitus type II, and hypertension have been reported as independent risk factors, with odds ratios (OD) of 5.97, 3.89, 2.47, and 2.29, respectively [76, 77]. Smokers with COPD, along with decreased lung function, show increased ACE2 expression, providing an even higher risk of complication [78, 79]. Hindered clearance of SARS-CoV-2, coupled with islet β-cell disruption, in diabetics as well as those with hypertension may result in more complicated disease states [76, 80]. Obesity has also been connected with worse outcomes with SARS-CoV-2 infection, primarily through increased activation of cytokines [81]. Interestingly, males have been shown to be more susceptible to COVID-19 compared to females, which may be due to linked activity of TMPRSS2 with androgen receptors and inherited vulnerabilities due to proximity of ACE2 and androgen gene loci on X chromosomes [82, 83]. Children have been described to be largely asymptomatic, which may be due to age-related differences in inflammatory response with lower pathogen-associated molecular pattern (PAMP) activation and less overall chronic inflammation [84, 85].

COVID-19-Induced Respiratory Failure

One of the most striking mysteries of the COVID-19 pandemic has been the phenotypic variation among patients infected with SARS-CoV-2. Hallmark symptoms have included fever, cough, and gustatory and olfactory loss; yet many patients have also been asymptomatic. Still, it would appear that the most feared manifestation of this disease is its progression to acute respiratory distress syndrome (ARDS).

The 2012 Berlin Definition of ARDS has provided a framework for distinguishing ARDS from other respiratory diseases [86]. According to this definition, ARDS must have an acute onset of 1 week or less. Computed tomography (CT) or a chest X-ray should demonstrate bilateral opacities consistent with pulmonary edema. The partial pressure of oxygen (PaO_2)-to-fraction of inspired oxygen (FiO_2) ratio must be less than 300 with a minimum of 5 cmH_2O positive end-expiratory pressure (PEEP), and the patient's symptoms must not be due to cardiac failure or fluid overload from another etiology.

Several studies have aimed to characterize COVID-induced ARDS (C-ARDS) phenotypes, but perhaps the most standardized is the distinction between type L-ARDS ("low" type) and type H-ARDS ("high" type). Marini et al. center their characterization around the functionality of elastance in the infected lung [87]. Elastance, the inverse of compliance, is the pressure required to inflate the lungs.

The type L-ARDS phenotype presents with characteristics embodied by low lung elastance. That is, the lungs will demonstrate nearly normal compliance, indicating that the amount of gas in the infected lung is similar to that of a normal, healthy lung. These patients will also show a low ventilation-to-perfusion (V/Q) ratio. With near-normal gas volume in the lungs, hypoxemia secondary to L-ARDS is most likely explained by a loss of hypoxic vasoconstriction in the lungs and resulting loss of perfusion regulation. Marini notes that type L patients will have low lung weight because the ground-glass densities seen on imaging are primarily subpleural or along lung fissures, allowing the lungs to maintain near-normal weight. Lastly, there will be low lung recruitability as gas volume is not severely impacted [87].

Patients with type L-ARDS will generally exhibit subpleural interstitial edema that gives rise to the ground-glass opacities seen on CT or chest radiograph. This rise in inflammation can lead to vasoplegia and later evolve into hypoxemia due to ineffective oxygen delivery through the vasculature. The body's instinctive response to hypoxemia is to increase minute ventilation, the amount of inhaled or exhaled gas per minute. Despite this evident hypoxemia, patients with type L phenotype may not show signs of dyspnea due to near-normal pulmonary compliance. That is, patients will have the sensation of inhaling an expected volume of gas per breath [87].

As the course of disease progresses, type L patients may experience further worsening of symptoms characterized by increasing pulmonary edema and weight of the lungs, and decreased gas volume at a certain threshold. In this progressed stage, tidal volumes generated with each breath are decreased despite an increase in respiratory rate. At this point, patients would be noted to have progressed to type H phenotype.

Type H-ARDS is illustrated by high lung elastance and low lung compliance. These patients also have a high right-to-left shunt, as a portion of their cardiac output perfuses edematous lung tissue and imposes increased retrograde pressure within the pulmonary vasculature. High lung weight, as a result of increased edema and inflammation, may become more apparent in imaging studies. Lastly, there will be greater lung recruitment in response to the evident hypoxemia [87].

As the pandemic progressed, it became clearer that vascular complications played a significant role in pulmonary dysfunction. These complications were especially seen in patients with thrombotic tendencies and hypercoagulable states [88]. Preliminary data demonstrates a 30% increase in venous and arterial thrombotic events among COVID-19 patients in the intensive care unit despite prophylaxis [89]. Postmortem evaluation of vasculature among COVID-19 patients provided evidence of endothelial cell injury and pulmonary vessel thrombosis, which was associated with a 5.4 times higher mortality risk for patients infected with the virus [47].

SARS-CoV-2 is known to drive an acute inflammatory response, which becomes responsible for the activation of platelets, disruption of endothelium (inner lining of blood vessels), and increasing coagulability [90]. While these features share obvious similarities to disseminated intravascular coagulation (DIC), which often has a bacterial etiology, there are notable differences that distinguish this from COVID-19-induced coagulopathy. Patients with SARS-CoV-2 have increased D-dimer levels with fibrinogen levels similar to those with DIC. However, in the former, prothrombin time and platelet count are largely maintained rather than depleted [91]. This becomes a critical marker for distinguishing coagulopathies of varying etiologies to that produced by COVID-19.

SARS-CoV-2 has a predilection for infecting endothelial cells within the pulmonary vascular bed. As previously described, SARS-CoV-2 gains entry into endothelial cells through angiotensin-converting enzyme 2 (ACE2) and a transmembrane protease serine 2 (TMPRSS-2) [92–96]. Once infected, endothelial cells are not able to maintain homeostatic functioning, including antithrombotic capabilities [92, 96]. Antithrombosis is achieved through endothelial synthesis of nitric oxide (NO), which prevents platelet and leukocyte adhesion and margination of inflammatory cells. Through infection with SARS-CoV-2, endothelial cells ultimately become damaged and undergo apoptosis (cell death) [92]. With such damage, the inherent and protective antithrombotic properties of the endothelium are compromised. Additionally, this damage increases the levels of von Willebrand factor (vWF) and factor VIII of the clotting cascade. This increase in clotting factors secondary to SARS-CoV-2 infection leads to thrombus formation in the pulmonary microcirculation and further respiratory dysfunction [93].

Arterial thrombosis is another coagulopathy associated with COVID-19. While this is an uncommon manifestation of most viral infections, a study of COVID-19 patients in Italy determined that 2.5% suffered ischemic stroke and 1.1% experienced acute coronary syndrome secondary to infection [94]. While the underlying cause of these arterial thrombi is still not fully understood, some have hypothesized that platelet activation as a result of large vWF multimers may be involved. Others have postulated a correlation with increased antiphospholipid antibodies [95].

Conflicts of Interest   No relevant conflicts of interest.

Funding   No funding was obtained.

References

1. Lauer SA, Grantz KH, Bi Q, Jones FK, Zheng Q, Meredith HR, Azman AS, Reich NG, Lessler J. The incubation period of coronavirus disease 2019 (COVID-19) from publicly reported confirmed cases: estimation and application. Ann Intern Med. 2020;172(9):577–82. https://doi.org/10.7326/M20-0504.
2. Nelemans T, Kikkert M. Viral innate immune evasion and the pathogenesis of emerging RNA virus infections. Viruses. 2019;11:E961. https://doi.org/10.3390/v11100961.
3. Prompetchara E, Ketloy C, Palaga T. Immune responses in COVID-19 and potential vaccines: Lessons learned from SARS and MERS epidemic. Asian Pac J Allergy Immunol. 2020;38:4401–9. https://doi.org/10.12932/AP-200220-0772.
4. Mokhtari T, Hassani F, Ghaffari N, Ebrahimi B, Yarahmadi A, Hassanzadeh G. COVID-19 and multiorgan failure: a narrative review on potential mechanisms. J Mol Histol. 2020;51(6):613–28. https://doi.org/10.1007/s10735-020-09915-3.
5. Loganathan S, Kuppusamy M, Wankhar W, et al. Angiotensin-converting enzyme 2 (ACE2): COVID 19 gate way to multiple organ failure syndromes. Respir Physiol Neurobiol. 2021;283:103548. https://doi.org/10.1016/j.resp.2020.103548.
6. Hoffmann M, Kleine-Weber H, Schroeder S, Krüger N, Herrler T, Erichsen S, et al. SARS-CoV-2 cell entry depends on ACE2 and TMPRSS2 and is blocked by a clinically proven protease inhibitor. Cell. 2020;181:271–80. https://doi.org/10.1016/j.cell.2020.02.052.

7. Organization W.H. Coronavirus disease 2019 (COVID-19): situation report; 2020. p. 73.
8. Zarrilli G, Angerilli V, Businello G, et al. The immunopathological and histological landscape of COVID-19-mediated lung injury. Int J Mol Sci. 2021;22(2):974. https://doi.org/10.3390/ijms22020974.
9. Gupta A, Madhavan MV, Sehgal K, Nair N, Mahajan S, Sehrawat TS, Bikdeli B, Ahluwalia N, Ausiello JC, Wan EY, et al. Extrapulmonary manifestations of COVID-19. Nat Med. 2020;26:1017–32. https://doi.org/10.1038/s41591-020-0968-3.
10. Li G, et al. Coronavirus infections and immune responses. J Med Virol. 2020;92:424–32. https://doi.org/10.1002/jmv.25685.
11. Naqvi AAT, et al. Insights into SARS-CoV-2 genome, structure, evolution, pathogenesis and therapies: structural genomics approach. Biochim Biophys Acta Mol basis Dis. 1866;2020:165878. https://doi.org/10.1016/j.bbadis.2020.165878.
12. Diaz JH. Hypothesis: angiotensin-converting enzyme inhibitors and angiotensin receptor blockers may increase the risk of severe COVID-19. J Travel Med. 2020; https://doi.org/10.1093/jtm/taaa041.
13. Belouzard S, Millet JK, Licitra BN, Whittaker GR. Mechanisms of coronavirus cell entry mediated by the viral spike protein. Viruses. 2012;4:1011–33. https://doi.org/10.3390/v4061011.
14. Zhou P, Yang X-L, Wang X-G, Hu B, Zhang L, Zhang W, Si H-R, Zhu Y, Li B, Huang C-L, Chen H-D, Chen J, Luo Y, Guo H, Jiang R-D, Liu M-Q, Chen Y, Shen X-R, Wang XI, Zheng X-S, Zhao K, Chen Q-J, Deng F, Liu L-L, Yan B, Zhan F-X, Wang Y-Y, Xiao G-F, Shi Z-L. A pneumonia outbreak associated with a new coronavirus of probable bat origin. Nature. 2020;579(7798):270–3. https://doi.org/10.1038/s41586-020-2012-7.
15. Walls AC, Park Y-J, Tortorici MA, Wall A, McGuire AT, Veesler D. Structure, function, and antigenicity of the SARS-CoV-2 spike glycoprotein. Cell. 2020;181(2):281–292.e6. https://doi.org/10.1016/j.cell.2020.02.058.
16. Verdecchia P, Cavallini C, Spanevello A, Angeli F. The pivotal link between ACE2 deficiency and SARS-CoV-2 infection. Eur J Intern Med. 2020;76:14–20. https://doi.org/10.1016/j.ejim.2020.04.037.
17. Ruimboom L. SARS-CoV 2; possible alternative virus receptors and pathophysiological determinants. Med Hypotheses. 2021;146:110368. https://doi.org/10.1016/j.mehy.2020.110368.
18. Radzikowska U, Ding M, Tan G, et al. Distribution of ACE2, CD147, CD26 and other SARS-CoV-2 associated molecules in tissues and immune cells in health and in asthma, COPD, obesity, hypertension, and COVID-19 risk factors. Allergy. 2020; https://doi.org/10.1111/all.14429.
19. Sungnak W, Huang NI, Bécavin C, et al. SARS-CoV-2 entry factors are highly expressed in nasal epithelial cells together with innate immune genes. Nat Med. 2020;26(5):681–7.
20. Ziegler CGK, Allon SJ, Nyquist SK, et al. SARS-CoV-2 receptor ACE2 is an interferon-stimulated gene in human airway epithelial cells and is detected in specific cell subsets across tissues. Cell. 2020;181(5):1016–1035.e19. https://doi.org/10.1016/j.cell.2020.04.035.
21. Qi F, Qian S, Zhang S, Zhang Z. Single cell RNA sequencing of 13 human tissues identify cell types and receptors of human coronaviruses. Biochem Biophys Res Commun. 2020;526(1):135–40.
22. Hibino T, Sakaguchi M, Miyamoto S, et al. S100A9 is a novel ligand of EMMPRIN that promotes melanoma metastasis. Cancer Res. 2013;73(1):172–83.
23. Sungnak W, Huang N, Bécavin C, Berg M, Queen R, Litvinukova M, Talavera-López C, Maatz H, Reichart D, Sampaziotis F, Worlock KB, Yoshida M, Barnes JL, Banovich NE, Barbry P, Brazma A, Collin J, Desai TJ, Duong TE, Eickelberg O, Falk C, Farzan M, Glass I, Gupta RK, Haniffa M, Horvath P, Hubner N, Hung D, Kaminski N, Krasnow M, Kropski JA, Kuhnemund M, Lako M, Lee H, Leroy S, Linnarson S, Lundeberg J, Meyer KB, Miao Z, Misharin AV, Nawijn MC, Nikolic MZ, Noseda M, Ordovas-Montanes J, Oudit GY, Pe'er D, Powell J, Quake S, Rajagopal J, Tata PR, Rawlins EL, Regev A, Reyfman PA, Rozenblatt-Rosen O, Saeb-Parsy K, Samakovlis C, Schiller HB, Schultze JL, Seibold MA, Seidman CE, Seidman JG, Shalek AK, Shepherd D, Spence J, Spira A, Sun X, Teichmann SA, Theis FJ, Tsankov AM, Vallier L, van den Berge M, Whitsett J, Xavier R, Xu Y, Zaragosi L-E, Zerti D, Zhang

H, Zhang K, Mauricio Rojas Figueiredo F. SARS-CoV-2 entry factors are highly expressed in nasal epithelial cells together with innate immune genes. Nat Med. 2020;26(5):681–7.

24. Sokolowska M, Lukasik ZM, Agache I, et al. Immunology of COVID-19: mechanisms, clinical outcome, diagnostics, and perspectives-a report of the European academy of allergy and clinical immunology (EAACI). Allergy. 2020;75(10):2445–76. https://doi.org/10.1111/all.14462.

25. Channappanavar R, Perlman S. Pathogenic human coronavirus infections: causes and consequences of cytokine storm and immunopathology. Semin Immunopathol. 2017;39:529–39. https://doi.org/10.1007/s00281-017-0629-x.

26. Lei F, et al. Longitudinal association between markers of liver injury and mortality in COVID-19 in China. Hepatology. 2020;72:389–98. https://doi.org/10.1002/hep.31301.

27. Zhang C, Wu Z, Li J-W, Zhao H, Wang G-Q. The cytokine release syndrome (CRS) of severe COVID-19 and Interleukin-6 receptor (IL-6R) antagonist Tocilizumab may be the key to reduce the mortality. Int J Antimicrob Agents. 2020;55(5):105954.

28. Lillicrap D. Disseminated intravascular coagulation in patients with 2019-nCoV pneumonia. J Thromb Haemost. 2020;18:786–7. https://doi.org/10.1111/jth.14781.

29. Quirch M, Lee J, Rehman S. Hazards of the cytokine storm and cytokine-targeted therapy in patients with COVID-19. J Med Int Res. 2020;22:e20193.

30. Hojyo S, Uchida M, Tanaka K, Hasebe R, Tanaka Y, Murakami M, Hirano T. How COVID-19 induces cytokine storm with high mortality. Inflamm Regen. 2020;40:37. https://doi.org/10.1186/s41232-020-00146-3.

31. Lu R, Zhao X, Li J, et al. Genomic characterisation and epidemiology of 2019 novel coronavirus: implications for virus origins and receptor binding. Lancet. 2020;395:565–74.

32. Diao B, Wang C, Tan Y, et al. Reduction and functional exhaustion of T cells in patients with coronavirus disease 2019 (COVID-19). MedRxiv. 2020. https://doi.org/10.1101/2020.02.18.20024364. (Epub ahead of print).

33. Okabayashi T, Kariwa H, Yokota SI, et al. Cytokine regulation in SARS coronavirus infection compared to other respiratory virus infections. J Med Virol. 2006;78(4):417–24.

34. Wan S, Yi Q, Fan S, et al. Characteristics of lymphocyte subsets and cytokines in peripheral blood of 123 hospitalized patients with 2019 novel coronavirus pneumonia (NCP). MedRxiv. 2020. https://doi.org/10.1101/2020.02.10.20021832. (Epub ahead of print).

35. Liu F, Li L, Xu M, et al. Prognostic value of interleukin-6, C-reactive protein, and procalcitonin in patients with COVID-19. J Clin Virol. 2020;127:104370.

36. Han H, Ma Q, Li C, et al. Profiling serum cytokines in COVİD-19 patients reveals IL-6 and IL-10 are disease severity predictors. Emerg Microbes Infect. 2020;9(1):1123–30.

37. Wang D, et al. Clinical characteristics of 138 hospitalized patients with 2019 novel coronavirus-infected pneumonia in Wuhan, China. JAMA. 2020;323:1061–9. https://doi.org/10.1001/jama.2020.1585.

38. Zhang H, Penninger JM, Li Y, Zhong N, Slutsky AS. Angiotensin-converting enzyme 2 (ACE2) as a SARS-CoV-2 receptor: molecular mechanisms and potential therapeutic target. Intensive Care Med. 2020;46(4):586–90. https://doi.org/10.1007/s00134-020-05985-9.

39. Mukherjee A, Ahmad M, Frenia D. A coronavirus disease 2019 (COVID-19) patient with multifocal pneumonia treated with hydroxychloroquine. Cureus. 2020;12:–e7473. https://doi.org/10.7759/cureus.7473.

40. Yi Y, Lagniton PNP, Ye S, Li E, Xu R-H. COVID-19: what has been learned and to be learned about the novel coronavirus disease. Int J Biol Sci. 2020;16:1753–66. https://doi.org/10.7150/ijbs.45134.

41. Robles A, et al. Viral vs bacterial community-acquired pneumonia: Radiologic features. Eur Respir Soc. 2011;38:2507.

42. Chung M, et al. CT imaging features of 2019 novel coronavirus (2019-nCoV). Radiology. 2020;295:202–7.

43. Shi H, Han X, Zheng C. Evolution of CT manifestations in a patient recovered from 2019 novel coronavirus (2019-nCoV) pneumonia in Wuhan, China. Radiology. 2020;295:20. https://doi.org/10.1148/radiol.2020200269.

44. Hamming I, Timens W, Bulthuis ML, Lely AT, Navis G, van Goor H. Tissue distribution of ACE2 protein, the functional receptor for SARS coronavirus. A first step in understanding SARS pathogenesis. J Pathol. 2004;203:631–7. https://doi.org/10.1002/path.1570.
45. Pyrc K, Berkhout B, van der Hoek L. The novel human coronaviruses NL63 and HKU1. J Virol. 2007;81:3051–7. https://doi.org/10.1128/jvi.01466-06.
46. Bernstein KE, Khan Z, Giani JF, Cao DY, Bernstein EA, Shen XZ. Angiotensin-converting enzyme in innate and adaptive immunity. Nat Rev Nephrol. 2018;14:325–36. https://doi.org/10.1038/nrneph.2018.15.
47. Ackermann M, Verleden SE, Kuehnel M, Haverich A, Welte T, Laenger F, Vanstapel A, Werlein C, Stark H, Tzankov A, et al. Pulmonary vascular endothelialitis, thrombosis, and angiogenesis in Covid-19. N Engl J Med. 2020;383:120–8. https://doi.org/10.1056/NEJMoa2015432.
48. Deshmukh V, Motwani R, Kumar A, Kumari C, Raza K. Histopathological observations in COVID-19: A systematic review. J Clin Pathol. 2020; https://doi.org/10.1136/jclinpath-2020-206995.
49. Varga Z, Flammer AJ, Steiger P, Haberecker M, Andermatt R, Zinkernagel AS, Mehra MR, Schuepbach RA, Ruschitzka F, Moch H. Endothelial cell infection and endotheliitis in COVID-19. Lancet. 2020;395:1417–8. https://doi.org/10.1016/S0140-6736(20)30937-5.
50. Calabrese F, Pezzuto F, Fortarezza F, Hofman P, Kern I, Panizo A, von der Thüsen J, Timofeev S, Gorkiewicz G, Lunardi F. Pulmonary pathology and COVID-19: Lessons from autopsy. The experience of European Pulmonary Pathologists. Virchows Arch. 2020;477:359–72. https://doi.org/10.1007/s00428-020-02886-6.
51. Barton LM, Duval EJ, Stroberg E, Ghosh S, Mukhopadhyay S. COVID-19 Autopsies, Oklahoma, USA. Am J Clin Pathol. 2020;153:725–33. https://doi.org/10.1093/ajcp/aqaa062.
52. Fox SE, Akmatbekov A, Harbert JL, Li G, Quincy BJ, Vander Heide RS. Pulmonary and cardiac pathology in African American patients with COVID-19: an autopsy series from New Orleans. Lancet Respir Med. 2020;8:681–6. https://doi.org/10.1016/S2213-2600(20)30243-5.
53. Buja LM, Wolf DA, Zhao B, Akkanti B, McDonald M, Lelenwa L, Reilly N, Ottaviani G, Elghetany MT, Trujillo DO, et al. The emerging spectrum of cardiopulmonary pathology of the coronavirus disease 2019 (COVID-19): Report of 3 autopsies from Houston, Texas, and review of autopsy findings from other United States cities. Cardiovasc Pathol. 2020;48:107233. https://doi.org/10.1016/j.carpath.2020.107233.
54. Menter T, Haslbauer JD, Nienhold R, Savic S, Hopfer H, Deigendesch N, Frank S, Turek D, Willi N, Pargger H, et al. Postmortem examination of COVID-19 patients reveals diffuse alveolar damage with severe capillary congestion and variegated findings in lungs and other organs suggesting vascular dysfunction. Histopathology. 2020;77:198–209. https://doi.org/10.1111/his.14134.
55. Hanley B, Naresh KN, Roufosse C, Nicholson AG, Weir J, Cooke GS, Thursz M, Manousou P, Corbett R, Goldin G, et al. Histopathological findings and viral tropism in UK patients with severe fatal COVID-19: a post-mortem study. Lancet Microbe. 2020;1:e245–e53. https://doi.org/10.1016/S2666-5247(20)30115-4.
56. Burchfield J. Renin-Angiotensin-Aldosterone system: double-edged sword in COVID-19 infection; 2020.
57. Jiang F, Deng L, Zhang L, Cai Y, Cheung CW, Xia Z. Review of the clinical characteristics of coronavirus disease 2019 (COVID-19). J Gen Intern Med. 2020;35:1545. https://doi.org/10.1007/s11606-020-05762-w.
58. Turner AJ, Hiscox JA, Hooper NM. ACE2: from vasopeptidase to SARS virus receptor. Trends Pharmacol Sci. 2004;25:291–4. https://doi.org/10.1016/j.tips.2004.04.001.
59. Zheng Y-Y, Ma Y-T, Zhang J-Y, Xie X. COVID-19 and the cardiovascular system. Nat Rev Cardiol. 2020;17(5):259–60. https://doi.org/10.1038/s41569-020-0360-5. PMID: 32139904; PMCID: PMC7095524.
60. Zou X, Chen K, Zou J, Han P, Hao J, Han Z. Single-cell RNA-seq data analysis on the receptor ACE2 expression reveals the potential risk of different human organs vulnerable to 2019-nCoV infection. Front Med. 2020;14(2):185–92. https://doi.org/10.1007/s11684-020-0754-0. Epub 2020 Mar 12. PMID: 32170560; PMCID: PMC7088738.

61. Gheblawi M, et al. Angiotensin-converting enzyme 2: SARS-CoV-2 receptor and regulator of the renin-angiotensin system: celebrating the 20th anniversary of the discovery of ACE2. Circ Res. 2020;126:1456–74. https://doi.org/10.1161/CIRCRESAHA.120.317015.

62. Bradley BT, et al. Histopathology and ultrastructural findings of fatal COVID-19 infections in Washington State: a case series. Lancet. 2020; https://doi.org/10.1016/S0140-6736(20)31305-2.

63. Wu C et al. Heart injury signs are associated with higher and earlier mortality in coronavirus disease 2019 (COVID-19). medRxiv. 2020.

64. Gu J, et al. Multiple organ infection and the pathogenesis of SARS. J Exp Med. 2005;202:415–24. https://doi.org/10.1084/jem.20050828.

65. Zhang T, et al. CaMKII is a RIP3 substrate mediating ischemia-and oxidative stress-induced myocardial necroptosis. Nat Med. 2016;22:175. https://doi.org/10.1038/nm.4017.

66. Mohanty SK, Satapathy A, Naidu MM, Mukhopadhyay S, Sharma S, Barton LM, Stroberg E, Duval EJ, Pradhan D, Tzankov A, et al. Severe acute respiratory syndrome coronavirus-2 (SARS-CoV-2) and coronavirus disease 19 (COVID-19)—anatomic pathology perspective on current knowledge. Diagn Pathol. 2020;15:103. https://doi.org/10.1186/s13000-020-01017-8.

67. Liu PP, Blet A, Smyth D, Li H. The science underlying COVID- 19: Implications for the cardiovascular system. Circulation. 2020; https://doi.org/10.1161/circulationaha.120.047549.

68. Zhou B, Zhao W, Feng R, Zhang X, Li X, Zhou Y, Peng L, Li Y, Zhang J, Luo J, et al. The pathological autopsy of coronavirus disease 2019 (COVID-2019) in China: a review. Pathog Dis. 2020;78 https://doi.org/10.1093/femspd/ftaa026.

69. Cao X. COVID-19: immunopathology and its implications for therapy. Nat Rev Immunol. 2020;20:269–70. https://doi.org/10.1038/s41577-020-0308-3.

70. Unsinger J, McDonough JS, Shultz LD, Ferguson TA, Hotchkiss RS. Sepsis-induced human lymphocyte apoptosis and cytokine production in "humanized" mice. J Leukoc Biol. 2009;86:219–27. https://doi.org/10.1189/jlb.1008615.

71. Li H, et al. SARS-CoV-2 and viral sepsis: observations and hypotheses. Lancet. 2020; https://doi.org/10.1016/s0140-6736(20)30920-x.

72. Hayashi Y, Wagatsuma K, Nojima M, et al. The characteristics of gastrointestinal symptoms in patients with severe COVID-19: a systematic review and meta-analysis. J Gastroenterol. 2021:1–12. https://doi.org/10.1007/s00535-021-01778-z.

73. Tabary M, Khanmohammadi S, Araghi F, Dadkhahfar S, Tavangar SM. Pathologic features of COVID-19: a concise review. Pathol Res Pract. 2020;216:153097. https://doi.org/10.1016/j.prp.2020.153097.

74. Suchonwanit P, Leerunyakul K, Kositkuljorn C. Cutaneous manifestations in COVID-19: lessons learned from current evidence. J Am Acad Dermatol. 2020;83:e57–60. https://doi.org/10.1016/j.jaad.2020.04.094.

75. El Hachem M, Diociaiuti A, Concato C, Carsetti R, Carnevale C, Ciofi Degli Atti M, Giovannelli L, Latella E, Porzio O, Rossi S, et al. A clinical, histopathological and laboratory study of 19 consecutive Italian paediatric patients with chilblain-like lesions: Lights and shadows on the relationship with COVID-19 infection. J Eur Acad Dermatol Venereol. 2020;34:2620–9. https://doi.org/10.1111/jdv.16682.

76. Wang B, Li R, Lu Z, Huang Y. Does comorbidity increase the risk of patients with COVID-19: evidence from meta-analysis. Aging (Albany NY). 2020;12(7):6049–57.

77. Dong X, Cao Y-Y, Lu X-X, et al. Eleven faces of coronavirus disease 2019. Allergy. 2020;75(7):1699–709. https://doi.org/10.1111/all.14289.

78. Wang J, Luo Q, Chen R, Chen T, Li J. Susceptibility analysis of COVID-19 in smokers based on ACE2. Preprintsorg. 2020; preprint.

79. Leung JM, Yang CX, Tam A, et al. ACE-2 expression in the small airway epithelia of smokers and COPD patients: implications for COVID-19. European Respiratory Journal. 2020;55(5):2000688.

80. Yang JK, Lin SS, Ji XJ, Guo LM. Binding of SARS coronavirus to its receptor damages islets and causes acute diabetes. Acta Diabetol. 2010;47(3):193–9.

81. Michalovich D, Rodriguez-Perez N, Smolinska S, et al. Obesity and disease severity magnify disturbed microbiome-immune interactions in asthma patients. Nat Commun. 2019;10(1):5711.
82. Wambier CG, Goren A. Severe acute respiratory syndrome coronavirus 2 (SARS-CoV-2) infection is likely to be androgen mediated. J Am Acad Dermatol. 2020;83(1):308–9.
83. Wang LS, Williamson SR, Zhang SB, et al. Increased androgen receptor gene copy number is associated with TMPRSS2-ERG rearrangement in prostatic small cell carcinoma. Mol Carcinogen. 2015;54(9):900–7.
84. Jones TC, Mühlemann B, Veith T, et al. An analysis of SARS-CoV-2 viral load by patient age. Submitted. 2020. https://doi.org/10.1101/2020.06.08.20125484.
85. Maddux AB, Douglas IS. Is the developmentally immature immune response in paediatric sepsis a recapitulation of immune tolerance? Immunology. 2015;145(1):1–10.
86. The ARDS. Definition Task force*. acute respiratory distress syndrome: the berlin definition. JAMA. 2012;307(23):2526–33. https://doi.org/10.1001/jama.2012.5669.
87. Marini JJ, Gattinoni L. Management of COVID-19 respiratory distress. JAMA. 2020;323(22):2329–30. https://doi.org/10.1001/jama.2020.6825.
88. Han H, Yang L, Liu R, Liu F, Wu KL, Li J, Liu XH, Zhu CL. Prominent changes in blood coagulation of patients with SARS-CoV-2 infection. Clin Chem Lab Med. 2020;58(7):1116–20. https://doi.org/10.1515/cclm-2020-0188.
89. Klok FA, Kruip MJHA, van der Meer NJM, Arbous MS, Gommers DAMPJ, Kant KM, Kaptein FHJ, van Paassen J, Stals MAM, Huisman MV, Endeman H. Incidence of thrombotic complications in critically ill ICU patients with COVID-19. Thromb Res. 2020;191:145–7. https://doi.org/10.1016/j.thromres.2020.04.013.
90. Nicolai L, Leunig A, Brambs S, Kaiser R, Weinberger T, Weigand M, Muenchhoff M, Hellmuth JC, Ledderose S, Schulz H, Scherer C, Rudelius M, Zoller M, Höchter D, Keppler O, Teupser D, Zwißler B, von Bergwelt-Baildon M, Kääb S, Massberg S, Pekayvaz K, Stark K. Immunothrombotic dysregulation in COVID-19 pneumonia is associated with respiratory failure and coagulopathy. Circulation. 2020;142(12):1176–89. https://doi.org/10.1161/CIRCULATIONAHA.120.048488. Epub 2020 Jul 28. PMID: 32755393; PMCID: PMC7497892
91. Iba T, Levy JH, Levi M, Thachil J. Coagulopathy in COVID-19. J Thromb Haemost. 2020;18(9):2103–9. https://doi.org/10.1111/jth.14975. Epub 2020 Jul 21. PMID: 32558075; PMCID: PMC7323352
92. Lukassen S, Chua RL, Trefzer T, Kahn NC, Schneider MA, Muley T, Winter H, Meister M, Veith C, Boots AW, Hennig BP, Kreuter M, Conrad C, Eils R. SARS-CoV-2 receptor ACE2 and TMPRSS2 are primarily expressed in bronchial transient secretory cells. EMBO J. 2020;39(10):e105114. https://doi.org/10.15252/embj.20105114. Epub 2020 Apr 14. PMID: 32246845; PMCID: PMC7232010
93. Wichmann D, Sperhake JP, Lütgehetmann M, et al. Autopsy findings and venous thromboembolism in patients with COVID-19: a prospective cohort study. Ann Intern Med. 2020;173(4):268–77. https://doi.org/10.7326/M20-2003.
94. Lodigiani C, Iapichino G, Carenzo L, Cecconi M, Ferrazzi P, Sebastian T, Kucher N, Studt JD, Sacco C, Bertuzzi A, Sandri MT, Barco S, Humanitas COVID-19 Task Force. Venous and arterial thromboembolic complications in COVID-19 patients admitted to an academic hospital in Milan, Italy. Thromb Res. 2020;191:9–14. https://doi.org/10.1016/j.thromres.2020.04.024. Epub 2020 Apr 23. PMID: 32353746; PMCID: PMC7177070
95. Connell NT, Battinelli EM, Connors JM, Coagulopathy of COVID-19 and antiphospholipid antibodies. J Thromb Haemost. 2020; https://doi.org/10.1111/jth.14893.
96. Wiersinga WJ, Rhodes A, Cheng AC, Peacock SJ, Prescott HC. Pathophysiology, transmission, diagnosis, and treatment of coronavirus disease 2019 (Covid-19): a review. JAMA. 2020;324(8):782–93. https://doi.org/10.1001/jama.2020.12839.

Chapter 9
Spread of COVID-19 and Personal Protective Equipment

Ario D. Ramezani, Nikhil A. Crain, and Taizoon Dhoon

Spread of COVID-19

As a member of the *Coronaviridae* family, severe acute respiratory syndrome coronavirus 2 (SARS-CoV-2) shares similar characteristics as other coronaviruses, which are enveloped, single-stranded RNA viruses with signature "crown-like" surface structures [1–3]. The illness caused by SARS-CoV-2, known as COVID-19, has emerged as a highly transmissible disease which reached pandemic status in March 2020 [4]. Respiratory droplets transmitted via cough to a person's mouth, nose, and eyes are the major source of transmission for COVID-19 [5–7]. However, evidence has shown that SARS-CoV-2 can persist in a variety of channels, including fomites and surfaces [6–8] and human feces and urine [9–15]. Given the many routes of transmission, both communities and hospitals can be high-risk environments for the spread of SARS-CoV-2; thus, frequent handwashing, protective shields, and physical distancing have been employed to help curb the transmission between individuals [9].

Transmission via respiratory secretions, saliva, or droplets via direct, indirect, or close contact is the primary mode of viral spread [16, 17]. Specifically, SARS-CoV-2 transmission via direct contact occurs when a healthy and infected person is within close contact, while indirect contact can happen when respiratory droplets are deposited onto surfaces or fomites [18]. Close contact is defined as a distance within 1 m in which an infected individual may disseminate respiratory droplets through coughing, sneezing, talking, and singing to a susceptible individual through the mouth, nose, or eyes [18–20].

It is important to distinguish the difference between transmission by respiratory droplets and aerosols (i.e., airborne transmission via droplet nuclei). Respiratory

A. D. Ramezani · N. A. Crain · T. Dhoon (✉)
Irvine Medical Center, University of California, Orange, CA, USA
e-mail: tdhoon@hs.uci.edu

© The Author(s), under exclusive license to Springer Nature Switzerland AG 2022
A. A. Hakimi et al. (eds.), *Mechanical Ventilation Amid the COVID-19 Pandemic*,
https://doi.org/10.1007/978-3-030-87978-5_9

droplets, primarily spread by the respiratory actions described above, are defined to have diameters greater than 5–10 µm, while aerosols are less than or equal to 5 µm propagated by aerosol-generating actions [21, 22]. Airborne transmission has unique meaning in that droplet nuclei stay suspended in the air for prolonged periods of time. Although experimentally driven studies were able to detect airborne SARS-CoV-2 ranging from 3 to 16 h with qualitative integrity there is debate on the infectious viral dose required for aerosol transmission under realistic conditions (i.e., normal coughing) [22]. Studies performed in routine hospital settings without aerosol-generating procedures have shown mixed results; while some have shown SARS-CoV-2 RNA in air samples [23–28], others found no viable viral particles [29–36].

Epidemiological data on COVID-19 favors the explanation that viral spread is through close contact transmission (i.e., short-range travel measuring less than 6 ft. of respiratory droplets) versus airborne transmission. Unlike *Varicella zoster* (chicken pox), *Mycobacterium tuberculosis* (tuberculosis), and *Rubeola* (measles) which have higher attack rates and can infect susceptible people present in an airspace after an infectious individual has left for up to several hours, SARS-CoV-2 spreads more like other respiratory viruses [37]. Nevertheless, uncommon circumstances in which respiratory droplets were transmitted further than 6 ft. and lasting after the departure of an infectious individual have been documented. In these well-documented scenarios (e.g., choir practice, fitness classes), crowded spaces involving extended expiratory effort without proper ventilation and masking could have facilitated the spread, as well as concurrent droplet and fomite transmission [37–41].

Temperature can play a role in viral transmission by impacting the stability of viral proteins and genome [42]. It has been shown that most enveloped viruses are inactivated at temperatures greater than 60 °C for more than 1 h, barring the caveat that there likely exists some protective influence that a surrounding material (e.g., saliva) provides insulation against environmental changes [43–45]. While extreme sustained temperatures of 60 °C are unrealistic in typical ambient climates across the globe, lower temperatures that facilitate viral stability may play a role in viral spread with World Health Organization (WHO) reports indicating that European and Northern American regions confirmed with the largest count of COVID-19 cases [5, 46]. Moreover, relative humidity can play a role in viral survivability due to denaturing of phospholipid-protein complexes of enveloped viruses [47]. While COVID-19 has certainly been prevalent in tropical regions, there is evidence suggesting that high humidity can shorten the duration of enveloped virus survival as well as accelerate the speed of droplet settling, thus limiting transmission [48, 49]. Both SARS-CoV and MERS-CoV have been shown to have increased survival in low humidity and temperatures, including the typical indoor office environment [50–52]. Along with higher temperatures and dry air, prior research has demonstrated that ultraviolet light (UV), and in particular UVC, can inactivate coronaviruses; therefore, outdoor environments may serve a role in mitigating the spread of SARS-CoV-2 [53–56].

Surface- and fomite-mediated transmissions are important points of discussion for COVID-19. Contaminated surfaces, particularly when dry, serve as a viable point source of infection, especially as one milliliter of sputum can contain over 108

SARS-CoV-2 copies [57, 58]. Surface stability was first demonstrated by van Doremalen et al. involving ten experiments across a variety of environmental surface types [22]. Plastic demonstrated the longest median half-life of surface presence (6.8 h), followed by stainless steel (5.6 h), cardboard (3 h), and copper (1 h) [22]. Additional studies showed that the texture of inert surfaces, such as those that are smooth, provides greater stability for SARS-CoV-2, in comparison to more porous materials (e.g., latex, fabrics) [59]. Further studies support the survivability of SARS-CoV-2 on various surfaces, indicating that this potential reservoir of viral presence should be a target of sanitization [59–62]. Alcohol-based cleaning agents and biocides have been shown to significantly reduce the survivability of SARS-CoV-2 [63–65]. The WHO has provided recommendations on how to most effectively clean surfaces with water, detergents, and disinfectants in order to reduce viral transmission [66].

Research has also shown that SARS-CoV-2 can exist in feces and urine samples [10–15]. One study showed that SARS-CoV-2 was expelled in human feces 33 days after a patient's negative confirmation for viral RNA [34]. Given large viral loads, SARS-CoV-2 present in feces may be transmitted to soil and water sources in the environment [67–71]. Despite such evidence of viral load presence in feces and urine, there is scarcity of published data on infectious transmission through these routes. Therefore, because other coronaviruses were previously shown to exist in water and sewage system sources, there is likely the need to further explore the fecal-oral route via environmental studies to elucidate the characteristics of such transmission [72–74].

Regarding viral behavior during the perinatal period, there are only a few cases of vertical or intrauterine transmission of SARS-CoV-2 from mother to infant, with another study demonstrating that breast milk samples showed low likelihood of viable virus [75–77]. In turn, the WHO recommends that mothers continue to breastfeed infants [78].

Personal Protective Equipment and Its Role in Preventing Spread Among Healthcare Workers and Communities

The COVID-19 pandemic has reached over 200 countries, spanning nearly every continent. Numerous measures have been initiated globally to combat this disease and curtail its spread, with interventions at the community and environmental levels. Personal protective equipment (PPE) has served as a cornerstone of defense for healthcare providers and the public alike. Since the onset of the pandemic, communities and hospitals adopted heightened strategies of defense against the virus. Among the different measures, such as social distancing and home isolation, the final barrier of individual defense against SARS-CoV-2 is PPE.

Transmission of SARS-CoV-2 primarily occurs via respiratory droplets measuring anywhere from 5 to 50 μm in diameter, which may be spread through direct contact of mucosal membranes or with contaminated fomites. However, transmission may also occur through aerosols measuring smaller than 5 μm in diameter [79]. These particles can be created through aerosol-generating procedures, such as endotracheal intubation or tracheostomy, or through an individual coughing or sneezing.

Upon infecting a host, SARS-CoV-2 begins to replicate and increase its viral load. It is this viral load that is often correlated with patient symptoms and transmissibility. Studies have shown the viral load to be highest, and thus the most contagious, during the first week following symptom onset [80]. Infectivity is also maintained during the virus's latency period regardless of whether the host is symptomatic or not [80].

Current research has demonstrated that each SARS-CoV-2 exposure results in 2.1–4 subsequent transmissions, while healthcare workers (HCWs) have demonstrated a 3.5–20% infection rate [81]. Procedures and policies to limit transmission—including general hygiene, PPE, and surface decontamination—have become paramount to curbing the spread of COVID-19.

The mask and respirator selection criteria for each individual should depend on the prevalence of COVID-19 within his or her community, availability of PPE, and risk of exposure. In this section, we highlight the strengths and limitations of these crucial PPE.

Surgical masks filter bacteria, large respiratory droplets, and other particulates. They are not considered protective against small respiratory droplets or aerosols as the lack of a tight seal allows unfiltered air to flow through the sides of the mask [79]. Additionally, surgical masks can vary in efficacy depending on the manufacturer, with some options providing excellent protection and others providing very little.

At the onset of the pandemic in March 2020, the Centers for Disease Control (CDC) only recommended that masks be worn by two groups: those exhibiting symptoms of COVID-19 and those who are caring for somebody sick. This recommendation also came at a time when there was a shortage of PPE, allowing the current stock of limited PPE to be prioritized for HCWs while manufacturing was increased. A few weeks later, the CDC changed their recommendation, stating that everyone, regardless of the symptom status, should wear a mask in public. This staunch shift in recommendations followed increased evidence demonstrating that SARS-CoV-2 can be transmitted by asymptomatic individuals [82]. When worn by HCWs, surgical masks typically protect the wearer from infectious bodily fluids or large droplets in nosocomial environments that may otherwise infect workers via direct contact to the nose or mouth. Surgical masks worn by patients reduce the concentration and trajectory of aerosolized particles, thereby limiting viral transmission [79, 83].

The efficacy of a face mask or respirator is dependent on both the quality of filtration and the fit of the device. According to the Food and Drug Administration (FDA) guidelines, medical grade masks are divided into American Society for Testing Materials (ASTM) levels 1, 2, or 3 depending on each mask's fluid resistance efficiency. While different countries utilize unique mask nomenclature, the United States' National Institute for Occupational Safety and Health (NIOSH) characterizes masks based on their resistance to oil. N-series masks are not oil resistant,

R-series are oil resistant, and P-series are oilproof. Respirators are also classified based on their filtration efficacy, determined by their effectiveness in preventing particles less than 5 μm in diameter from passing through the filter. The three standard filtration efficacy classifications are 95%, 99%, and 99.75% [84].

For respirator manufacturers to acquire NIOSH certification, several tests are performed to evaluate efficacy, including sodium chloride (NaCl) aerosol challenge, dioctyl phthalate (DOP) test, valve leak test, and inhalation and exhalation tests. In the NaCl aerosol challenge, a controlled amount of aerosolized NaCl is exposed to the respirator. The amount that passes through the filter is utilized to determine filtration efficacy. The DOP test challenges respirators with particles of 0.3 μm in diameter to assess penetration beyond the filter as well as airflow resistance. To assess for leaks through the exhalation valve, the respirator is placed on a soft medium, simulating the face of the wearer. This is later attached to a hose and vacuum apparatus used to simulate respirations and assess for leaks within the valve. These inhalation and exhalation tests are performed to evaluate the breathability of the respirator. This is performed by measuring the resistance of gas flow, which cannot exceed 35 mm of water column height pressure during inhalation and 25 mm of water column height pressure with exhalation [84].

Several mechanisms for particulate filtration have been engineered into respirators such as the N95 and N99. These mechanisms include fibrous filtration membranes, gravity settling, inertial impaction, and diffusion via electrostatic attraction [85]. Since the twentieth century, the most common fibrous membranes in masks and respirators include polypropylene glycol (PP), woolen felt, and glass papers. Respirators are commonly manufactured with four layers: an inner layer of spunbound PP, a second layer of melt-blown PP, a third layer of cellulose and polyester, and an outer layer of spun-bound PP [85].

The mechanism in which particulate is filtered through the respirator is first dependent on its size. Larger particulates (greater than 0.3 μm in diameter) typically travel along a linear path due to their size. Contact with a fibrous membrane will capture the particle via inertial impact [83]. Smaller particles (less than 0.3 μm in diameter) are more susceptible to external forces as they move through the environment, randomly altering their trajectory. The random trajectory of these smaller particles translates to a theoretical uncertainty regarding whether the particle will make contact with the fibrous material and thus be filtered [83]. To combat this, respirators are created with a melt-blowing technique, which charges the fibrous membranes to form a quasi-permanent electrical field that can attract smaller particles via electrostatic attraction [86, 87]. Respirators are manufactured to deliver a tight seal around the face so that the flow of air is directed through the mask as opposed to its perimeter. Therefore, each user should undergo a fit test to determine the custom size that provides the safest seal for their face.

High-efficiency particulate air (HEPA) filters and ultralow penetration air (ULPA) filters are devices that were originally designed to be used in laboratory and factory settings to maintain controlled environments free of dust and other airborne particles. Today, they can also be found in a myriad of products including automobiles, vacuum cleaners, and air purifiers. These filters have been very efficacious in filtering air and thus combating the spread of SARS-CoV-2 [88]. HEPA and ULPA filters are designed to trap particles that are 0.3 µm in diameter, which is referred to by scientists as the most penetrating particle size (MPPS) because of their ability to evade capture in air filters compared to smaller or larger particles. HEPA filters have a minimum efficiency of 99.97% by the DOP test, whereas ULPA filters have a minimum efficiency of 99.99% by the DOP test.

HEPA and ULPA filters are generally constructed from paper media, although newer designs using fine fiber technology in a nonwoven media have also been introduced for manufacturing. The paper media continues to be more widely used and is made of matted glass fiber, such as borosilicate microfiber. The filtration efficiency demonstrated by these two filters is largely due to the small fiber diameter and high packing density of the media [87]. As air passes through the fibrous filter, particulate is collected onto the media through mechanisms such as inertial impact, interception, diffusion, and sieving.

The HEPA and ULPA filter media is also pleated to increase the surface area-to-volume flow rate [87]. While this is the reason that these filters are often referred to as "extended media filters," pleating the media too closely during manufacturing can cause collected particulate to bridge pleats together, reducing the surface area and the filtration efficiency. In general, most filters will have 12–16 pleats per inch and each pleat will be 1 in. to 16 in. deep.

The airflow capacity through the filter is a function of resistance, which in this scenario is the pressure drop across the filter and particulate matter loading. When dust and other particles are collected onto the filter surface, the resistance to airflow increases, thus decreasing gas flow [87, 88]. When airflow is decreased and filtration efficiency is not met, the filter needs to be disposed of and replaced by a new one.

The use of HEPA and ULPA filters in preventing the spread of SARS-CoV-2 has become a point of interest amid the growing COVID-19 pandemic. While meticulous measures and protocols have been adopted by HCWs and global communities to reduce the risk of viral transmission, the risk of infection remains in environments where prolonged contact with people of confirmed or unknown infection status routinely takes place. Air filters may reduce airborne viral particles, risk of particulate buildup on inanimate objects, and threat of fomite creation [88]. The judicious use of PPE, HEPA, and ULPA filters can reduce infection rates even in the highest-risk settings.

Fluid droplets from coughing or sneezing are typically 5 µm in diameter or greater and can be reliably captured by HEPA filters [88]. Smaller particles, such as a single virion that measures approximately 0.12 µm in diameter, are filtered more reliably by ULPA filters, which have a higher filtration efficiency. This points to the possibility of purifying patients' hospital room air by use of a portable air filter. This is particularly useful among hospitals who have reached capacity in their Airborne Infection Isolation Rooms (AIIRs), designed to maintain negative pressure. Studies have demonstrated the benefits of portable air filters in the operating room during nasal surgical interventions, a case especially susceptible to aerosol formation [89]. As viral surges continue to strike worldwide, the demand for AIIRs may increase. In this scenario, HEPA and ULPA filters may help mitigate shortfalls in AIIR availability.

Fig. 9.1 Masks and respirators. (**a**) Surgical mask . (**b**) N95 respirator. (**c**) Powered air-purifying respirator (PAPR)

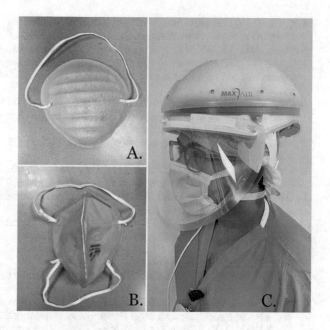

Although many healthcare workers utilize respirator masks or powered air-purifying respirators (PAPR), some have proposed the use of additional filtration to purify the surrounding air rather than simply respired air. One of the highest-risk activities in terms of transmission of SARS-CoV-2 virions is the removal of used PPE. The addition of portable HEPA and ULPA filtration systems in healthcare settings has the potential to limit virion presence on hands, clothing, medical equipment, and PPE (Fig. 9.1).

Conflicts of Interest   No relevant conflicts of interest.

Funding   No funding was obtained.

References

1. Harapan H, Itoh N, Yufika A, Winardi W, Keam S, Te H, et al. Coronavirus disease 2019 (COVID-19): a literature review. J Infect Public Health. 2020;13:667–73.
2. Naddco V, Liu H. Editorial perspectives: 2019 novel coronavirus (SARS-CoV-2): what is its fate in urban water cycle and how can the water research community respond? Environ Sci: Water Res Technol. 2020;6:1213–6.
3. La Rosa G, Fratini M, Libera SD, Iaconelli M, Muscillo M. Emerging and potentially emerging viruses in water environments. Ann Ist Super Sanita. 2012;48:397–406.

4. Cucinotta D, Vanelli M. WHO declares COVID-19 a pandemic. Acta Biomed. 2020;91(1):157–60. https://doi.org/10.23750/abm.v91i1.9397. Published 2020 Mar 19.
5. Manigandan AS, Wu MT, Ponnusamy VK, Raghavendra VB, Pugazhendhi A, Brindhadevi K. A systematic review on recent trends in transmission, diagnosis, prevention and imaging features of COVID-19. Process Biochem. 2020;98:233–40. https://doi.org/10.1016/j.procbio.2020.08.016.
6. Chan JF-W, Yuan S, Kok K-H, To KK-W, Chu H, Yang J. A familial cluster of pneumonia associated with the 2019 novel coronavirus indicating person-to-person transmission: a study of a family cluster. Lancet. 2020;395:514–23.
7. Meselson M. Droplets and aerosols in the transmission of SARS-CoV-2. N Engl J Med. 2020;382:2063.
8. Chin AWH, Chu JTS, Perera MRA, Hui KPY, Yen H-L, Chan MCW. Stability of SARS-CoV-2 in different environmental conditions. Lancet Microbe. 2020;1:e10.
9. Gormley M, Aspray TJ, Kelly DA. COVID-19: mitigating transmission via wastewater plumbing systems. Lancet Glob Health. 2020;8:e643.
10. Guan WJ, Ni ZY, Hu Y, Liang WH, Ou CQ, He JX, et al. Clinical characteristics of coronavirus disease 2019 in china. New Engl J Med. 2020;382:1708–20.
11. Pan Y, Zhang D, Yang P, Poon LLM, Wang Q. Viral load of SARS-CoV-2 in clinical samples. Lancet Infect Dis. 2020;20(4):411–2.
12. Wang W, Xu Y, Gao R, Lu R, Han K, Wu G, et al. Detection of SARS-CoV-2 in different types of clinical specimens. JAMA. 2020;323(18):1843–4.
13. Wu Y, Guo C, Tang L, Hong Z, Zhou J, Dong X, et al. Prolonged presence of SARS-CoV-2 viral RNA in faecal samples. Lancet Gastroenterol Hepatol. 2020;5(5):434–5.
14. Zheng S, Fan J, Yu F, Feng B, Lou B, Zou Q, et al. Viral load dynamics and disease severity in patients infected with SARS-CoV-2 in Zhejiang province, China, January–March 2020: retrospective cohort study. BMJ. 2020;369:m1443.
15. Sun J, Zhu A, Li H, Zheng K, Zhuang Z, Chen Z, et al. Isolation of infectious SARS-CoV-2 from urine of a COVID-19 patient. Emerg Microbes Infect. 2020;9:991–3.
16. WHO. Transmission of SARS-CoV-2: implications for infection prevention precautions; July 2020. WHO/2019-nCoV/Sci_Brief/Transmission_modes/2020.3.
17. Kutter JS, Spronken MI, Fraaij PL, Fouchier RA, Herfst S. Transmission routes of respiratory viruses among humans. Curr Opin Virol. 2018;28:142–51. https://doi.org/10.1016/j.coviro.2018.01.001.
18. Morawska L, Cao J. Airborne transmission of SARS-CoV-2: the world should face the reality. Environ Int. 2020;139:105730. https://doi.org/10.1016/j.envint.2020.105730.
19. Jones RM, Brosseau LM. Aerosol transmission of infectious disease. J Occup Environ Med. 2015;57:501–8. https://doi.org/10.1097/JOM.0000000000000448.
20. WHO Advice on the use of masks in the context of COVID-19: interim guidance. World Health Organization. 2020. https://doi.org/10.1093/jiaa077.
21. WHO. World Health Organization; 2020. Transmission of SARS-CoV-2 – Implications for Infection Prevention Precautions: Scientific Brief [WWW Document]. URL: https://www.who.int/news-room/commentaries/detail/transmission-of-sars-cov-2-implications-for-infection-prevention-precautions.
22. van Doremalen N, Bushmaker T, Morris DH, Holbrook MG, Gamble A, Williamson BN, Tamin A, Harcourt JL, Thornburg NJ, Gerber SI, Lloyd-Smith JO, de Wit E, Munster VJ. Aerosol and surface stability of SARS-CoV-2 as compared with SARS-CoV-1. N Engl J Med. 2020;382:1564–7. https://doi.org/10.1056/NEJMc2004973.
23. Chia PY, for the Singapore Novel Coronavirus Outbreak Research T, Coleman KK, Tan YK, Ong SWX, Gum M, et al. Detection of air and surface contamination by SARS-CoV-2 in hospital rooms of infected patients. Nat Comm. 2020;11(1):2800.
24. Guo Z-D, Wang Z-Y, Zhang S-F, Li X, Li L, Li C, et al. Aerosol and Surface Distribution of Severe Acute Respiratory Syndrome Coronavirus 2 in Hospital Wards, Wuhan, China, 2020. Emerg Infect Dis. 2020;26(7):1583–91.
25. Santarpia JL, Rivera DN, Herrera V, Morwitzer MJ, Creager H, Santarpia GW, et al. Transmission potential of SARS-CoV-2 in viral shedding observed at the University of

Nebraska Medical Center (pre-print). MedRxiv 2020. https://doi.org/10.1101/2020.03.2 3.20039446.

26. Zhou J, Otter J, Price JR, Cimpeanu C, Garcia DM, Kinross J, et al. Investigating SARS-CoV-2 surface and air contamination in an acute healthcare setting during the peak of the COVID-19 pandemic in London (pre-print). MedRxiv. 2020. https://doi.org/10.1101/2020.0 5.24.20110346.

27. Liu Y, Ning Z, Chen Y, Guo M, Liu Y, Gali NK, et al. Aerodynamic analysis of SARS-CoV-2 in two Wuhan hospitals. Nature. 2020;582:557–60.

28. Ma J, Qi X, Chen H, Li X, Zhan Z, Wang H, et al. Exhaled breath is a significant source of SARS-CoV-2 emission (pre-print). MedRxiv. 2020. https://doi.org/10.1101/2020.05.3 1.20115154.

29. Faridi S, Niazi S, Sadeghi K, Naddafi K, Yavarian J, Shamsipour M, et al. A field indoor air measurement of SARS-CoV-2 in the patient rooms of the largest hospital in Iran. Sci Total Environ. 2020;725:138401.

30. Cheng VC-C, Wong S-C, Chan VW-M, So SY-C, Chen JH-K, Yip CC-Y, et al. Air and environmental sampling for SARS-CoV-2 around hospitalized patients with coronavirus disease 2019 (COVID-19). Infect Control Hosp Epidemiol. 2020:1–32. https://doi.org/10.1017/ ice.2020.282.

31. Ong SWX, Tan YK, Chia PY, Lee TH, Ng OT, Wong MSY, et al. Air, surface environmental, and personal protective equipment contamination by severe acute respiratory syndrome coronavirus 2 (SARS-CoV-2) from a symptomatic patient. JAMA. 2020;323(16):1610–2.

32. Taskforce for the COVID-19 Cruise Ship Outbreak, Yamagishi T. Environmental sampling for severe acute respiratory syndrome coronavirus 2 (SARS-CoV-2) during a coronavirus disease (COVID-19) outbreak aboard a commercial cruise ship (pre-print). MedRxiv. 2020.

33. Döhla M, Wilbring G, Schulte B, Kümmerer BM, Diegmann C, Sib E, et al. SARS-CoV-2 in environmental samples of quarantined households (pre-print). MedRxiv. 2020. https://doi. org/10.1101/2020.05.02.20088567.

34. Wu S, Wang Y, Jin X, Tian J, Liu J, Mao Y. Environmental contamination by SARS-CoV-2 in a designated hospital for coronavirus disease 2019. Am J Infect Control. 2020;48:910–4.

35. Ding Z, Qian H, Xu B, Huang Y, Miao T, Yen H-L, et al. Toilets dominate environmental detection of SARS-CoV-2 virus in a hospital (pre-print). MedRxiv. 2020. https://doi.org/10.110 1/2020.04.03.20052175.

36. Cheng VCC, Wong SC, Chen JHK, Yip CCY, Chuang VWM, Tsang OTY, et al. Escalating infection control response to the rapidly evolving epidemiology of the coronavirus disease 2019 (COVID-19) due to SARS-CoV-2 in Hong Kong. Infect Control Hosp Epidemiol. 2020;41:493–8.

37. CDC Oct 5 2020. Science Brief: SARS-CoV-2 and Potential Airborne Transmission. https:// www.cdc.gov/coronavirus/2019-ncov/science/science-briefs/scientific-brief-sars-cov-2.html.

38. Hamner L, Dubbel P, Capron I, Ross A, Jordan A, Lee J, et al. High SARS-CoV-2 attack rate following exposure at a choir practice — Skagit County, Washington, March 2020. MMWR Morb Mortal Wkly Rep. 2020;69:606–10.

39. Leclerc QJ, Fuller NM, Knight LE, Funk S, Knight GM, Group CC-W. What settings have been linked to SARS-CoV-2 transmission clusters? Wellcome Open Res. 2020;5(83):83.

40. Jang S, Han SH, Rhee J-Y. Cluster of coronavirus disease associated with fitness dance classes, South Korea. Emerg Infect Dis. 2020;26(8):1917–20.

41. Adam D, Wu P, Wong J, Lau E, Tsang T, Cauchemez S, et al. Clustering and superspreading potential of severe acute respiratory syndrome coronavirus 2 (SARS-CoV-2) infections in Hong Kong (pre-print). Res Sq. 2020. https://doi.org/10.21203/rs.3.rs-29548/v1

42. Price RHM, Graham C, Ramalingam S. Association between viral seasonality and meteorological factors. Sci Rep. 2019;9:1–11. https://doi.org/10.1038/s41598-018-37481-y.

43. Tang JW. The effect of environmental parameters on the survival of airborne infectious agents. J R Soc Interface. 2009;6 https://doi.org/10.1098/rsif.2009.0227.focus.

44. Pan M, Carol L, Lednicky JA, Eiguren-Fernandez A, Hering S, Fan ZH, Wu CY. Determination of the distribution of infectious viruses in aerosol particles using water-based condensational

growth technology and a bacteriophage MS2 model. Aerosol Sci Technol. 2019;53:583–93. https://doi.org/10.1080/02786826.2019.1581917.

45. Woo MH, Grippin A, Anwar D, Smith T, Wu CY, Wander JD. Effects of relative humidity and spraying medium on UV decontamination of filters loaded with viral aerosols. Appl Environ Microbiol. 2012;78:5781–7. https://doi.org/10.1128/AEM.00465-12.

46. W.H. Organization. Vol. 72. 2020. (Coronavirus Disease 2019 (COVID-19): Situation Report).

47. da Silva PG, Nascimento MSJ, Soares RRG, Sousa SIV, Mesquita JR. Airborne spread of infectious SARS-CoV-2: moving forward using lessons from SARS-CoV and MERS-CoV. Sci Total Environ. 2021;764:142802. https://doi.org/10.1016/j.scitotenv.2020.142802.

48. Sobsey MD, Meschke JS. Virus survival in the environment with special attention to survival in sewage droplets and other environmental media of fecal or respiratory origin; 2003.

49. Yang W, Marr LC. Dynamics of airborne influenza a viruses indoors and dependence on humidity. PLoS One. 2011;6 https://doi.org/10.1371/journal.pone.0021481.

50. Chan KH, Peiris JSM, Lam SY, Poon LLM, Yuen KY, Seto WH. The effects of tempera-ture and relative humidity on the viability of the SARS coronavirus. Adv Virol. 2011;2011:7. https://doi.org/10.1155/2011/734690.

51. van Doremalen N, Bushmaker T, Munster VJ. Stability of Middle East respiratory syndrome coronavirus (MERS-CoV) under different environmental conditions. Eur Secur. 2013;18:1–4. https://doi.org/10.2807/1560-7917.ES2013.18.38.20590.

52. Pyankov OV, Bodnev SA, Pyankova OG, Agranovski IE. Survival of aerosolized coronavirus in the ambient air. J Aerosol Sci. 2018;115:158–63.

53. Darnell MER, Subbarao K, Feinstone SM, Taylor DR. Inactivation of the coronavirus that induces severe acute respiratory syndrome, SARS-CoV. J Virol Methods. 2004;121:85–91. https://doi.org/10.1016/j.jviromet.2004.06.006.

54. Walker CM, Ko G. Effect of ultraviolet germicidal irradiation on viral aerosols. Environ Sci Technol. 2007;41:5460–5. https://doi.org/10.1021/es070056u.

55. Ratnesar-Shumate S, Williams G, Green B, Krause M, Holland B, Wood S, Bohannon J, Boydston J, Freeburger D, Hooper I, Beck K, Yeager J, Altamura LA, Biryukov J, Yolitz J, Schuit M, Wahl V, Hevey M, Dabisch P. Simulated sunlight rapidly inactivates SARS-CoV-2 on surfaces. J Infect Dis. 2020;222:214–22. https://doi.org/10.1093/infdis/jiaa274.

56. Schuit M, Ratnesar-Shumate S, Yolitz J, Williams G, Weaver W, Green B, Miller D, Krause M, Beck K, Wood S, Holland B, Bohannon J, Freeburger D, Hooper I, Biryukov J, Altamura LA, Wahl V, Hevey M, Dabisch P. Airborne SARS-CoV-2 is rapidly inactivated by simulated sunlight. J Infect Dis. 2020;222:564–71. https://doi.org/10.1093/infdis/jiaa334.

57. Kampf G, Todt D, Pfaender S, Steinmann E. Persistence of coronaviruses on inanimate sur-faces and their inactivation with biocidal agents. J Hosp Infect. 2020;104:246–51.

58. Rothe C, Schunk M, Sothmann P, Bretzel G, Froeschl G, Wallrauch C. Transmission of 2019-nCoV infection from an asymptomatic contact in Germany. N Engl J Med. 2020;382:970–1.

59. Gerlier D, Martin-Latil S. Persistence of infectious SARS-CoV-2 on inert surfaces and hand-mediated transmission. Virologie. 2020;24:162–4. https://doi.org/10.1684/vir.2020.0849.

60. Marquès DM, Domingo JL. Contamination of inert surfaces by SARS-CoV-2: persistence, stability and infectivity. A review. Environ Res. 2021;193:110559. https://doi.org/10.1016/j.envres.2020.110559.

61. Aboubakr HA, Sharafeldin TA, Goyal SM. Stability of SARS-CoV-2 and other coronaviruses in the environment and on common touch surfaces and the influence of climatic conditions: a review. Transbound Emerg Dis. 2020:1–17. https://doi.org/10.1111/tbed.13707.

62. Chin AWH, Chu JTS, Perera MRA, Hui KPY, Yen HL, Chan MCW, Peiris M, Poon LLM. Stability of SARS-CoV-2 in different environmental conditions. Lancet Microbe. 2020;1:e10. https://doi.org/10.1016/S2666-5247(20)30003-3.

63. Suman R, Javaid M, Haleem A, Vaishya R, Bahl S, Nandan D. Sustainability of coronavi-rus on different surfaces. J Clin Exp Hepatol. 2020;10:386–90. https://doi.org/10.1016/j.jceh.2020.04.020.

64. Dev KG, Mishra A, Dunn L, Townsend A, Oguadinma IC, Bright KR, Gerba CP. Biocides and novel antimicrobial agents for the mitigation of coronaviruses. Front Microbiol. 2020;11:1351. https://doi.org/10.3389/fmicb.2020.01351.
65. Gerlach M, Wolff S, Ludwig S, Schäfer W, Keiner B, Roth NJ, Widmer E. Rapid SARS-CoV-2 inactivation by commonly available chemicals on inanimate surfaces. J Hosp Infect. 2020;106:633–4. https://doi.org/10.1016/j.jhin.2020.09.001.
66. WHO. 2020. Coronavirus Disease (COVID-19): Cleaning and Disinfecting Surfaces in Non-health Care Settings. https://www.who.int/news-room/q-a-detail/coronavirus-disease-covid-19-cleaning-and-disinfecting-surfaces-in-non-health-care-settings Available at: [Google Scholar] [Ref list].
67. Ahmed W, Angel N, Edson J, Bibby K, Bivins A, O'Brien JW. First confirmed detection of SARS-CoV-2 in untreated wastewater in Australia: a proof of concept for the wastewater surveillance of COVID-19 in the community. Sci Total Environ. 2020;728:138764.
68. Arora S, Nag A, Sethi J, Rajvanshi J, Saxena S, Shrivastava SK. Sewage surveillance for the presence of SARS-CoV-2 genome as a useful wastewater based epidemiology (WBE) tracking tool in India. medRxiv. 2020. https://doi.org/10.1101/2020.06.18.20135277.
69. Kocamemi BA, Kurt H, Hacioglu S, Yarali C, Saatci AM, Pakdemirli B. First data-set on SARS-CoV-2 detection for Istanbul wastewaters in Turkey. medRxiv. 2020. https://doi.org/10.1101/2020.05.03.20089417.
70. Kocamemi BA, Kurt H, Sait A, Sarac F, Saatci AM, Pakdemirli B SARS-CoV-2 detection in Istanbul wastewater treatment plant sludges. medRxiv. 2020. https://doi.org/10.1101/2020.05.12.20099358.
71. Medema G, Heijnen L, Elsinga G, Italiaander R, Brouwer A. Presence of SARS-Coronavirus-2 RNA in sewage and correlation with reported COVID-19 prevalence in the early stage of the epidemic in the Netherlands. Environ Sci Technol Lett. 2020;7:511–6.
72. Hung IFN, Cheng VCC, Wu AKL, Tang BSF, Chan KH, Chu CM. Viral loads in clinical specimens and SARS manifestations. Emerg Infect Dis. 2004;10:1550.
73. Leung WK, To K-F, Chan PKS, Chan HLY, Wu AKL, Lee N. Enteric involvement of severe acute respiratory syndrome-associated coronavirus infection. Gastroenterology. 2003;125:1011–7.
74. Yeo C, Kaushal S, Yeo D. Enteric involvement of coronaviruses: is faecal–oral transmission of SARS-CoV-2 possible? Lancet Gastroenterol Hepatol. 2020;5:335–7.
75. Liu H, Wang L-L, Zhao S-J, Kwak-Kim J, Mor G, Liao A-H. Why are pregnant women susceptible to viral infection: an immunological viewpoint? J Reprod Immunol. 2020;139:103122.
76. Li Y, Zhao R, Zheng S, Chen X, Wang J, Sheng X, Zhou J, Cai H, Fang Q, Yu F. Lack of vertical transmission of severe acute respiratory syndrome coronavirus 2, China. Emerg Infect Dis. 2020;26:1335–6.
77. Chen H. Clinical characteristics and intrauterine vertical transmission potential of COVID-19 infection in nine pregnant women: a retrospective review of medical records. Lancet. 2020; https://doi.org/10.1016/S0140-6736(20)30360-3.A.
78. Breastfeeding and COVID-19. Geneva: World Health Organization; 2020 (available at https://www.who.int/news-room/commentaries/detail/breastfeeding-and-covid-19).
79. Ha JF. The COVID-19 pandemic, personal protective equipment and respirator: a narrative review. Int J Clin Pract. 2020;74(10):e13578. https://doi.org/10.1111/ijcp.13578.
80. Yu P, Zhu J, Zhang Z, Han Y, Huang L. A familial cluster of infection associated with the 2019 novel coronavirus indicating potential person-to-person transmission during the incubation period. J Infect Dis. 2020;
81. Bedford J, Enria D, Giesecke J, Heymann DL, Ihekweazu C, Kobinger G, et al. COVID-19: towards controlling of a pandemic. Lancet. 2020;
82. Bai Y, Yao L, Wei T, Tian F, Jin DY, Chen L, Wang M. Presumed Asymptomatic carrier transmission of COVID-19. JAMA. 2020;323(14):1406–7. https://doi.org/10.1001/jama.2020.2565. PMID: 32083643; PMCID: PMC7042844.
83. Bischoff W, Reid T, Russell GB, et al. Transocular entry of seasonal influenza-attenuated virus aerosols and the efficacy of N95 respirators, surgical masks, and eye protection in humans. J Infect Dis. 2011;204:193–9.

84. O'Dowd K, Nair KM, Forouzandeh P, et al. Face masks and respirators in the fight against the COVID-19 pandemic: a review of current materials, advances and future perspectives. Materials (Basel). 2020;13(15):3363. https://doi.org/10.3390/ma13153363.
85. Bien C, Revoir WH. Respiratory protection handbook. Oxforshire: Taylor & Francis Limited; 2019.
86. Ekabutr P, Chuysinuan P, Suksamrarn S, Sukhumsirichart W, Hongmanee P, Supaphol P. Development of antituberculosis melt-blown polypropylene filters coated with mangosteen extracts for medical face mask applications. Polym Bull. 2018;76:1985–2004.
87. Robert AH. Selection and uses of HEPA and ULPA filters. Heating/Piping/Airconditioning 1986:119–123.
88. Hyttinen M, Rautio A, Pasanen P, Reponen T, Earnest GS, Streifel A, Kalliokoski P. Airborne infection isolation rooms – a review of experimental studies. Indoor Built Environ. 2011;20(6):584–94.
89. Wong BJF, Hakimi AA, Elghobashi S. Smoke evacuator use with ultra-low particulate air filtration in rhinoplasty and sinus surgery. Facial Plast Surg Aesthet Med. 2020;22(6):404–5. https://doi.org/10.1089/fpsam.2020.0434.

Chapter 10
An Overview of Personal Protective Equipment and Disinfection

Ario D. Ramezani, Nikhil A. Crain, and Taizoon Dhoon

Protection of Personnel

Effective protection against COVID-19 for medical personnel, hospital patients, and general population has been a leading concern amid the pandemic. While there remains controversy on the most effective type of mask, there is robust evidence to suggest that all cotton, surgical, and N95 masks can provide some protection against the transmission of SARS-CoV-2, especially when the mask is worn by an infectious individual [1, 2]. Both the World Health Organization (WHO) and Centers for Disease Control (CDC) recommend that the general public wear face masks in public where they will be in close proximity with people such as in public transportation, airports and trains, events, and gatherings [3, 4]. In the hospital setting, protection for staff, particularly in patient-facing roles, has emerged as a major area of discussion. As described by the Occupational Safety and Health Administration (OHSA), there are three major guards against airborne biothreats: engineering measures, administrative controls, and personal protective equipment (PPE) [5].

Currently, general agreement on the minimum standards for PPE in suspected COVID-19 cases includes eye protection (e.g., goggles, safety glasses), gloves, gown, and mask (e.g., N95, PFF2) [6]. Specifically, aerosol-generating procedures (AGPs) with potential exposure to COVID-19 have been the focus of safety discussions; nevertheless, recommended protocols have varied across the globe [7, 8]. To complicate matters further, AGPs vary greatly in risk profile depending on many factors [9]. The type of surgery (e.g., endoscopic sinus surgery has greater

Ario D. Ramezani and Nikhil A. Crain have contributed equally to this work.

A. D. Ramezani · N. A. Crain · T. Dhoon (✉)
Irvine Medical Center, University of California, Orange, CA, USA
e-mail: tdhoon@hs.uci.edu

© The Author(s), under exclusive license to Springer Nature Switzerland AG 2022   115
A. A. Hakimi et al. (eds.), *Mechanical Ventilation Amid the COVID-19 Pandemic*,
https://doi.org/10.1007/978-3-030-87978-5_10

particulate release from forceful drilling), duration of aerosol production, and length and proximity of aerosol exposure by healthcare workers may increase the hazards of AGPs [10, 11]. Moreover, COVID-19 patients suffering from advanced illness have been shown to carry viral loads up to 60 times greater than those with mild symptoms. It is also important to note that some protective equipment, such as face filtering pieces (FFP), may have a possible time limit on effectiveness, thus making longer procedures riskier [11].

With variable clinical circumstances and characteristics of masks, it has been suggested that hospitals design multiple protocols that can utilize reusable respirators, including elastomeric air-purifying respirators (APRs) and powered air-purifying respirators (PAPRs), and disposable respirators, such as the standard N95 [12]. FFP level 2 or 3 has also been recommended to have effective filtration efficacy for disposable masks when compared to N95s []. While N95s have a minimum filtration capacity of particles larger than 0.3 mm equal to 95%, FFP2 and FFP3 have efficacies of 94% and 99%, respectively []. The CDC has endorsed the use of either PAPRs or N95 FFR with face shields to ensure thorough protection of vulnerable areas, including the eyes, mouth, and nose from SARS-CoV-2 exposure [13]. PAPRs were granted emergency authorization by the CDC in March 2020, leading to increasing availability to healthcare workers, though the CDC offered no preference towards PAPRs over N95s [13, 14]. Nonetheless, PAPRs warrant a particular focus on evaluating the benefits, drawbacks, and potential strategies for their use.

By definition, PAPRs provide clean air to the masked, hooded, or helmeted user by filtering out contaminants via a battery-powered blower, resulting in a superior air protection factor (AFP) [15]. AFP is the ratio of external to internal pollutants (e.g., APF equal to 50 indicates that the wearer will inhale 1/50 of environmental pollutants), when compared to reusable respirators, such as APRs and N95s [8]. PAPRs utilize high-efficiency particulate air (HEPA) filters, which achieve 99.7% filtration of particles greater than 0.3 mm in diameter [16]. The most popular PAPRs are produced by two US manufacturers 3M (St. Paul, Minnesota) and Bullard (Cynthiana, NY) [10]. While there are a variety of PAPR devices approved by the CDC's National Institute for Occupational Safety and Health (NIOSH), the newest CleanSpace Halo model can be used without the attachment of a hose [17].

There are both pros and cons to consider when integrating the use of PAPRs in care protocols. Studies have demonstrated that PAPRs achieve greater APFs compared to N95s ($\leq$100 vs. 10) and more effective filtration [18–21]. Because PAPRs can maintain an outward positive pressure while filtering air, they may be more protective, especially in lengthy, potentially hazardous AGPs like tracheostomy [9, 22, 23]. Nevertheless, there are some disadvantages to PAPR utilization. Surgical procedures that require equipment like surgical headlights and loupes may limit the use of PAPRs [18, 24]. Similarly, communication has been noted to be more challenging with PAPRs compared with disposable masks [9]. In addition, high infection rates have been reported in the absence of proper training on PAPR use and disposal [9, 25, 26].

The original use of PAPRs was in the industrial setting. In turn, PAPRs work to limit exposure via inhalation rather than filter-expired air [8, 9]. Therefore, caution has been placed by some manufacturers on PAPR use in sterile surgical fields [12]. Studies investigating the impact of PAPRs on sterility report favorable results, indicating no increase in particulate count under laminar flow environments and lower colony-forming units (CFU) when compared to N95s [27, 28]. Several otolaryngology societies have indicated the preference of PAPR use, especially for endoscopic procedures which require drilling [11, 29, 30]. PAPR utilization has also been recommended during intubation and extubation, as well as in the management of COVID-19 patients with severe illness [31]. Ultimately, hospitals should adopt an individualized approach respirator selection based upon patient presentations, diversity of procedures, care workflow, and resource availability [9, 12, 29, 30].

Environmental Protection

Prior studies have outlined the persistence and stability of the SARS-CoV-2 virus on different types of surfaces [31]. Even with properly donned PPE and hygienic precautions, contaminated surfaces still pose a risk. Therefore, recognizing factors that support viral presence and methods of decontamination are important.

Several common biocidal agents were evaluated for their efficacy in disinfecting surfaces that had collected dried viral particles. These agents include both chemical disinfectants, such as ethanol, and physical agents, including ultraviolet radiation and heat. Alcohol-based disinfectants are the most common and widely used of these agents in public communities. Ethanol and isopropanol are commonly utilized for viral, bacterial, and fungal decontamination. Their efficacy is dependent on concentration. Ethanol (78–95%), 2-propanol (70–100%), and a mixture of 45% 2-propanol with 30% 1-propanol demonstrated inactivation of coronaviruses by greater than 4 log10 [32]. These biocidal solvents denature viral proteins by breaking their intramolecular hydrogen bonds and disrupting the viral protein's tertiary structure. Alcohol also works as a disinfectant by damaging cellular membranes. However, it is important that alcohol-based disinfectants are formulated to be between 60% and 90% alcohol (v/v) to be most effective [31, 33, 34]. Alcohol disinfectants less than 60% demonstrated limited efficacy in virion penetration while those greater than 90% evaporate more quickly than lower concentrations, limiting their exposure time with the pathogen. Moreover, higher concentrations of alcohol avidly coagulate proteins, which can create a barrier between the solvent and other proteins, protecting them from coagulation, thus hindering the effectiveness of the disinfectant [33].

Another common household disinfectant is bleach. At an acidic pH, bleach contains sodium hypochlorite and hypochlorous acid. The hypochlorous acid is an oxidizing agent which serves as an effective biocidal agent due to its ability to disrupt cellular membranes. Kampf et al. found that the minimally required concentration of sodium hypochlorite to actively disinfect coronaviruses is 0.21% [32]. Other solvents, such as formaldehyde and glutaraldehyde, have also been identified as effective biocidal agents that work by alkylating proteins and nucleic acids, thereby disturbing their functionality. In the same study, formaldehyde (0.7–1%) and glutardialdehyde (0.5–2.5%) inactivated coronaviruses by greater than 4 log10. The use of these aldehydes has, however, been limited in varying communities due to their carcinogenic properties. Hydrogen peroxide was also found to be an effective biocidal agent when used at a concentration of at least 0.5% and given a 1-min incubation period. Povidone-iodine at concentrations between 0.23% and 7.5% was also highly effective in inactivating coronaviruses (Table 10.1).

While disinfection is paramount in the prevention of SARS-CoV-2 transmission by self-inoculation, there was previously little information on the impact of common disinfectants on the filtration efficacy of respirators. Different studies investigated the efficacy of these biocidal agents on face filtering respirators. Table 10.2 summarizes the effects of oven-drying, microwaving, chlorinated disinfectant,

Table 10.1 Efficacy of different biocidal agents on coronavirus inactivation (adapted from Akram, 2020) [34]

Disinfectant	Concentration (%)	Incubation period (min)	Infectivity reduction (log 10)
Ethanol	78–95	30 s	Greater than 5.5
2-Propanol	70–100	30 s	Greater than 4
2-Propanol with 1-propanol	45 with 30	30 s	Greater than 4
Sodium hypochlorite	0.21	30 s	Greater than 4
Formaldehyde	0.7–1	2 min	Greater than 3
Glutaraldehyde	0.5–2.5	2–5 min	Greater than 4
Hydrogen peroxide	0.5	1 s	Greater than 3
Povidone-iodine	0.23–7.5	15–60 s	4.6

Table 10.2 Impact of various methods of disinfection on facial respirator performance and pathogen activity (adapted from Jung et al., 2020) [36]

Method of disinfection	Impact on filtration	Decontamination efficacy
Oven-dry	Filtration performance maintained with 75–100-°C treatment, but decreased at 125 °C	5-log10 decrease of SARS-CoV-2 after 5 min of 95 °C treatment
Microwaving	No change in filtration performance after 2.5-min treatment	Greater than 4-log10 decrease in *E. coli* after 2.5 min under 500 W
Chlorinated disinfectant	No change in filtration performance after hypochlorite wipe use	1-log10 decrease in *S. aureus*
Ethanol	Up to 18% decrease in performance	Complete biocidal activity after 5-min treatment
Isopropanol	Approximately 5% decrease in performance	N/A
Laundering	Up to 39% decrease in performance	N/A

N/A: Not available

alcohol-based solvents, and detergent laundering on both reducing the pathogenic infectivity and filtration performance of facial respirators. Respirators that were oven-dried at 95 degree Celsius showed a 5-log10 decrease in SARS-CoV-2 activity after 5 min. The filtration performance of oven-dried respirators was maintained when treated at temperatures between 75 and 100 °C but decreased in performance at temperatures above 125 °C [35]. No studies were found that directly evaluated the correlation between microwaving and reduction of SARS-CoV-2 viral activity. However, one study reported greater than 4-log10 reduction of *E. coli* from respirators after 2.5-min exposure under 500-watt power [36]. Filtration performance was also maintained in this environment. When using chlorinated disinfectants, such as a hypochlorite wipe, filtration performance of the respirator was maintained, but a decrease of only 1-log10 in *S. aureus* was observed [37]. As previously discussed, ethanol does exhibit notable biocidal activity against SARS-CoV-2. In a study by Ullah et al., the application of ethanol suppressed bacterial growth after a 5-min immersion. However, this resulted in up to an 18% decrease in respirator filtration efficiency [38]. Isopropanol application resulted in a 5% decrease in efficiency. Laundering masks with detergent also significantly decreased (up to 39%) the filtration performance of face respirators [39].

In response to the strategic recommendation of reusing respirators, the CDC and NIOSH announced guidelines for disinfection via ultraviolet (UV) light irradiation, vaporous hydrogen peroxide, and moist heat. Of these methods, UV irradiation has been widely studied. Most studies have evaluated the efficacy of UV irradiation of either UVC at 254 nm, UVA at 365 nm, or a combination of the two [40]. Results indicated that the combination of UVC and UVA irradiation resulted in total inactivation of SARS-CoV-2 after 9 min of exposure. The same result was derived with UVC alone, whereas UVA alone was found to be less effective. The authors concluded that UVC irradiation is a reliable method for inactivating SARS-CoV-2.

Despite this landmark finding, UVC poses a known threat to the safety of human skin and eyes, especially at the studied wavelength (254 nm) [41]. More recent studies have evaluated the effectiveness of "far-UVC" (222 nm) on inactivating SARS-CoV-2, as this wavelength is less harmful since it has limited penetration in the skin or eyes. Cells in the study were cultured with SARS-CoV-2 to achieve a virus titer of 50% tissue culture infectious dose. These cultured cells were then suspended and loaded onto a polystyrene plate that was subject to exposure to 222 nm UVC irradiation. This study revealed a 99.7% reduction in viable SARS-CoV-2, demonstrating the effectiveness of this decontamination modality and its potential for use in greater communities [41].

Airborne infection isolation rooms (AIIRs) have been another pivotal tool in environmental protection measures during the COVID-19 pandemic. These single-occupancy patient rooms were previously used for cases of tuberculosis prior to the pandemic but were quickly adapted for use due to increased hospital demand for isolation measures. AIIRs are designed essentially to prevent the spread of droplet nuclei beyond the perimeter of the room, protecting hospital personnel and other patients from exposure to infectious airborne particles. These specialized rooms are a product of the facility's heating, ventilation, and air-conditioning (HVAC) system.

In this capacity, airflow that is supplying the room is balanced with air through an exhaust, creating a negative pressure difference [42]. When operating properly, these rooms maintain this negative pressure relative to other parts of the hospital. When the doors to an AIIR open, the negative pressure results in air flowing into the AIIR rather than the reverse. Air that has been circulating in the infected patient's room is now less likely to escape to the rest of the facility, limiting additional unintended exposures. Further, the air from AIIRs does not reenter the HVAC system. Rather, either it can be exhausted to the outdoor environment where virial droplets will be diluted by the surrounding air or the air from the room can be passed through a HEPA filter which, as previously discussed, has a filtration efficiency of 99.97%. Currently, AIIRs have been recommended by the CDC to be prioritized for COVID-19 patients who will be undergoing aerosol-generating procedures [43–45].

Conflicts of Interest No relevant conflicts of interest.

Funding No funding was obtained.

References

1. Fouladi Dehaghi B, Ghodrati-Torbati A, Teimori G, Ibrahimi Ghavamabadi L, Jamshidnezhad A. Face masks vs. COVID-19: a systematic review. Invest Educ Enferm. 2020;38(2):e13. https://doi.org/10.17533/udea.iee.v38n2e13.
2. Ueki H, Furusawa Y, Iwatsuki-Horimoto K, et al. Effectiveness of face masks in preventing airborne transmission of SARS-CoV-2. mSphere. 2020;5(5):e00637–20. https://doi.org/10.1128/mSphere.00637-20. Published 2020 Oct 21
3. WHO. Coronavirus disease (COVID-19) advice for the public: When and how to use masks. December 2020. https://www.who.int/emergencies/diseases/novel-coronavirus-2019/advice-for-public/when-and-how-to-use-masks
4. CDC. Guidance on Face Masks. Feb 2021. https://www.cdc.gov/coronavirus/2019-ncov/prevent-getting-sick/about-face-coverings.html
5. 1910.134 - respiratory protection: occupational safety and health administration. Available at: https://www.osha.gov/laws-regs/regulations/standardnumber/1910/1910.134. Accessed 4 Apr 2021.
6. Hojaij FC, Chinelatto LA, Boog GHP, Kasmirski JA, Lopes JVZ, Medeiros VMB. Head and neck practice in the COVID-19 pandemics today: a rapid systematic review. Int Arch Otorhinolaryngol. 2020;24(4):e518–26. https://doi.org/10.1055/s-0040-1715506.
7. Guidance. COVID-19 personal protective equipment (PPE) 2020. Available at: https://www.gov.uk/government/publications/wuhan-novel-coronavirus-infection-prevention-and-control/covid-19-personal-protective-equipment-ppe#ppe-guidance-by-healthcare-context. Accessed 4 Apr 2021.
8. Powered Air-Purifying Respirators Strategy: Centers for Disease Control; 2020. Available at: https://www.cdc.gov/coronavirus/2019-ncov/hcp/ppe-strategy/powered-air-purifying-respirators-strategy.html. Accessed 4 Apr 2021.
9. Licina A, Silvers A. Use of powered air-purifying respirator(PAPR) as part of protective equipment against SARS-CoV-2-a narrative review and critical appraisal of evidence. Am J Infect Control. 2021;49(4):492–9. https://doi.org/10.1016/j.ajic.2020.11.009.
10. Roberts V. To PAPR or not to PAPR? Can J Respir Ther. 2014;50:87–90.

11. Howard BE. High-risk aerosol-generating procedures in COVID-19: respiratory protective equipment considerations. Otolaryngol Head Neck Surg. 2020;163:98–103.
12. Board on Health Sciences P, Institute of M. National Academies Press (US) Copyright 2015 by the National Academy of Sciences; Washington DC: 2015. The National Academies Collection: Reports funded by National Institutes of Health. The Use and Effectiveness of Powered Air Purifying Respirators in Health Care: Workshop Summary.
13. Wizner K, Nasarwanji M, Fisher E, Steege AL, Boiano JM. Exploring respiratory protection practices for prominent hazards in healthcare settings. J Occup Environ Hyg. 2018;15:588–97.
14. Food and Drug Administration Emergency Authorization for Respirator Use [cited 2020 September]. Available at: https://www.fda.gov/media/135763/download. Accessed 30 Nov 2020.
15. The Use and Effectiveness of Powered Air Purifying Respirators in Health Care. National Academies Press (US); 2015. Workshop Summary Washington (DC). https://www.ncbi.nlm.nih.gov/books/NBK294217/ [Institute of Medicine: [Based on Health Sciences Policy]. Available at: [Google Scholar].
16. Guo ZD, Wang ZY, Zhang SF. Aerosol and surface distribution of severe acute respiratory syndrome coronavirus 2 in hospital wards, Wuhan, China, 2020. Emerg Infect Dis. 2020;26:1583–91.
17. Chughtai AA, Seale H, Rawlinson WD, Kunasekaran M, Macintyre CR. Selection and use of respiratory protection by healthcare workers to protect from infectious diseases in hospital settings. Ann Work Expo Health. 2020;64:368–77.
18. Givi B, Schiff BA, Chinn SB, et al. Safety recommendations for evaluation and surgery of the head and neck during the COVID-19 pandemic. JAMA Otolaryngol Neck Surg. 2020;146:579–84.
19. Hsieh TY, Dedhia RD, Chiao W, et al. A guide to facial trauma triage and precautions in the COVID-19 pandemic. Facial Plast Surg Aesthet Med. 2020;22(03):164–9.
20. Vukkadala N, Qian ZJ, Holsinger FC, Patel ZM, Rosenthal E. COVID-19 and the otolaryngologist: preliminary evidence-based review. Laryngoscope. 2020;130:2537–43.
21. Parikh SR, Bly RA, Bonilla-Velez J, et al. Pediatric otolaryngology divisional and institutional preparatory response at Seattle children's hospital after COVID-19 regional exposure. Otolaryngol Neck Surg. 2020;162:800–3.
22. Rengasamy A, Zhuang Z, Berryann R. Respiratory protection against bioaerosols: literature review and research needs. Am J Infect Control. 2004;32:345–54.
23. Rengasamy S, Eimer BC, Shaffer RE. Comparison of nanoparticle filtration performance of NIOSH-approved and CE-marked particulate filtering facepiece respirators. Ann Occup Hyg. 2009;53:117–28.
24. Day AT, Sher DJ, Lee RC, et al. Head and neck oncology during the COVID-19 pandemic: Reconsidering traditional treatment paradigms in light of new surgical and other multilevel risks. Oral Oncol. 2020;105:104684.
25. Kulcsar MA, Montenegro FL, Arap SS, Tavares MR, Kowalski LP. High Risk of COVID-19 Infection for Head and Neck Surgeons. Int Arch Otorhinolaryngol. 2020;24(02):e129–30.
26. Frauenfelder C, Butler C, Hartley B, et al. Practical insights for paediatric otolaryngology surgical cases and performing micro-laryngobronchoscopy during the COVID-19 pandemic. Int J Pediatr Otorhinolaryngol. 2020;134:110030.
27. Kim Y, Hale M. Pilot study to examine the use of a powered air purifying respirator (PAPR) in the operating room. Am J Infect Control. 2017;45:S84.
28. Church T. Bacterial contamination study of loose-fitting power air purifying respirators (PAPR) compared to N-95 FFR and surgical mask, in a simulated sterile environment; 2019.
29. Vukkadala N, Qian ZJ, Holsinger FC, Patel ZM, Rosenthal E. COVID-19 and the otolaryngologist: preliminary evidence-based review. Laryngoscope. 2020;130:2537–43.
30. Takhar A, Walker A, Tricklebank S. Recommendation of a practical guideline for safe tracheostomy during the COVID-19 pandemic. Eur Arch Otorhinolaryngol. 2020;277:2173–84.

31. Ti LK, Ang LS, Foong TW, Ng BSW. What we do when a COVID-19 patient needs an operation: operating room preparation and guidance. Can J Anesth. 2020;67:756–8.
32. Chin AWH, Chu JTS, Perera MRA, Hui KPY, Yen HL, Chan MCW, Peiris M, Poon LLM. Stability of SARS-CoV-2 in different environmental conditions. Lancet Microbe. 2020;1(1):e10. https://doi.org/10.1016/S2666-5247(20)30003-3. Epub 2020 Apr 2. PMID: 32835322; PMCID: PMC7214863
33. Kampf G, Todt D, Pfaender S, Steinmann E. Persistence of coronaviruses on inanimate surfaces and their inactivation with biocidal agents. J Hosp Infect. 2020;104(3):246–51.
34. Reynolds SA, Levy F, Walker ES. Hand sanitizer alert. Emerg Infect Dis. 2006;12(3):527–9. https://doi.org/10.3201/eid1203.050955.
35. Akram MZ. Inanimate surfaces as potential source of 2019-nCoV spread and their disinfection with biocidal agents. Virusdisease. 2020;31(2):94–6. https://doi.org/10.1007/s13337-020-00603-0. Epub 2020 Jun 5. PMID: 32656305; PMCID: PMC7274069
36. Campos RK, Jin J, Rafael GH, Zhao M, Liao L, Simmons G, Chu S, Weaver SC, Chiu W, Cui Y. Decontamination of SARS-CoV-2 and other RNA viruses from N95 level melt-blown polypropylene fabric using heat under different humidities. ACS Nano. 2020;14:14017–25.
37. Jung S, Hemmatian T, Song E, Lee K, Seo D, Yi J, Kim J. Disinfection treatments of disposable respirators influencing the bactericidal/bacteria removal efficiency, filtration performance, and structural integrity. Polymers (Basel). 2020;13(1):45. https://doi.org/10.3390/polym13010045. PMID: 33374397; PMCID: PMC7796291
38. Heimbuch BK, Wallace WH, Kinney K, Lumley AE, Wu C-Y, Woo M-H, Wander JD. A pandemic influenza preparedness study: use of energetic methods to decontaminate filtering facepiece respirators contaminated with H1N1 aerosols and droplets. Am J Infect Control. 2011;39:e1–9.
39. Ullah S, Ullah A, Lee J, Jeong Y, Hashmi M, Zhu C, Joo KI, Cha HJ, Kim IS. Reusability comparison of melt-blown vs nanofiber face mask filters for use in the coronavirus pandemic. ACS Appl Nano Mater. 2020:acsanm.0c01562. https://doi.org/10.1021/acsanm.0c01562. PMCID: PMC7323055
40. Lin TH, Chen CC, Huang SH, Kuo CW, Lai CY, Lin WY. Filter quality of electret masks in filtering 14.6–594 nm aerosol particles: effects of five decontamination methods. PLoS One. 2017;12(10):e0186217. https://doi.org/10.1371/journal.pone.0186217. PMID: 29023492; PMCID: PMC5638397
41. Heiligloh CS, Aufderhorst UW, Schipper L, Dittmer U, Witzke O, Yang D, Zheng X, Sutter K, Trilling M, Alt M, Steinmann E, Krawczyk A. Susceptibility of SARS-CoV-2 to UV irradiation. Am J Infect Control. 2020;48(10):1273–5. https://doi.org/10.1016/j.ajic.2020.07.031. Epub 2020 Aug 4. PMID: 32763344; PMCID: PMC7402275
42. Kitagawa H, Nomura T, Nazmul T, Omori K, Shigemoto N, Sakaguchi T, Ohge H. Effectiveness of 222-nm ultraviolet light on disinfecting SARS-CoV-2 surface contamination. Am J Infect Control. 2021;49(3):299–301. https://doi.org/10.1016/j.ajic.2020.08.022. Epub 2020 Sep 4. PMID: 32896604; PMCID: PMC7473342
43. Hyttinen M, Rautio A, Pasanen P, Reponen T, Earnest GS, Streifel A, Kalliokoski P. Airborne infection isolation rooms—a review of experimental studies. Indoor Built Environ. 2011;20(6):584–94.
44. Shiu Eunice YC, Leung NHL, Cowling BJ. Controversy around airborne versus droplet transmission of respiratory viruses: implication for infection prevention. Curr Opin Infect Dis. 2019;32(4):372–9.
45. Tran K, Cimon K, Severn M, Pessoa-Silva CL, Conly J. Aerosol generating procedures and risk of transmission of acute respiratory infections to healthcare workers: a systematic review. PLoS One. 2012;7(4):e35797.

Part III
Bridge Ventilator Design and Components

Chapter 11
What Is a Bridge Ventilator? Basic Requirements, the Bag Valve Mask, and the Breathing Circuit

Amir A. Hakimi, Govind Rajan, Brian J. F. Wong, Thomas E. Milner, and Austin McElroy

One of the most important components of any ventilator device is how it provides oxygen to the patient. Conventional ventilators are considered *flow source* meaning that a healthcare provider sets a certain oxygen flow rate. Many bridge ventilator designs are centered upon a handheld self-inflating manual resuscitator known as a bag valve mask (BVM). The BVM is comprised of a flexible air chamber which is attached to a face mask by a shutter valve (Fig. 11.1). The face mask is tightly sealed

A. A. Hakimi (✉)
Department of Otolaryngology – Head and Neck Surgery, Medstar Georgetown University Hospital, Washington, DC, USA

Beckman Laser Institute & Medical Clinic, University of California – Irvine, Irvine, CA, USA
e-mail: amir.a.hakimi@medstar.net

G. Rajan
Department of Anesthesiology and Perioperative Care, University of California – Irvine, Orange, CA, USA
e-mail: grajan@hs.uci.edu

B. J. F. Wong
Beckman Laser Institute & Medical Clinic, University of California – Irvine, Irvine, CA, USA

Department of Biomedical Engineering, University of California - Irvine, Irvine, CA, USA

Department of Otolaryngology – Head & Neck Surgery, University of California – Irvine, Orange, CA, USA
e-mail: bjwong@uci.edu

T. E. Milner
Beckman Laser Institute & Medical Clinic, University of California – Irvine, Irvine, CA, USA

A. McElroy
University of Texas at Austin, Austin, TX, USA

© The Author(s), under exclusive license to Springer Nature Switzerland AG 2022
A. A. Hakimi et al. (eds.), *Mechanical Ventilation Amid the COVID-19 Pandemic*,
https://doi.org/10.1007/978-3-030-87978-5_11

Fig. 11.1 Operation of the BVM. The flexible air chamber is held and squeezed with one hand while the second hand tightly seals the mask around the patient's face. *Graphic by Pearson Scott Foresman—Archives of Pearson Scott Foresman*

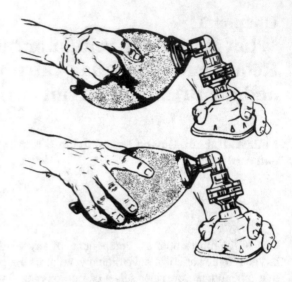

to a patient's face and the air chamber is squeezed circumferentially with a single hand. This forces air through the patient's lungs, and upon release the chamber self-inflates by drawing in ambient air or low-pressure oxygen flow (Fig. 11.1).

Unlike a conventional ventilator, the BVM is a *pressure source*: a certain external force is applied to the bag which then produces a pressure. Providing consistent flow to patients requiring ventilatory support requires important considerations in BVM bag compression. Variables including how hard the bag is pressed, the duration of bag depression, and the frequency in which the bag is compressed are critical to providing safe ventilatory support. Numerous groups have devised innovative means of controlling one or more of these variables through a cam-based system, actuating arm, negative pressure, and more. The ultimate goal is to replace the human hand with an automated "machine hand." The strengths and limitations of these mechanisms are discussed in a later chapter. It is important to note that these BVMs were not designed for prolonged use or for forceful actuation. Given the variable mechanisms of applying force to the BVM, it is critical to test the longevity and time to failure for each of these bags when succumbing to the forces of a bridge ventilator.

The basic requirements for any bridge ventilator were heavily discussed during our BVC meetings. Our expert panel ultimately selected the following minimum necessities:

- Able to generate a tidal volume of 200–800 cc to meet the ventilatory needs of most adults.
- Able to apply positive end-expiratory pressure (PEEP) of 5–20 cmH$_2$O: This can be conveniently achieved by applying a PEEP valve to the expiratory end of the BVM.
- Able to deliver a breath with inspiratory time of 0.5–2 s.

- Able to deliver a respiratory rate of 10–30 breaths/min.
- Includes a heat moisture exchanger (HME) filter to humidify and act as a bacterial/viral filter. Can be attached between the endotracheal tube and BVM.
- Corrugated extension tubing should be added to move the ventilatory bellows a convenient distance away from the patient.
- Able to deliver varying concentrations of oxygen (this is a preconfigured element of the BVM apparatus).
- Includes a high-inspiratory pressure pop-off device with alarm and a failed ventilation alarm.

An instructional video for breathing circuit assembly is available on our website, www.bli.uci.edu/bvc.

Conflicts of Interest The authors have no relevant conflicts of interest to disclose.

Funding This work was not funded.

Chapter 12
Hardware Considerations

Austin McElroy, Nitesh Katta, Scott F. Jenney, Tim B. Phillips,
and Thomas E. Milner

Evolution of the Actuating Arm

The following hardware descriptions and instructions are based on the experiences of the University of Texas at Austin's Automated Bag Breathing Unit (ABBU) bridge ventilator device. Regardless of the final arm design, the windshield wiper motor served as a constant. Power requirement of a healthy lung with the additional resistance of the breathing circuit was calculated at around 1.35 W/breath (Appendix A). A Toyota Corolla wiper motor (Cardone 85–3000) was selected for both its availability and mechanical power. This is a DC brushed motor which sells for approximately $40, and operates at 12 V at 2.5 A, for an approximate input electrical power of 30 W.

Once the motor has been identified, the next challenge is to determine how the motor will interface with the bag. A bag-valve mask is intended to be compressed using a human hand, typically with five fingers and the palm, roughly 0.54 m^2 for a typical male hand [1]. Moreover, the bag is compressed in a C-shaped pattern with circumference of the hand changed and "sliding" over the bag with little friction.

The most obvious and simple solution involved actuating the bag with a metal arm attached to the motor. However, this solution had limited surface area and caused increased bag failures such that it was quickly abandoned. The next approach involved securing a ball (e.g., tennis ball) to the end of the metal rod. Although this

A. McElroy (✉) · T. B. Phillips
University of Texas at Austin, Austin, TX, USA

N. Katta · T. E. Milner
University of Texas at Austin, Austin, TX, USA

Beckman Laser Institute and Medical Clinic, Irvine, CA, USA
e-mail: nkatta@uci.edu

S. F. Jenney
Beckman Laser Institute and Medical Clinic, Irvine, CA, USA

© The Author(s), under exclusive license to Springer Nature Switzerland AG 2022
A. A. Hakimi et al. (eds.), *Mechanical Ventilation Amid the COVID-19 Pandemic*,
https://doi.org/10.1007/978-3-030-87978-5_12

worked better than the naked arm, the ball could not traverse on the arm leading to issues with increased friction against the bag.

The ball was then replaced by a caster wheel with a rubber "tire." This modification provided a larger surface area as well as an arm that can "slide" when interacting with the bag. In turn, this design reduces wear on the bag and provides a larger surface area for the arm to interact with the bag, thus maximizing the volume which can be delivered to the patient.

Printed Circuit Board (PCB) Design

It is important that the PCB be designed to be as easy to manufacture as possible, to keep with the original goals of the project—an emergency device with easy-to-get parts that could be assembled in most settings. This means through hole components, as soldering is much more straightforward compared to surface-mount parts. The layout does not need to have high speed or precision analog signals that need special routing, impedance-matched traces, or special attention to ground-plane impedance.

Optical Reflectors

Open-loop control of the actuating arm, such that the arm is commanded to move forward and backward without feedback to a microcontroller, may lead to complications if the unit was not operating under optimal conditions. To combat this issue, bands can be painted along the arm like zebra stripes and a reflective optical encoder (e.g., OPB745) may be mounted on the chassis to help determine arm location. It is important to note that glossy paint should be avoided as the optical element cannot differentiate between white and black gloss. Rather, the optical signal should be binary as it is used on the Arduino as a digital interrupt. Matte paint is a viable alternative.

Pulse with Modulation (PWM) Board

The Cardone wiper motor can run with both positive and negative voltages such that a positive voltage moves the arm forward and a negative voltage moves the arm backward. A set DC voltage at ± 12 V moves the arm at a fixed speed. It is important to note that the resuscitator should accommodate not only changes in the rate at which the patient breathes (breaths per minute), but also the length of the breath (inspiratory time) and the speed at which the arm would return to home.

One such solution to account for these parameters involves driving the motor with a PWM signal. A PWM signal consists of two parts: the duration or period of

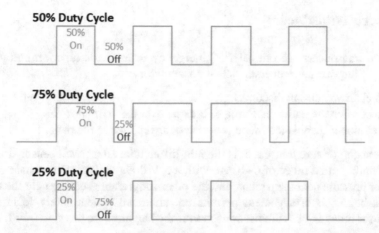

Fig. 12.1 The PWM signal consists of two parts: the duration or period of the pluses and the duty cycle of a pulse. Duty cycles are demonstrated

the pulses and the duty cycle of a pulse (Fig. 12.1). Regardless of the period, the longer the duty cycle, the faster the motor will operate until it reaches ±12 V. Similarly, regardless of the period, a 0% duty cycle will stop the motor.

The Cytron MD13S met the power and voltage requirements of the Cardone motor and is also easy to procure in large quantities (Appendix D). This board also works at both 3.3 V and 5 V logic levels. Finally, the Cytron MD13S had a large range of periods that it operated over. The Cytron MD13S and Cardone motor were originally operated using the Arduino PWM library, which has a period of around 1 kHz. The Cardone performance was enhanced for a faster period, which required the use of a custom software timer instead of the Arduino-supplied PWM library. The software timer allows for an interrupt function to be called after a period of time so the PWM functionality can be extended beyond the 1 kHz PWM supplied by Arduino.

Power Supply

A computer power supply serves as an inexpensive and readily available option for emergency resuscitators. They generally provide 12 V and at least 180 W of power which is more than sufficient for the Cardone wiper motor. However, if the device is to be considered for use in the clinical setting, it is important to use a compatible power supply that is approved by local regulatory bodies. This may include units with a strain relief locking mechanism like the Inventus MWA220, a 12 V, 220 W supply with a six-pin Molex connector that has a lip so the supply cannot be unintentionally disconnected.

Pressure Transducers

Pressure transducers are critical for emergency resuscitator function and safety. Incorporating two transducers makes it possible to:

- Detect airway circuit disconnects
- Detect when the patient is trying to breathe over the ventilator
- Determine if there is too much pressure being applied to the patient

One such pressure transducer is the non-differential Honeywell sensor from the NBP family with a range of 0–1 PSI, with a 5 V drive voltage. One sensor can be used for pressure near the patient, and the other for pressure sensing near the resuscitation bag. This arrangement permits an additional patient safety feature that checks for breathing circuit disconnection if the bag pressure drops to 0 PSI.

User Input Controls

There should be a focus on ensuring that emergency resuscitators are easy to use and include a simple user interface (Fig. 12.2). We found that the five essential knobs would control for the following parameters:

- Tidal volume—amount of air volume actuated per cycle.

  - This can range from 200 to 800 mL. The upper limit is fixed by the resuscitation bag, while the lower limit is derived by consensus among the Bridge Ventilator Consortium's expert respiratory panel.

- Respiration rate—number of times the arm actuates the resuscitation bag per minute.

  - Note that this time also includes the inspiration time. Turning this knob all the way to the left stops the arm from moving.

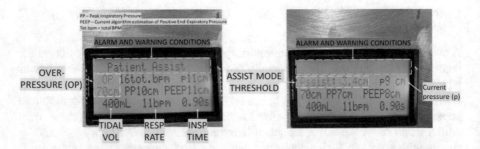

Fig. 12.2 Example of a simple user interface displaying key parameters for ventilatory support

- Inspiratory time—time over which the tidal volume is delivered.

  - This can be adjusted from 0.5 to 1.5 s and is included in the calculation of the respiration rate.

- Overpressure—pressure value deemed damaging to the patient.

  - This is a pressure setting adjustable between 50 and 70 cmH_2O.
  - If the air pressure at the patient exceeds the overpressure value, the arm retracts. This feature helps prevent damage to the patient's lungs.

- Assist mode threshold—the pressure limit that would trigger a patient-assisted breath (this is covered in more detail in a subsequent chapter).

  - This is a pressure adjustable between −1 and −10 cmH_2O.
  - The patient pressure is directed into an algorithm to determine the peak end-expiratory pressure (PEEK).
  - If the patient pressure falls below $P_{PEEK} + P_{assist}$, the patient is determined to be trying to draw a breath and a breath is delivered.
  - Setting the assist to −10 cmH_2O effectively disables the assist feature.

High-Priority Alarms

High-priority alarms signal a critical, damaging, or life-threatening condition. A high-priority alarm may be indicated by a flashing LED and/or audio alarm. Alarms should continue notifying the user until a corrective action is taken or the emergency resuscitator device is turned off. The software implementation is further discussed in the Software chapter.

Overpressure

This alarm activates when the patient pressure transducer measures a pressure that is higher than the pressure set using the overpressure knob. This could mean that the patient's airway or patient breathing circuit has an obstruction. The user must inspect the breathing circuit and/or the patient to identify the underlying obstruction or increase the overpressure setting to clear the alarm.

Underpressure

This alarm is typically tied to an improper breathing circuit. If the bag pressure transducer measures a pressure less than 3 cmH_2O, the alarm will trigger. The corrective action is to check for breaks or leaks in the breathing circuit and the resuscitation bag.

Loss of Power

The emergency resuscitator should operate from a standard electrical wall outlet, which in the United States is 120 V AC at 60 Hz. If power is lost, the lever arm will cease operation, leaving the patient in a critical state. A 9 V backup battery should be installed that can run the microcontroller and alarms for at least 7 min to alert the user that power has been lost. This alarm will clear only after power is restored or the 9 V battery discharges.

The 9 V backup battery *must* be replaced as soon as power is restored and the patient is safe, as future power losses on the same battery will decrease the likelihood that the alarm will function as intended.

Low-Priority Alarms

Low-priority alarms are intended to alert the user to an issue that is likely not critical for patient care or safety, but should be assessed.

Tidal Volume Out of Spec

This can happen if the tidal volume is very large, but the patient's lungs may not be able to handle the actuated air. In this scenario, the requested encoder count would not be met, as the arm stalls on the bag. The corrective action would be to check for obstructions or reduce the tidal volume.

Motor End of Life

This warning should be displayed after the motor has reached a set number of arm cycles. Using the aforementioned Cardone motor, it is recommended to set the warning to 7,000,000 arm cycles. The only way to remove this notification is to send the unit back to the manufacturer to have the motor replaced.

Conflicts of Interest None

Funding Information This work was not funded.

Outline of Motor Power Requirement Estimate

Energy/Power/Pressure Conversions:

- 1 cmH_2O = 98.06 Pa
- 1 cmH_2O × ml = 0.098 mJ
- 1 cmH_2O × ml/s = 0.098 mW

Energy/Power into Ambu Bag

- Change in pressure is 3 kg over 1″ diameter. This converts to 5.808 Pa of pressure.
- Compliance estimate of Ambu bag is delta_V/delta_P = 800 ml/5.808 Pa = 137.74 ml/Pa or 1.38 × 10–4 m 3/Pa.
- Energy to eject 800 ml from Ambu bag: E(Ambu bag) = 0.5 × V_2^2/C = 232 3.217 ml Pa = 2.31 mJ.
- Over 0.5 s this is a power of 4.646 mW.

Power Loss In 10 ft. Long Tube

- Resistance of the tube is 8 $\mu L/(\pi R^4)$.
- Parameters:

  - **Dynamic viscosity of air**: 1.825 10–5 kg/(m s)
  - **Length**: 10′ is 3.048 m
  - **πR^4**: R = 9 mm; $\pi R 4$ = 2.0612 10 $^{-8}$ m⁴
  - **Resistance**: 8 (1.825 × 10⁻⁵) 3.048/(2.0612 × 10⁻⁸) = 2.159 × 10⁴ [kg/(s m⁴)] or (Pa s/m³)
  - **Resistance in pulmonary units**: 2.159 × 10⁴ (Pa s/m²) (1 cmH_2O/98.06 Pa) (m/100 cm)² = 0.022 (cmH_2O s/cm)
  - **Instantaneous power loss**: P = Q^2R = 0.0016² (m⁶/s²) 2.159 × 10⁴ (Pa s/m³) = 0.05527 W or 55.27 mW
  - **Instantaneous energy loss over 0.5 s**: 27.64 mJ

Power/Energy Loss in Pulmonary Resistance

- **Lung and airway resistance**: 1.5 cmH_2O/(L/s), converting to MKS 1.5 cmH_2O/(L/s) (98.06 Pa/cmH_2O) (1 L/s)/(0.001 m³/s) = 1.471 × 10⁵ (Ps s/m³).
- **Instantaneous power loss**: P = Q^2R = 0.0016 2 (m⁶/s²) 1.471 × 10⁵ (Pa s/m³) = 0.3766 W.
- **Instantaneous energy loss over 0.5 s**: 188 mJ.

Energy/Power for Lung Compliance

$$V = a + \left[\frac{b}{1 + e^{-\frac{P-c}{d}}} \right].$$

$a = 10$ ml, $b = 1200$ ml, $c = 20$ cmH$_2$O, and $d = 3$ cmH$_2$O.

Linear compliance: delta_V/delta_P = 1500 ml/(14.5 cmH$_2$O) = 103.45 (ml/cmH$_2$O).

Converting to MKS: 103.45 (ml/cmH$_2$O) (10^{-6} m^3/ml) (1 cmH$_2$O/98.06 Pa) = 1.055 × 10^{-6} m^3/Pa.

Energy to inject 800 ml into lung: E(Lung) = 0.5 × ($V\_2^2 - V\_1^2$)/C = 0.5 × ($0.001^2 - 0.0002^2$)/($1.055 × 10^{-6}$ m^3/Pa) = 0.454 J.

Instantaneous power: 0.91 W.

Total energy: 672 mJ.

Total instantaneous power: 1.344 W.

Reference

1. Kaye R, Konz S. Volume and surface area of the hand. In: Proceedings of the Human Factors Society Annual Meeting, Vol. 30.4. Los Angeles, CA: SAGE Publications Sage CA; 1986. pp. 382–384.

Chapter 13
Software Considerations

Austin McElroy, Nitesh Katta, Scott F. Jenney, Tim B. Phillips, and Thomas E. Milner

Software Overview

The following software descriptions and instructions are based on the experience of the University of Texas at Austin's Automated Bag Breathing Unit (ABBU) bridge ventilator device. C and C++ programming was performed, with C style being preferred, and C++ being used predominantly for the **std::string** library and for organizing code into a **class**. Memory was statically allocated at compile time using the **#define** options in **settings.h**. The goal was to avoid using **malloc** and **free** so as to avoid long-term memory fragmentation and non-determinism.

The programming environment was Microsoft Studio Community with the Visual Micro plug-in. Visual Micro provided a clean interface between Visual Studio and the Arduino compiler, GCC 7.3.0. The plug-in also provided a **JTAG** interface for programming and debugging the Arduino Due with an Atmel-ICE-C for SAM processors. This was invaluable and the project could not have been completed through typical Arduino debugging techniques such as serial logging.

The pins discussed in the following section are referenced to the Arduino pin map, which is common across nearly all Arduino families with the same footprint. One advantage of the Arduino Due over the Arduino Mega is that only certain digital pins could be used on the Arduino Mega for digital interrupts whereas almost any digital pin can be assigned as a digital interrupt trigger on the Due.

A. McElroy (✉) · T. B. Phillips
University of Texas at Austin, Austin, TX, USA

N. Katta · T. E. Milner
University of Texas at Austin, Austin, TX, USA

Beckman Laser Institute and Medical Clinic, Irvine, CA, USA
e-mail: nkatta@uci.edu

S. F. Jenney
Beckman Laser Institute and Medical Clinic, Irvine, CA, USA

© The Author(s), under exclusive license to Springer Nature Switzerland AG 2022
A. A. Hakimi et al. (eds.), *Mechanical Ventilation Amid the COVID-19 Pandemic*,
https://doi.org/10.1007/978-3-030-87978-5_13

Analog Input Acquisition

Several of the tasks were responsible for collecting data from the outside world, via either user input knobs, pressure transducers, or power supply. The data acquisition shared a common set of reusable functions. Each signal input was acquired by one of several 10-bit data acquisition pins mapped to the Arduino analog-to-digital converters as outlined below:

- Respiration rate → Pin 0
- Patient assist → Pin 1
- Inspiration time → Pin 2
- Bag pressure → Pin 3
- Patient pressure → Pin 4
- Voltage sense → Pin 5
- Overpressure → Pin 8
- Tidal volume → Pin 9

The analog input values were acquired using an AnalogInput class which provided a common platform for analog acquisition and linearly mapping the acquired voltages to physical values. Creating an AnalogInput object required the pin that was to be acquired as well as an optional history size parameter used for keeping a running history of prior values.

Once the voltage was acquired, it was kept in 10-bit digitally quantized form and had a dead zone applied to it. This is useful for preventing quantization error at either the lowest or the highest setting of the potentiometer. The ABBU set the acquired value to zero if the quantized voltage was below 32, or maximized the acquired value if the quantized value was above 992. The quantized value was mapped to a physical value using a struct LinearMap, which contains slope, intercept, and zero _if_ below parameters. The zero _if_ below variable was used in the case of respiration knob, and provided a means of setting the mapped value to zero if the quantized count was below a certain value. In production, the zero _if_ below count was 128 only for the respiration knob. All of these values can then be easily modified in **settings.h**.

Linear maps can be created using the AnalogInput::createLinearMap static method, which could be fed into an AnalogInput object using setLinearMap static method, which could be fed into an AnalogInput object using setLinearMap. On the original Arduino Mega, an 8-bit microcontroller applying a floating-point linear map required a substantial amount of CPU time. To minimize the processing time, the linear map was applied only when calling the AnalogInput::acquire Measurement method, which cached the computed value and could be quickly recalled using AnalogInput::getMeasurement. The quantized value in volts could also be fetched using AnalogInput::getVoltage, which was useful when monitoring the power supply to check for power loss conditions.

Hardware and Timer Interrupts

There are several time-critical operations of bridge ventilators that require the use of hardware interrupts. These special functions should supersede almost all other operations and can be called a few clock cycles after being triggered. The triggering event can happen initially, as is the case with a hardware timer, or externally, as is the case for optical encoders. The main benefit of interrupts and hardware timers is that they take next to no processing power and the functions tied to the interrupts are only called when the interrupt event happens. The interrupt-related pins for the ABBU system are as follows:

- Home optical encoder → Digital Pin 2
- Motor PWM → Digital Pin 3
- Motor direction → Digital Pin 4
- Lid limit switch → Digital Pin 5
- Arm optical encoder → Digital Pin 10
- Alarm buzzer → Digital Pin 11
- Blue alarm LED → Digital Pin 12
- Red alarm LED → Digital Pin 13

It is important to note that when the interrupt occurs, the CPU registers may or may not hold the values that the interrupt function needs to operate on. When the compiler optimizes code, it can leave variables in CPU registers, a phenomenon known as **caching**. It is critical that any variable that is used in an interrupt routine be marked *volatile*, so that the compiler can create the proper instructions to pull the value from memory instead of maybe or maybe not a cached value in a register.

PWM Timer and Encoder Interrupts

The most important timer section is the timer to control the PWM signal to the motor driver (Cytron MD13S—see "Hardware Considerations" section). The traditional AnalogWrite function through the Arduino code may be ineffective and cause the motor to behave sluggishly due to the 1000 Hz maximum PWM frequency. One way to counter this is to move the PWM to a 10 μs time base with a period of 255 ticks per period, for an overall PWM period of 2.5 ms (and 10 μs resolution). The 225 value is an efficient number as it is represented by the unit8_t value that over flows to zero; thus the only value that needs to be updated is the number of ticks high and low. No bounds checking is needed. The main class that interacts with the motor should encapsulate the timer, encoder interrupts, and a digital output to control the direction.

Motor Control Task

The motor control task is one of the most complicated of the tasks and is responsible for all actuation arm-related motion, interfacing with patient assist mode, actuation arm calibration, and disabling the arm. The task was designed as a state machine: after completion of each task, the state is either changed or maintained as needed. This task also keeps track of how long the state has been running. Prior to entering the state machine, a few checks are made that may force an override of the prior state decision. These possible overrides are as follows:

- Overpressure—if the pressure reading was measured to be above the set overpressure value, the arm would retract to home and wait for the next breath.
- Motor off—if the respiration knob was turned all the way to the left, the motor would enter an "off" state and move to the home position.
- Patient assist—if the patient assist algorithm identified the patient trying to breathe, the motor will move forward, regardless of the set respiration frequency.

If none of the override conditions are met, the motor control task should maintain normal operation, moving forward and backward based on the control knobs.

Alarm Class

The Alarm Class is responsible for managing the alarm state and the timers associated with the tone generation and blinking or static LED lights. Alarms can be encoded in an unsigned integer number, with each alarm occupying a bit location. This was preferred over a more traditional Queue because it is deterministic, and a switch-case statement allows developers to rank the alarms in order of priority. It is suggested that each alarm case be blocked for 3 s, so that only a single alarm can be active at a given time. Once the alarm finishes, the bit associated with the error is cleared and the next alarm may be activated. If no alarm was active, built-in delay of 100 ms can be incorporated.

Display Class

The Display Class is the main interface between the software and the display, and can be created using the **LiquidCrystal** library provided by Arduino. Most of the tasks have values that need to be displayed, but calling the display update functions could impact performance. To avoid this, each task could cache a method variable in the Display Class that needs to be updated, and the display task would execute every 100 ms and update the display with the cached values. The exception to this is in the case of an alarm. An Alarm Class update should be allowed to update the first row of the display, which should be dedicated to alarms.

Flash Storage

Flash storage is a small amount of memory on a processor that is nonvolatile, meaning its flash memory retains its value regardless of the device's power state. However, flash memory can only be written when the unit is powered. The SAM3X processor provides 512 kB of flash memory, divided into program space and user space. The defaults, which are sufficient for use, are half of the flash for program space and half for user space, which can be used to record the motor count (number of times the motor left and returned home), how many times a watchdog error occurred, and how many times a watchdog error was reset.

This amounts to approximately 7 bytes of data recorded, a fraction of the space provided. Waveforms and other diagnostic data could be recorded in the remaining space.

Watchdog Timer

A watchdog timer is a specialized timer, either internal or external, that is periodically reset when software and hardware are running as intended. If the timer is not reset, it usually indicates that an error has occurred and a fail-safe action is necessary. On the SAM3X processor, this functionality runs on separate hardware from the main code loop. If the watchdog timer is not reset, the processors reboot and the software restarts.

For bridge ventilators that rely on an actuating arm, one of the worst events that could happen would be that the arm fails to move, either because it is stuck or detached from the motor or the motor has failed. This is a critical life-threatening event and represents a perfect use of a watchdog timer. This also introduces a natural watchdog reset such that the watchdog timer is reset when the actuation arm returns home. If the arm is disabled, the watchdog timer should also reset.

A watchdog error occurs if the watchdog timer was not reset after 14 s. A status register is checked when the software starts to detect whether the unit was reset due to the watchdog, and if so nonvolatile counter was incremented. If this occurs three times, the bridge ventilator should be "bricked" and should not be used.

Since this may often occur during testing and assembly, a unit can be "unbricked" by setting the input knobs to a certain orientation prior to executing the startup code. If a unit was "unbricked" in this manner, a counter can be incremented in nonvolatile memory and can be displayed at startup. This way manufacturers can see if the units are being reset or improperly used in the field.

Doxygen Documentation

Doxygen is a de facto standard tool for generating documentation from annotated C++ sources, but also supports other popular programming languages. It is programmed to open a file and look for specifically formatted comments, pull them out, and compile them into a monolithic document. Thus, the final document is only as good as the comments provided by the programmers. Once all of the code is commented, Doxygen may be configured to generate LATEX and HTML documentation. The LATEX documents can then be swiftly converted into a PDF which will be submitted to the Food and Drug Administration as part of the Emergency Use Authorization package (Figs. 13.1 and 13.2).

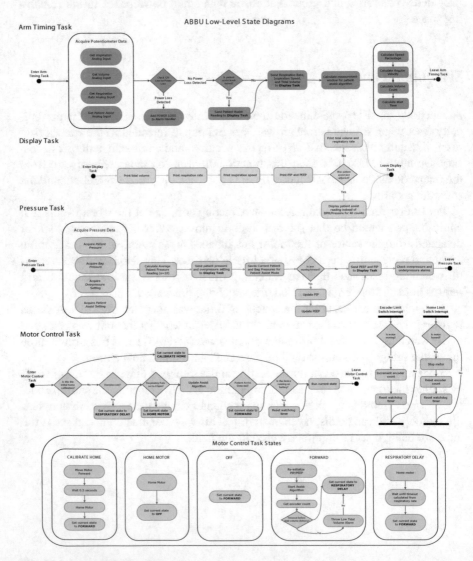

Fig. 13.1 Low-level state diagram

ABBU High-Level State Diagram

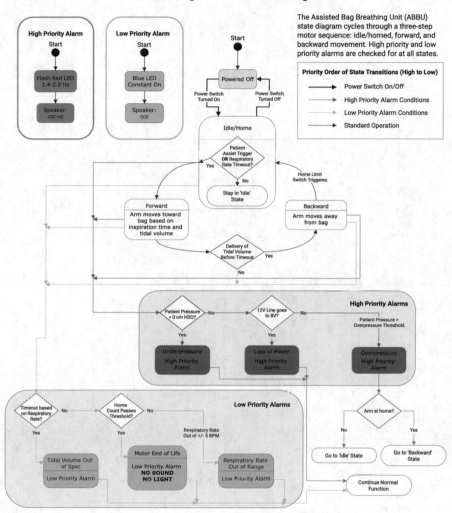

Fig. 13.2 High-level state diagram

Conflicts of Interest   None

Funding Information   This work was not funded.

Chapter 14
Development of Emergency Resuscitators: Considerations for Mechanical and Electrical Components

Shijun Sung

Introduction

In 2010, a student team from the Massachusetts Institute of Technology (MIT) introduced a novel concept for low-cost, portable ventilators utilizing a manual resuscitator. Breaths are delivered by compressing a conventional bag-valve mask (BVM) with an automated mechanism [1]. This automated manual resuscitator (AMR) device does not depend on the availability of external pressurized air and sophisticated pneumatic control system which are required for conventional medical ventilators. Rather, it is designed to be produced at a significantly low cost and to be used in dire emergency situations in resource-strapped environments.

The original design featured a pivoting cam arm to compress an Ambu BVM bag (Ambu USA, Ballerup, Denmark). The AMR device is able to adjust tidal volume, number of breaths per minute, and positive end-expiratory pressure (PEEP). Using pressure sensors, the device prototype can also monitor breath attempts by the patient and operate in assist-control mode. Additional features include an alarm to indicate overpressurization of the system.

In 2020, MIT Emergency Ventilator Project revisited this concept and developed an emergency resuscitator device which refined resuscitator operation with improved mechanical/electrical systems, incorporation of a respiratory system physiology model, and a revised breathing circuit [2]. The developers of the project performed careful analysis of the resulting airflow from the action of pushing the bag, and developed a control mechanism to deliver airflow waveforms similar to what a conventional ventilator can deliver. This design posed several inherent limitations, including difficulties in interrupting/adjusting breath delivery and undetermined risk for barotrauma. However, AMRs were considered one of the few methods

S. Sung (✉)
Irvine School of Medicine, University of California, Irvine, CA, USA
e-mail: shijuns1@hs.uci.edu

© The Author(s), under exclusive license to Springer Nature Switzerland AG 2022
A. A. Hakimi et al. (eds.), *Mechanical Ventilation Amid the COVID-19 Pandemic*,
https://doi.org/10.1007/978-3-030-87978-5_14

viable for clinical deployment, and several other emergency resuscitator devices approved by the United States Food and Drug Administration for emergency use adopted/resembled this design. Coventor Adult Manual Resuscitator Compressor developed by the University of Minnesota Medical School and Boston Scientific Corporation, and LifeMech, developed by LifeMech, Inc., used refined bag pushing mechanisms and implemented additional features such as adjustable inspiratory:expiratory (I:O) ratios, positive-pressure ventilation, volume-control ventilation, and respiratory rate. While these devices are designed for use in triage situations and cannot provide certain operations such as pressure-control mode or comprehensive measurement of ventilation parameters [3], they incorporate various sensors and safety features such as pressure-relief valves. Developers of some of these devices later implemented feedback mechanisms to monitor pressure for controlled operation and for patient monitoring.

Each of the teams that developed these automated resuscitators sought to come up with a low-cost, portable, and mass-producible design that can be applied in emergency and resource-poor environments so that more full-capacity ventilators can be freed. While there is no ground to compromise the reliability and safety of the device, these devices required careful considerations for cost and operation requirements.

This chapter provides an introduction and overview of the most fundamental components of ventilator/resuscitator devices: motor, controller, power supply, and control system. These components are among the most critical hardware components of AMR devices, and account for much of the manufacturing cost.

Motor Systems

When developing AMR devices, there is a need for several critical reliability and fail-safe features. Developers of all of the aforementioned devices generated design requirements that included stand-alone operation, robust mechanical and electrical systems, portability, and continuous operation without failure—for example, for 14 days, 24 h/day [2].

Another important reliability feature is the ability to recover from errors. If the actuating arm is displaced due to obstruction or unexpected interruption of the breathing circuit (e.g., changing connectors, patient coughing), the end-expiratory and end-inspiratory pressures must not consequently drift. Errors in delivered tidal volume (TV), when they occur, must not accumulate with every breath delivered. In both of these scenarios, the actuating system not only needs to sense that the error has occurred, but also needs to reset itself. In order to do so, the system needs to sense the position of the motor and mount an appropriate response.

These tasks can be accomplished by two most used motor types in automation: stepper motors and servomotors. Their operational characteristics and motor system components are discussed in the following sections.

Stepper Motor

Stepper motors have a unique operating mechanism that is advantageous in many applications for precision and complex motion control. Unlike other types of motors that turn continuously from applied electrical current, a stepper motor's shaft only moves in a discrete angular amount at a time. This type of motion can be controlled accurately without additional feedback mechanisms required in other motor systems. Stepper motors can be programmed to turn by desired direction, speed, and amount with a relatively simple command, and are highly responsive without having to use a high-performance control mechanism. For these reasons, stepper motors are well suited for automation applications for medical devices including scanners, samplers, fluid pumps , respirators, and laboratory automation machinery [4].

Basic Principles of Operation

A stepper motor is constructed with multiple electromagnets ("stators") around a central rotating element ("rotor"). Sending electrical current through a stator produces a magnetic field that exerts force on the rotor, which rotates to align itself to the magnetic field. When the adjacent set of stators are energized, the rotor further rotates to the next position, thereby creating a rotary motion. Repeating these actions drives the rotor, which continues to rotate by a specific angle.

In a stepper motor, these stators are arranged such that each positioning of the rotor is stable and precise, and the transition of rotor positions is facilitated when the next set of stators are active. In order to produce a magnetic field strong enough to move the rotor and quickly transition to the next set, the stators require relatively high current with quick rise and fall times. Such requirements are best achieved by synchronized electrical pulses provided by a driver circuit or a microcontroller. These specialized circuits are required to operate stepper motors. A block diagram of a typical stepper motor system is shown in Fig. 14.1. The controller interfaces high-level commands (e.g., acceleration, deceleration, steps per second, and distance) provided by the user with synchronized current output to the motor.

Stepper Motor Operation

The most basic method of operation described in the previous section is not commonly used anymore. Rather, there are several advanced methods to "drive" the stepper motor that enhances torque, resolution, and operating noise [4]. There are also different subtypes of stepper motors based on the types of magnets used as highlighted below. Stepper motor control engineering has advanced greatly in design and sophistication, and now there are many commercially available controller circuits for a wide range of applications with prices ranging from a few dollars

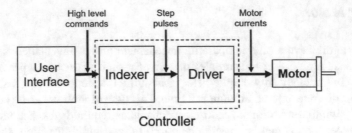

Fig. 14.1 A typical stepper motor system architecture. In the controller circuit, the indexer receives high-level commands from the user or operating program and generates the necessary step and direction pulses to the driver. The driver sends out currents that operate the motor. The controller also often features the ability to incorporate auxiliary input/output with external sensors such as limit switch

to hundreds of dollars [5, 6]. The LifeMech resuscitator device, which has received FDA emergency use authorization (EUA), uses a stepper motor with 1.8° step angle with holding torque of 1.06 N-m.

Encoders

An encoder is a sensor that tracks the angular position and speed of the motor. A type of encoder called "incremental encoder" is shown in Fig. 14.2. It looks like a disc with a spoke attached to the motor shaft so that the disc turns with it. An LED light sensor captures light signal modulated by the turning spokes as the motor turns. The motor's control system can interpret the resulting signal to a precise position and speed of the motor. Although a stepper motor does not need to have an encoder, it is essential for AMR devices and many medical devices because accurate motor positioning is critical. For example, the MIT Emergency Ventilator Project modeled its device operation and analysis based on the direct correlation between the encoder position and amount of air delivered (Fig. 14.3). The encoder also allows operators to "zero" the position of the motor so that the motor position does not drift with missed steps, overshoot, or inadvertently displace the position (e.g., the actuating component is stuck).

Servomotor

Servomotors are another widely used motor system that are versatile and commercially available and vary in performance and cost. A servomechanism (servo) broadly describes a control system that uses a closed-loop feedback mechanism to modulate output. A servomotor uses a position and speed feedback to achieve the desired position and speed of the motor.

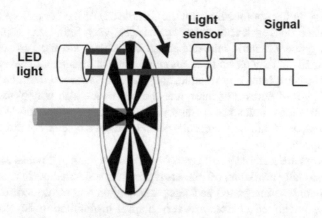

Fig. 14.2 Motor encoder

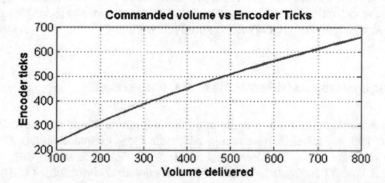

Fig. 14.3 Volume delivered (*x*-axis) versus motor position by encoder tick count (*y*-axis) in MIT Emergency Ventilator Version 3 [2]. This is an illustrative example of how precise motor position is used for ventilator operation. This curve is calibrated specifically to this device and was used to deliver desired tidal volume. Figure adapted from MIT Emergency Ventilator Project [7]

A rotary encoder, identical to the one shown in Fig. 14.2, provides the position and speed of the motor. Most commonly, a proportional–integral–derivative (PID) controller [8, 9] is used to achieve precise control of motor position and speed. In place of an encoder, a potentiometer attached to the motor can provide analog signals to indicate position only, which results in slower achievement of a stable position.

It is common to operate servomotors with an external device that contains both a PID controller and driver circuit that provide current to the motor. Much like the controller circuit used in stepper motor control (Fig. 14.1), a specialized servomotor driver interfaces high-level commands with currents that are supplied to the motor. Unlike stepper motors, a servomotor's responsiveness and speed-torque relationship depend on the parameters of the PID controller.

Depending on the components and the complexity of the control system, servomotors' construction, cost, and performance highly vary. Small servos using simple DC motors, potentiometers, and embedded controllers are used in radio-control (RC) toys, small appliances, and various automation components. These motors can be very inexpensive, relatively reliable, and simple to control with microprocessors and only a few lead wires. For these reasons, servos are also widely used in small robotics applications. Industrial grade servomotors may employ complex gear systems, encoders, and additional control system to achieve precise control of position, power, and speed.

Servomotors are a staple of all types of electromechanical devices and there are many commercially available, off-the-shelf products at desired performance parameters. There are also integrated packages that contain a control module within the motor. These integrated devices are very helpful in facilitating development and manufacturing, and they have a price range of tens of dollars to hundreds of dollars. The United States Food and Drug Administration Emergency Use Authorization-approved Coventor device, for example, used an integrated servomotor system capable of delivering the peak torque of 7.4 N-m and continuous (RMS) torque of 1.7 N-m within the device's operating speed range [3].

Motor System Considerations and Comparison

At a reasonable upper limit of operation, the AMR device would deliver tidal volumes of 200–800 mL at 30 breaths/min. Mechanical load of modulating Ambu bags at this rate depends on the mechanical design of the actuation mechanism. As an example, the MIT Emergency Ventilator Project's device design requires 12.18 N-m of torque to be supplied by the motor coupled with gears to the actuating arm [2]. Although this calculation does not take into account the dynamic load of lung compliance, overall pneumatic load resistance should not exceed 40 mmH$_2$O of pressure gradient. It is also reasonable to operate actuators and sensors within 5% of correct reading [10]. These requirements do not demand the highest levels of precision or speed, and are well within the limitations of a small stepper or servomotor system.

While stepper motors and servomotors are both readily available, programmable, and versatile devices, there are advantages and disadvantages of using one of these motors depending on the application. These two motor types also have special functions and characteristics stemming from their construction and mechanisms of operation. A general comparison between the stepper motor and servomotor is provided in Table 14.1.

For AMR devices, the main advantage of stepper motors is the great reliability with torque, especially at low speed. High-holding torque at rest is especially useful when the device operates at a lower breathing rate and the actuating arm is frequently at rest. These advantages contribute to a more consistent bag pushing mechanism and allow operators to choose smaller motors (compared to servomotors) that have less power consumption and cost. Stepper motors are also very robust and

Table 14.1 General comparison between stepper motor and servomotor

	Stepper motor	Servomotor
Power efficiency	Low	Moderate
Feedback control	Optional; open-loop operation typical	Position feedback required
Speed range	Low—typically 200–2000 RPMs	High
Torque-speed relationship	High torque at low speed	Higher torque at higher speed
Accuracy	Limited by step angle	Excellent
Responsiveness	Excellent response to starting, stopping, and reversing	Varies by the servo bandwidth
Cost[a]	Varies by performance	Varies by performance
Special functions	High-holding torque: Full torque when the motor is not in motion due to motor's inherent design	Torque limiting: Servomotors can control motor torque through precise monitoring of the current provided to the motor
Other characteristics/ pitfalls	Noisy due to fast stepping Runs hot (typically 50–90 °C) Potential missed steps	

[a]Stepper motors are generally less expensive than a comparable servomotor

require low maintenance due to brushless operation. However, they dissipate a lot of power, and therefore its low efficiency should be considered when designing a battery-operable device.

Servomotors constructed with brushless motor types are reasonable alternative to stepper motor with the advantage of better power efficiency and quieter operation. Torque-limiting capability may be used as an additional safety feature to prevent overpressurization, and may also be used as an error-recovery mechanism. Although servomotor systems are generally more expensive, servomotors with comparable operating parameters (holding torque, speed, responsiveness) in this application do not cost much more. Both motor systems are readily available, their respective control modules provide excellent auxiliary input/output, and both motor types come in integrated packages.

Conclusion

Reliability and robustness are the most important operational requirements for ventilator/resuscitator devices that deliver mechanically powered breath. Stepper motors and servomotors are commercially available versatile devices that can be used for such devices from the development process to manufacturing stage. Important performance parameters to consider in this application are holding torque, responsiveness, accuracy, and power consumption.

While both motor systems use sophisticated control and drive mechanisms, there are many commercially available integrated systems that streamline the development and manufacturing process. Innovative minds who strive to develop low-cost, portable, and reliable emergency resuscitators may benefit from the basic knowledge of electromechanical components and their applications.

Conflicts of Interest None

Funding Information This work was not funded.

References

1. Abdul Mohsen Al Husseini HJL, Negrete J, Powelson S, Servi A, Slocum A, Saukkonen J. Design and prototyping of a low-cost portable mechanical ventilator. Proceedings of the 2010 Design of Medical Devices Conference, April 2010.
2. M. E. V. Project. (2020, 05/13/2021). MIT Emergency Ventilator Project - Design Toolbox. Available: https://emergency-vent.mit.edu/
3. U. O. Minnesota. Coventor Emergency Ventilator - Adult Manual Resuscitator Compressor design file; May 8, 2021.
4. A. M. Systems. Stepper Motor System Basics. Accessed on 06 Jan 2021. Available: http://stepcontrol.com/pdf/step101.pdf
5. Zribi M, Chiasson J. Position control of a PM stepper motor by exact linearization. IEEE Trans Autom Control. 1991;36(5):620–5.
6. D. J. Reston Condit. Stepping motors fundamentals. Accessed on 06 Jun 2021. Available: http://www.bristolwatch.com/pdf/stepper.pdf
7. M. E. V. Project. Figure 3 – MIT Emergency Ventilator Version 3 calibration curvy goal so, ed; 2020.
8. Kiam Heong A, Chong G, Yun L. PID control system analysis, design, and technology. IEEE Trans Control Syst Technol. 2005;13(4):559–76.
9. Hashimoto H, Yamamoto H, Yanagisawa S, Harashima F. Brushless servo motor control using variable structure approach. IEEE Trans Ind Appl. 1988;24(1):160–70.
10. Krishnamurthy L. Design requirements. LifeMech Open Source Project Materials. Accessed on 05 Jan 2021. Available: https://www.ovvp.org/avs

Chapter 15
Incorporating Patient Assist Mode: The ABBU Experience

Aleksandra B. Gruslova, Nitesh Katta, Andrew G. Cabe, Scott F. Jenney, Jonathan W. Valvano, Tim B. Phillips, Austin B. McElroy, Robert K. LaSalle, Aydin Zahedivash, Van N. Truskett, Nishi Viswanathan, Marc D. Feldman, Richard Wettstein, Thomas E. Milner, and Stephen Derdak

Synchronous mechanical ventilation is Automated Bag Breathing Unit's (ABBU) default operation that is used to maintain appropriate blood gas oxygenation and carbon dioxide clearance. The ABBU synchronous operation is defined by the patient assist algorithm. If the threshold is set very high or if the patient is not attempting to breathe, ABBU will periodically deliver breaths as set by the operator. In this case, we say that ABBU is running asynchronously. If the patient is

A. B. Gruslova · A. G. Cabe · M. D. Feldman
Department of Medicine, UT Health San Antonio, San Antonio, TX, USA
e-mail: gruslova@uthscsa.edu; cabe@uthscsa.edu; feldmanm@uthscsa.edu

N. Katta · T. E. Milner
Beckman Laser Institute, The University of California Irvine, Irvine, CA, USA

UT Austin Cockrell School of Engineering, The University of Texas, Austin, TX, USA
e-mail: nkatta@uci.edu

S. F. Jenney · J. W. Valvano (✉) · T. B. Phillips · A. B. McElroy · V. N. Truskett
UT Austin Cockrell School of Engineering, The University of Texas, Austin, TX, USA
e-mail: jonathan.valvano@engr.utexas.edu; valvano@mail.utexas.edu; vtruskett@utexas.edu

R. K. LaSalle
ThermoTek, Inc., Flower Mound, TX, USA
e-mail: rlasalle@thermotekusa.com

A. Zahedivash
Stanford Medical School, Palo Alto, CA, USA
e-mail: aydin@utexas.edu

N. Viswanathan
Dell Medical School, UT Austin, Austin, TX, USA
e-mail: nishi.viswanathan@utexas.edu

R. Wettstein · S. Derdak
UT Health San Antonio, San Antonio, TX, USA
e-mail: wettstein@utscsa.edu

© The Author(s), under exclusive license to Springer Nature Switzerland AG 2022
A. A. Hakimi et al. (eds.), *Mechanical Ventilation Amid the COVID-19 Pandemic*,
https://doi.org/10.1007/978-3-030-87978-5_15

attempting to breathe and ABBU correctly delivers breaths as desired, we say that ABBU is running synchronously. Figure 15.1 shows the patient assist algorithm.

An important element of the ABBU patient assist algorithm is the establishment of a **response window**, which is the time period when ABBU is measuring peak expiratory end pressure (PEEP) and searching to detect a patient effort to breathe. The ABBU supports a reliable hardware time marker during a respiratory cycle. In Fig. 15.1 , the **green Forward arrow** is the time when the ABBU mechanical arm

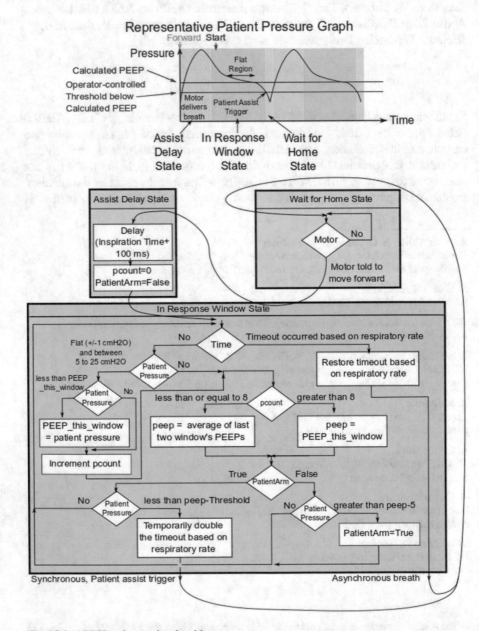

Fig. 15.1 ABBU patient assist algorithm

starts movement toward the bag-valve mask during a ventilated breath, whether the breath was initiated through patient effort or triggered automatically from the user-defined breaths per minute (BPM) potentiometer setting. In the figure, **Start** is the beginning of the response window, which begins after a blanking period (inspiration time plus 100 ms) after Forward. The blanking period means that the patient pressure (pp) measurements are not affected by electromechanical noise created by the ABBU motor. The response window can end in two ways: either a patient assist trigger occurs (synchronous) or a time-out occurs (asynchronous).

Patient assist has five features that reduce false positives and false negatives:

- First, the operator has control over the threshold parameter. This allows the operator to observe the patient and ABBU and adjust the threshold for maximum patient comfort.
- Second, the algorithm only considers the patient pressure to be PEEP if the patient pressure is flat for a long time (pcount > 8). This feature removes false positive caused by mechanical motion, and creates a reliable PEEP calculation.
- Third, during a disconnect or during a line suction, the patient pressure goes low and stays low. The algorithm has a **PatientArm** flag that is true once the pressure rises to near the last PEEP. If the patient pressure goes low and stays low, the **PatientArm** flag remains false and the algorithm will not trigger a synchronous breath.
- Fourth, the algorithm has a maximum rate at which it will supply synchronous breaths, implemented in the assist delay state, which reduces the possibility of breath stacking. This maximum rate is 60 BPM.
- Fifth, if the patient is trying to breathe at a rate similar to the operating setting, there is a potential for false positives (ABBU delivers breaths before the patient wants it). To eliminate false positives, the algorithm will temporarily extend the time-out period for asynchronous breaths so the patient can establish the rate. Once an asynchronous breath is delivered, the time-out period is restored to the operator setting.

ABBU measures patient pressure (pp) at a sampling rate of 100 samples/s in the breathing circuit near the patient. An 8-point averaging low-pass filter is applied in the measurement, with a group delay of 40 ms, to improve signal-to-noise ratio. Let $x(n)$ be the raw sampled pressure while $pp(n)$ contains the averaged pressures, which are used in the patient assist algorithm:

$$pp(n) = \left(\begin{array}{l} x(n) + x(n-1) + x(n-2) + x(n-3) + \\ x(n-4) + x(n-5) + x(n-6) + x(n-7) \end{array} \right) / 8$$

The algorithm calculates the change in pressure, dp, using four of the last eight pressure measurements. The algorithm considers the pressure to be flat if $-1.0 < dp < 1.0 \ \text{cmH}_2\text{O}$:

$$dp = pp(n) + 2pp(n-2) - 2pp(n-5) - pp(n-7)$$

pp measurements and *dp* calculations only occur in the response window. The flat criterion ($-1.0 < dp < 1.0$ cmH$_2$O) is an integral element of the ABBU patient assist algorithm to prevent missed triggers (false negatives), auto-triggers (false positives), and breath stacking. The selected forms to compute *pp(n)* and *dp* were derived from experimental testing (see below) and managing the trade-off between a short trigger delay (i.e., fast response) and minimization of missed triggers (false negatives), auto-triggers (false positives), and breath stacking. The time marker labeled Start in the figure is the beginning of the response window. If ABBU detects a patient effort, the ABBU actuator moves forward toward the bag resuscitator and will deliver a breath to assist the patient. If a patient effort to breathe was not detected, a time-out occurs and ABBU delivers a breath according to the operator-set breath rate determined by the BPM. The patient assist algorithm is governed by three activities that occur during the response window:

1. **Estimation of PEEP in response window**. If the pressure is flat, is more than 5 cmH$_2$O, and is less than 25 cmH$_2$O, the current *pp* is considered for the **peep_ this_window**. **peep_this_window** is the smallest *pp* value during the response window when *pp* is relatively flat. If a high-pressure cough event occurs, the high-pressure data are ignored. If a low-pressure patient inspiration event occurs, the low-pressure data are ignored. The *pp* calculation will only be included in PEEP estimations when $-1.0 < dp < 1.0$ cmH$_2$O.
2. **Calculation of PEEP**. If there is a long flat region (*pcount*>8), PEEP parameter is the smallest value of **peep_this_window**. If the pressure has not yet been flat during the response window, the PEEP parameter is averaged from two previous breaths with the most recent breath having a higher weighing.
3. **Patient assist trigger**. A threshold pressure set by the operator by a potentiometer on the ABBU enclosure labeled "assist mode threshold." The threshold pressure is operator-set between 1 cmH$_2$O and 20 cmH$_2$O. If *pp* goes below **PEEP threshold**, then a patient effort is triggered, shown as Trigger in the figure. Notice in the figure that at Trigger, the *pp* dropped 1 cmH$_2$O below PEEP (threshold pressure was set to -1 cmH$_2$O on the assist mode threshold on the ABBU enclosure).

One activity occurs at the start of each Forward state. The PEEP values for the last two breaths are updated. The **peep2**, **peep1**, and **peep_this_window** are shifted. If no flat periods in the last response window occurred, the PEEP values are not shifted, which allows coughs and suction to be ignored.

1. **peep1** is shifted into **peep2**.
2. **peep_this_window** is shifted into **peep1**.
3. 25.0 cm is shifted into **peep_this_window**.

ABBU Synchronous Operation Testing

ABBU synchronous operation utilizes the patient assist algorithm. The algorithm was developed and adjusted during a preliminary pig study (data not included). A "true positive" is defined as the patient initiating a breath resulting in the ABBU delivering an assist within 160 ms. 80 ms of this delay corresponds to the time it takes the patient to drop their airway pressure, and the other 80 ms is the time for ABBU to detect and move the arm initiating airflow from the bag. A "true negative" is defined as the patient failing to initiate a breath and the ABBU delivering a breath according to the manual settings. A "false positive" is defined as the ABBU delivering a breath at a time in which the patient did not initiate a breath. A number of innovative features were added to reduce false positives. A "false negative" is defined as the patient initiating a breath without the ABBU delivering an assisted breath.

The ability of ABBU to come in and out of patient assist mode was tested on a porcine model ($n = 2$). The assist mode threshold was set at -5 cmH$_2$O, and data were collected as the animal went from light anesthesia to heavier anesthesia. Tidal volume was adjusted from 200 mL to 800 mL and PEEP was set to 5 cmH$_2$O. Figure 15.2 shows six true-positive followed by three true-negative events.

In summary, the patient assist algorithm was tested over a wide range of anesthetic scenarios. Unless there was a disconnect or line suction, ABBU could effectively calculate PEEP. Once there was an accurate PEEP, the operator was able to set the threshold to minimize false positives and false negatives. Adjusting the manual PEEP valve quickly can cause false positives; however, adjusting the PEEP slowly

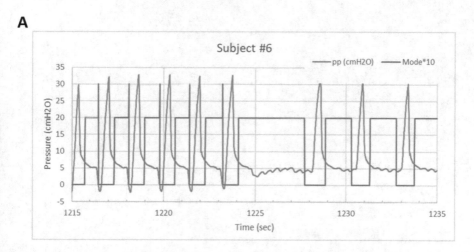

A

B

Porcine Study	True Positives	True Negatives	False Positives	False Negatives
Subject #5	612	456	0	0
Subject #6	64	117	0	2

Fig. 15.2 ABBU patient assist mode data in porcine model. (**a**) A representative trace of pressure data (blue) during the porcine experiment. Mode = 30 means that a patient assist was started, Mode = 0 means that a breath was delivered, and Mode = 20 means that ABBU is calculating PEEP. (**b**) The test summary of patient assist algorithm on porcine model ($n = 2$)

eliminates these false positives. The summary of all experiments is shown in Fig. 15.2b. Ultimately, the key to ABBU effectiveness is the ability of the operator to adjust the assist mode threshold.

Conflicts of Interest None

Funding Information No funding was obtained.

Chapter 16
A Qualitative Overview of Emergency Resuscitators Approved in the COVID-19 Pandemic

Karthik R. Prasad, Shijun Sun, and Scott F. Jenny

Introduction

Section 564 of the Federal Food, Drug, and Cosmetic Act empowers the US Secretary of Health and Human Services (HSS) special regulatory privileges to combat chemical, biological, radiological, and nuclear (CBRN) threats. In the face of CBRN threats, the HSS Secretary can issue an Emergency Use Authorization (EUA), allowing the Federal Drug Association (FDA) to authorize unapproved medical products or unapproved uses of approved medical products [1].

On March 24, 2020, the HSS Secretary issued an EUA in response to concerns about insufficient supply and availability of FDA-cleared ventilators for use in healthcare settings during the COVID-19 pandemic. Since that time, the FDA has approved over 86 different types of ventilators and resuscitators [1, 2]. This chapter provides an analytical overview of the 11 EUA-approved emergency resuscitators, examining their identified modes of actuation, design advantages, and trade-offs.

Resuscitators vs. Ventilators

At times used erroneously interchangeably in conventional conversation, resuscitators and ventilators are different but important devices for respiratory support in distressed patients. Ventilators are traditionally used for intubated patients who require prolonged respiratory support. These patients are often sedated, with

K. R. Prasad (✉) · S. Sun
UC Irvine School of Medicine, University of California, Irvine, CA, USA
e-mail: krprasad@hs.uci.edu; shijuns1@hs.uci.edu

S. F. Jenny
University of Texas at Austin Cockrell School of Engineering, The University of Texas, Austin, TX, USA

© The Author(s), under exclusive license to Springer Nature Switzerland AG 2022
A. A. Hakimi et al. (eds.), *Mechanical Ventilation Amid the COVID-19 Pandemic*,
https://doi.org/10.1007/978-3-030-87978-5_16

pharmacologically or physiologically suppressed respiratory effort. These ventilators can act in a supportive capacity (in addition to the patient's effort) or independently manage their ventilation function. Given the complex patient population, ventilators are equally complex medical devices, resulting in high costs per device, ranging between $25,000 and $50,000. Furthermore, their manufacturing requires specialized facilities that meet the FDA's Good Manufacturing Practice regulations [3, 4].

On the other hand, resuscitators are far less complex. Inherently, the design parameters for resuscitators focus on emergency intervention for patients who find themselves in sudden respiratory distress. Ideally, resuscitators would bridge patients' respiratory function until more permanent solutions are found. Thus, traits such as ease of use, low cost, and portability were viewed favorably, with early 1900s' resuscitators resembling bike pumps. However, the resuscitator has undergone several revisions since then.

The modern manual resuscitator is the bag-valve mask (BVM), but is also often known by popular manufacturing companies, like the Ambu bag [5]. BVMs are handheld devices that provide positive-pressure ventilation to patients via manual compression of a flexible air chamber. A series of valves provide unidirectional flow of air to an external mask. Some variations of the device incorporate the use of supplemental oxygen and/or use of positive end-expiratory pressure (PEEP) valves for better respiratory support. Rescuers commonly use BVMs in preference to mouth-to-mouth ventilation.

However, BVMs have several significant limitations. When used in isolation, they can control neither respiratory rate nor tidal volume through built-in safety adjustments. As a result, their effective use depends on the primary user's clinical expertise. Nevertheless, given their low cost, ease of use, and portability, BVMs have become widely adopted by healthcare providers and commercial customers.

During the early months of the COVID-19 pandemic, demand for ventilators far outstripped supply. Patients died as they awaited a free ventilator. As a result, the medical community looked for innovative ways to prolong the use of resuscitators as "bridge ventilators." Ideally, these devices would help manage low-acuity patients who may need mild-to-moderate respiratory support. In rare cases, they would substitute for a ventilator until one could be found, responsible for a patient's entire respiratory function. After the FDA announced the EUA for resuscitators, the subsequent response from the public and private communities was decisive. In less than a month, five different emergency resuscitators were approved by the FDA under the EUA. Around three months later a total of 11 different resuscitators were similarly approved. Below we examine each of them.

SecondBreath LLC

The first FDA EUA-approved resuscitator was created by SecondBreath LLC. It featured a pneumatically actuated arm that provided unilateral compression via a cylindrical puck on a manual resuscitator bag (MRB) (Fig. 16.1) [6]. The device is

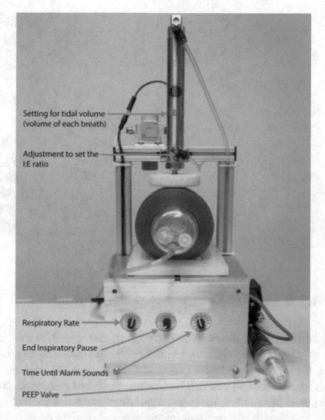

Setting for tidal volume
(volume of each breath)

Adjustment to set the
I:E ratio

Respiratory Rate

End Inspiratory Pause

Time Until Alarm Sounds

PEEP Valve

Fig. 16.1 Mark 1 Pneumatic Rapid Response Ventilator by SecondBreath LLC

controlled via a mix of dials and mechanical adjustment. It offered control over the following respiratory parameters:

- Respiratory rate
- Inspiratory pause
- Tidal volume
- Inspiratory-to-expiratory time (I:E) ratio
- Time until alarm sounds
- PEEP valve

However, its inventors stated that this device could only be used on sedated patients with paralyzed respiratory function. Furthermore, they mentioned that rebreathing in the inspiratory limb over time may cause CO_2 to build up. Thus, prolonged device use would require intermittent flushing of the inspiratory limb [7].

Undoubtedly, this device meets the requirement of low cost. However, it suffers in its ease of use and restricted patient population. It would not be of service to patients with mild-to-moderate respiratory distress who would otherwise not benefit from intubation. Also, it would require a clinician who is comfortable with crude mechanical adjustments of a clinically acute patient's respiratory support.

Fig. 16.2 Coventor

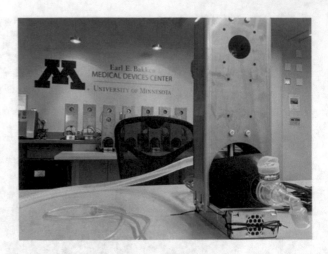

Coventor Adult Manual Resuscitator Compressor

Approved just a day later, the "Coventor" was an emergency manual resuscitator developed by the University of Minnesota Medical School and Boston Scientific Corporation. It used an electrically powered piston system to provide continuous unilateral compression of an MRB. The Coventor boasted a compact size, roughly the size of a cereal box, and an inexpensive production cost of $150 (Fig. 16.2) [8]. Additionally, this device did not require pressurized oxygen or air supply, unlike commercially available mechanical ventilators.

By using a single rotating arm, the device's design complexity was reduced. Moreover, it took steps to shield consumers from its moving parts. However, it lacked any capability to provide clinicians real-time clinical feedback information or failure alarms that are critical for safety. Thus, its ideal patient population, like SecondBreath, were patients with pathologically or pharmacologically paralyzed respiratory function. Overall, this device's strength was its low cost, small size, and ease of manufacturing [9].

Umbulizer

Approved on the same day as the "Coventor," the Umbulizer was created by a group of Harvard, MIT, and Boston university graduates (Fig. 16.3). Though approved for emergency use in 2020, Umbulizer had been under development for 3 years prior. Initially directed toward low-resource settings, it found new life in the COVID-19 pandemic and included several features that make it an attractive emergency resuscitator [10].

Fig. 16.3 Umbulizer

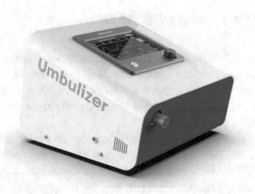

The Umbulizer used an electrically powered motor to actuate a convex paddle that applied unilateral compression on a strapped-in MRB. Furthermore, it incorporated sensors to track patient respiratory function dynamically, displayed it on a screen, and wirelessly transmitted the information to providers.

Regarding its actuation, Umbulizer's use of a convex paddle and strapped-in MRB is unique. A flat contact surface (like in Coventor and SecondBreath) deforms the bag in a nonlinear motion. Clinically, this means patients could experience a sudden jump in flow rate and pressure. Moreover, a flat contact surface creates stress concentrations at the edges of the driver and the folding area of the bag. This stress could lead to faster degradation of the bag and even critical leaks or tears over more extended periods. A convex surface offers linear deformation to the air chamber while limiting wear and tear by reducing stress concentrations. The strap limits the air chamber movement and provides higher fidelity in actuation [11].

Other features in this device include:

- Positive end-expiratory pressure (adjustable up to 25 cmH$_2$O)
- Programmable tidal volume: 200–800 mL
- Respiratory rate: 10–35
- I/E ratio: from 1.1 to 1.4
- 10-min battery backup power supply
- Wireless connectivity and patient monitoring

The main drawback is its cost of $2000 per unit. While cheaper than modern ventilators, this device is dramatically more expensive than its emergency resuscitator counterparts. Furthermore, this device is only designed for an intubated patient. However, Umbulizer's price tag and patient population limitation would be more appropriate if a clinician was looking for a low-cost ventilator [12].

PVA Prevent (RECALLED)

Approved on April 17, 2020, Prevent was developed by PVA. The company was the first nonmedical device company to receive FDA approval to design and manufacture ventilators under the COVID-19 EUA [13]. It uses an electrically powered servo stepper motor that drives two rigid flat arms that bilaterally compress a fixed MRB (Fig. 16.4).

Available videography of the device in action demonstrates a rapid release of the MRB. This action could lead to a rapid expiratory phase. In cases where the preset PEEP valve is insufficient, the sudden decrease in expiratory pressure could lead to airway collapse. Furthermore, the setup process involves a relatively long assembly and disassembly of the safety brackets which would not be ideal in an emergency setting.

Despite being developed by a precision engineering company, PVA Prevent was subject to Class 2 Device Recall due to errant false alarms, which caused incomplete movement of the paddles resulting in an impaired inhale/exhale cycle. However, with only three units in commercial use at the time, we expect that the impact was minimal [14]. Nevertheless, it serves as a stark reminder of the importance of thorough software testing before device deployment.

Fig. 16.4 PVA Prevent

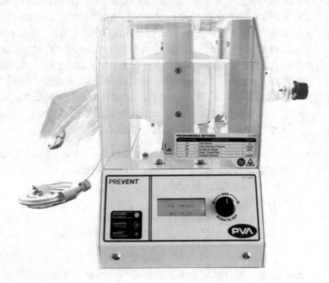

Spiro Wave

Approved on the same day as Prevent, Spiro Wave was inspired by the MIT Emergency Ventilator and designed to automate a manual resuscitator, expand functionality, and increase quality control. The device uses two electrically powered slightly convex paddles that apply synchronous bilateral compression to a fixed but easily detachable MRB (Fig. 16.5) [15]. The use of convex paddles confers the same advantages as previously discussed with Umbulizer. However, unlike Umbulizer, Spiro Wave uses bilateral compression and has the MRB in an accessible location. Moreover, it has a clear emergency stop button to halt function in less-than-optimal conditions.

Spiro Wave allows users to set the following three parameters:

- Tidal volume
- Respiratory rate
- Inspiration-to-expiration ratio

These settings are displayed on the accompanying LCD screen. The display also includes real-time clinical information from Spiro Wave's pressure sensors. In addition, these sensors help alert its users to low pressure, high pressure, high resistive pressure, and high driving pressure errors. Spiro Wave also has a dedicated battery backup that allows for 10 min of uninterrupted work during a power failure.

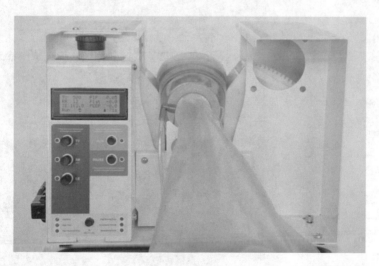

Fig. 16.5 Spiro Wave

However, given the plethora of features, Spiro Wave carries a relatively high cost of $5000. Also, the device's large shape and size raise portability concerns. However, like the Umbulizer, if this device is aimed toward a patient who would traditionally be on a ventilator, it is a cost-effective solution.

Virgin Orbit Resuscitator

Leveraging its manufacturing ingenuities born from rocketry, Virgin Orbit threw its hat in the resuscitator ring with the development of Virgin Orbit Resuscitator. While not performing rocket science, Virgin Orbit still held their device design to a high standard, emphasizing manufacturability and limiting the use of custom parts. Thus, this device uses a unique asymmetric rotatory cylinder that periodically actuates a convex paddle applying a unilateral compressive force on an MRB (Fig. 16.6).

The use of an asymmetric rotating cylinder is a simple but elegant solution to deliver a fixed periodic compressive force on an MRB. Its fully enclosed design provides safety from its moving parts. The convex paddle offers the same

Fig. 16.6 Virgin Orbit
Resuscitator

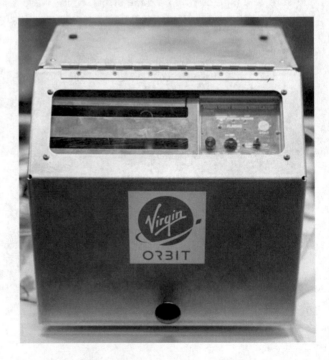

advantages as seen with Spiro Wave and Umbulizer. However, the device has several notable limitations. Users can only set the respiratory rate and adjust the high-pressure alarm threshold. Settings such as tidal volume and I:E ratio appear to be fixed. Moreover, it lacks a dynamic user display system and does not provide any real-time clinical information [16, 17].

Venti-Now

Approved on April 30, 2020, Venti-Now advertises itself as a low-cost portable resuscitator. Like SecondBreath, Venti-Now electrically drives a metal rod with an attached circular puck on its distal tip on an MRB, supplying a unilateral compressive force (Fig. 16.7). However, unlike SecondBreath, Venti-Now allows medical staff to set the inspiration time, I/E ratio, and respiration rate via the inspiration and expiration adjustment knobs *and* read the resulting inspiration time, I/E, and BPM on the LCD. Additionally, its suitcase-like design with a handle makes the device readily portable.

Venti-Now's choice of a single actuation arm reduces points of failure and complexity. However, the unilateral compression could cause asymmetric wear and tear on the MRB. Moreover, its inclusion of real-time clinical information has most likely driven up the unit price, with estimates putting it below $4000. Nevertheless, these devices have been actively shipped out and used in hospitals in Tanzania and Uganda [18, 19].

Fig. 16.7 Venti-Now

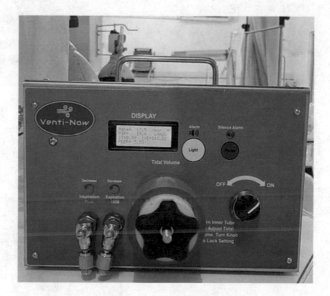

Fitbit Flow

Known more for their fitness products, Fitbit rose to meet the resuscitator demand by producing the Fitbit Flow. This device electorally drives two curved rectangular paddles, which supply a bilateral compressive force on a fixed but accessible MRB. Fitbit Flow supports conventional volume-control and pressure-control modes of ventilation and an "assist control" feature to support breaths triggered by the patient. The Fitbit Flow has many built-in safety features. It contains pressure and flow sensors that provide real-time clinical information on the LCD screen and alert users to less than optimal settings (Fig. 16.8).

Controls are provided for setting the following respiratory parameters:

- Respiratory rate
- I:E ratio
- Tidal volume
- Inspiratory pressure

While the Fitbit Flow contains many features, it has one glaring design oversight. It lacks an internal backup battery and cannot sound an alarm if its power is interrupted. Additionally, the authors raise question about ease of manufacturing with

Fig. 16.8 Fitbit Flow

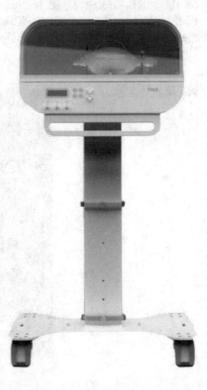

this device's judicious use of custom-cut parts, intricate overlays, and stylistically designed layout. As a result, it will come as no surprise to readers to learn that the Fitbit Flow comes with a $5000 price tag. Moreover, unlike several resuscitators we have discussed, it is unclear if this device has seen actual clinical use [20, 21].

Air Boost Austin P51

The Austin P51 derives its name from the WWII P-51 Mustang pursuit/fighter airplane designed and produced in just 102 days [22]. Similarly, the design development and prototype production of this device were completed in a mere 16 days. One month after the initial concept, the resuscitators were rolling down the production line [23].

Austin P51 works with two curved paddles that provide bilateral compression on an attached and accessible MRB (Fig. 16.9). What is more notable is the device's exterior. Austin P51 is housed in a rugged waterproof suitcase that contains a battery

Fig. 16.9 Austin P51

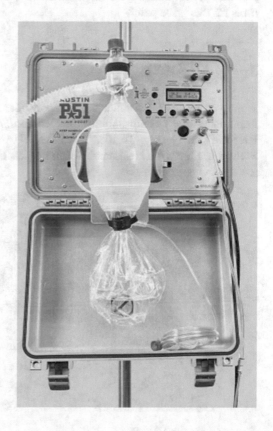

backup. Moreover, once opened, an Austin P51 can easily attach to a hospital intravenous pole. The device allows its users to adjust:

- Tidal volume (200–800 ml)
- I:E ratio
- Respiratory rate (8–40)
- Peep (0–20 cmH₂O)
- Peak pressure: 50 cmH₂O.

While it does not provide real-time continuous clinical information, clinicians can push the "measure button" which will provide point peak and plateau pressure values.

There are a few noticeable concerns. Like all devices that use a bilateral compression mechanism, it increases the device complexity and points of failure. Additionally, the Austin P51 appears to rely on custom software and device design. We surmise that this may pose some challenges for others to replicate without advanced manufacturing capabilities. Additionally, these features come in at an estimated cost of around $2000 [22–24]. However, given the range of features and portability, the authors were very impressed with the design considerations and features for this price point.

Apollo ABVMN

Approved by the FDA under the EUA on June 26, 2020, Apollo ABVMN was an iteration of a DIY controllable automated compressive system for BVM created by Rice University (Fig. 16.10). The FDA EUA-qualified device was finalized by Stewart & Stevenson Healthcare Technologies, LLC. The Apollo ABVMN uses two

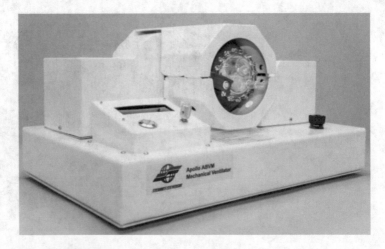

Fig. 16.10 Apollo ABVMN

independent servomotors that drive two bilateral arms on rack and pinion systems, exerting a bilateral compressive force on a fixed MRB. The enclosed model provides increased safety from actuating parts. Aiding in its ease of use, the inventors provided a clear red stop button and LCD.

The Apollo ABVMN allows for control of:

- Tidal volume
- Respiratory rate
- I:E volume

However, the leading cause of concern is its use of bilateral servomotors. Servo motors emit a large amount of heat. With continued use, this heat may damage sensitive parts. For prolonged use, the device would require a dedicated heat sink or cooling system. This feature would add to manufacturing complexity and cost. Second, the use of a rack and pinion system lends itself to gear slippages which may cause incorrect steppage. An error of this nature would lead to asymmetric MRB compression [25].

LifeMech A-VS

The most recently approved emergency resuscitator under the FDA EUA at the time of this analysis was LifeMech A-VS (Fig. 16.11). It uses an electrically powered motor to actuate a convex paddle that applies unilateral compression on an inserted MRB. Thus far, out of all the devices reviewed, it is the only one that uses a touchscreen to input ventilator settings and displays real-time clinical data. Its inventors claim that the manufacturing cost is around $400; however, there is no published final price.

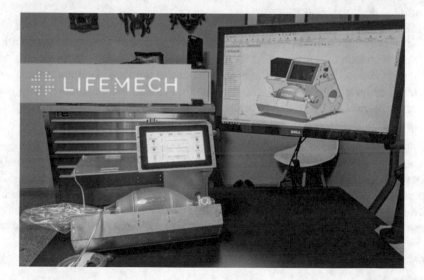

Fig. 16.11 LifeMech A-VS

As previously mentioned, using a single arm with a curved surface reduces device complexity and potentially reduces long-term wear and tear. However, this device does not appear as readily portable as Umbulizer, which uses a similar actuation mechanism. Secondly, the use of a touchscreen raises concerns about ease of use and affordability. Some touchscreens are pressure sensitive, while others require skin contact. In a healthcare setting, the latter would pose a challenge to healthcare providers who are often gloved. However, the screen is most impressive out of all the resuscitators approved under the EUA [26, 27].

Conclusions and Parting Design Considerations

Private and public enterprises provided a wide variety of emergency resuscitator models. In this cohort, there existed a broad spectrum of functionality and cost. A majority of these devices aimed toward functioning as a "bridge ventilator" to assist those with mild-to-moderate respiratory distress. From their designs, we can summarize key design considerations and common trade-offs:

- *Bilateral vs. unilateral compression trade-off:* Bilateral compression applies a balanced force on an MRB. However, it increases the number of moving parts, increasing manufacturing complexity and potential sites of failure.
- *Common user-adjustable settings.* The most common user-adjustable settings were tidal volume, respiratory rate, and I:E ratio.
- *Common safety features:* Low pressure and high pressure alerts.
- *Battery backup:* While Fitbit Flow system had the glaring error of failing to generate an alarm in the setting of power loss, most devices had a system that provided temporary support while alerting users of the issue. We view this as a critical design consideration.
- *Careful selection of target population.* Fundamentally, device design should aim to meet its communities' health needs in the context of their resource availability. Some device designs state that their target population is in a low-resource setting; however, they incorporate custom parts and wireless communications systems, or have high price points. Devices that aim to simultaneously help both resource-rich and resource-poor communities often end up too overpriced for low-resource settings or too functionally poor for resource-rich settings.

Finally, almost all models made the fundamental assumption that an MRB would be readily available. While that may be generally true, an MRB may be as valuable as a ventilator itself in resource-limited settings. Thus, there could be an avenue for future device development for emergency resuscitators that bring their infrastructure and minimize specialized hospital equipment use. Additional information regarding several of the aforementioned devices is highlighted in the table below.

Conflicts of Interest None.

Funding None.

	Power	Operation	AMBU bag actuation	Microcontroller	Tidal volume (ml)	Rate (BPM)	High-pressure valve (cm H_2O)	Patient assist mode	Open-source design?
LifeMech by *LifeMech, Inc.*	Input: Standard wall outlet Device input: 12 VDC Backup power: Battery, up to 60 min	VCV, SIMV with breathing assist; variable I:E ratio	Stepper motor + encoder	System: RASPBERRY PI 4 Motor: NANOTECH CL4-E-1-12-5VD1	150–800	5–35	40	Breath detection: Sense pressure of −1 to 5 cm H_2O	Yes
Apollo ABVMN by *Stewart & Stevenson Healthcare Technologies, LLC*	Input: Standard wall outlet Device input: 7.5 **VDC** Backup power: None	VCV, PCV with breathing assist; Variable I:E ratio	Stepper motor	Proprietary	200–700	8–40	40	No	No
Fitbit Flow by *Fitbit*	Input: 132 W medical-grade Class II power supply Device input: 12 VDC Backup power: Battery, up to 2 h	VCV, PCV with breathing assist; variable I:E ratio	Stepper motor	Proprietary	200–700	8–40	40	Breath detection: Sense pressure of −2 cmH_2O	No
Spiro Wave by *Spiro Devices LLC*	Modeled after MIT Emergency Ventilator	VCV, PCV with breathing assist; variable I:E ratio	Stepper motor	Proprietary	200–800	10–35	40	Breath detection: Sense pressure of −2 cmH_2O	No
Coventor Adult Manual Resuscitator Compressor by *University of Minnesota Medical School and Boston Scientific Corporation*	Input: Standard wall outlet Device input: 24VDC 180 W AC:DC Class I Adapter; battery backup: none	VCV, PCV Variable I:E ratio	Stepper motor		272–731	10–30	40	No	Yes
MIT Emergency Ventilator model	Power supply: Digikey 12 V 150 W power supply—LRS-150-12; battery backup: UPS (uninterruptible power supply)—BN450M	Modes: VCV, PCV with breathing assist; variable I:E ratio	Prototype: Andy Mark AM 3556 188:1 gearmotor with encoder; motor options: brushed DC motor with gearbox and position feedback; stepper motor	System: Arduino Mega Motor controller: RoboClaw Solo motor controller	200–800	6–40	40	Breath detection: Sense pressure of −2 cmH_2O	Yes

aStandard wall outlet: 100–240 VAC, 50–60 Hz

References

1. Commissioner O of the Emergency Use Authorization. FDA. Published online May 7, 2021. https://www.fda.gov/emergency-preparedness-and-response/mcm-legal-regulatory-and-policy-framework/emergency-use-authorization. Accessed 8 May 2021.
2. Health C for D and R. Ventilators and Ventilator Accessories EUAs. *FDA*. Published online April 28, 2021. https://www.fda.gov/medical-devices/coronavirus-disease-2019-covid-19-emergency-use-authorizations-medical-devices/ventilators-and-ventilator-accessories-euas. Accessed 8 May 2021.
3. Research C for DE and. Current Good Manufacturing Practice (CGMP) Regulations. *FDA*. Published online September 21, 2020. https://www.fda.gov/drugs/pharmaceutical-quality-resources/current-good-manufacturing-practice-cgmp-regulations. Accessed 8 May 2021.
4. High-Acuity Ventilator Cost Guide. https://hcpresources.medtronic.com/blog/high-acuity-ventilator-cost-guide. Accessed 8 May 2021.
5. Ambu® Resuscitators. https://www.ambuusa.com/emergency-care-and-training/clinical-evidence/ambu-resuscitator. Accessed 8 May 2021.
6. Photo Gallery. SecondBreath. https://secondbreathmed.com/photo-gallery/. Accessed 8 May 2021.
7. SecondBreath - Mark 1 Pneumatic Rapid Response Ventilators - Home. SecondBreath. https://secondbreathmed.com/. Accessed 8 May 2021.
8. Tribune JOS. University of Minnesota is going "full-on MacGyver" against COVID-19. Star Tribune. https://www.startribune.com/university-of-minnesota-is-going-full-on-macgyver-against-covid-19/569000032/. Accessed 8 May 2021.
9. adangol. COVID-19 Ventilator. Medical School - University of Minnesota. Published March 24, 2020. https://med.umn.edu/covid19Ventilator. Accessed 8 May 2021
10. Are portable ventilators the future? - The Boston Globe. https://www.bostonglobe.com/2020/06/01/metro/are-portable-ventilators-future/. Accessed 8 May 2021
11. Piracha SA, Gupta S, Jadeja R, Anwer W. Ventilation apparatus Published online November 7, 2019. https://patents.google.com/patent/US20190336713A1/en?assignee=Umbulizer&oq=Umbulizer. Accessed 8 May 2021.
12. Umbulizer: A reliable, portable, and low cost ventilator. Umbulizer. https://www.umbulizer.com. Accessed 8 May 2021.
13. PVA's PREVENT Receives FDA Approval Allowing a Safer, Affordable Emergency Ventilator Available Now. http://smt.iconnect007.com/index.php/article/122586/pvas-prevent-receives-fda-approval-allowing-a-safer-affordable-emergency-ventilator-available-now/122589/?skin=smt. Accessed 8 May 2021.
14. Class 2 Device Recall PVA, PREVENT. https://www.accessdata.fda.gov/scripts/cdrh/cfdocs/cfres/res.cfm?id=182621. Accessed 8 May 2021.
15. Newlab. *Spiro Wave Product Video*.; 2020. https://vimeo.com/408227658. Accessed 8 May 2021.
16. Virgin Orbit Designs New Mass-Producible Ventilator for COVID-19 Patients. Virgin Orbit. Published March 30, 2020. https://virginorbit.com/the-latest/virgin-orbit-uci-and-ut-austin-design-new-mass-producible-ventilator-for-covid-19-patients/. Accessed 8 May 2021.
17. Virgin Orbit Ventilators Granted Emergency Use Authorization, First Deliveries Expected to Begin Soon. Virgin Orbit. Published April 23, 2020. https://virginorbit.com/the-latest/virgin-orbit-ventilators-granted-emergency-use-authorization-first-deliveries-expected-soon/. Accessed 8 May 2021.
18. P&G retirees invent low-cost ventilator for COVID-19 patients. WCPO. Published May 1, 2020. https://www.wcpo.com/money/local-business-news/p-g-retirees-invent-low-cost-ventilator-for-covid-19-patients. Accessed 8 May 2021.
19. Venti-now | Cincinnati OH. Venti-Now. https://www.venti-now.org. Accessed 8 May 2021.

20. Fitbit Flow US Manual.pdf. https://help.fitbit.com/manuals/manual_fev_en_US.pdf. Accessed 8 May 2021.
21. How a Small Team of Researchers, Designers, and Engineers at Fitbit Created an Emergency Ventilator to Help Save Lives. Fitbit Blog. Published June 3, 2020. https://blog.fitbit.com/fitbit-flow/. Accessed 8 May 2021.
22. AustinP51+M3+Overview+Guide+−+Version+1.3.0.pdf.   https://static1.squarespace.com/static/5e98c9682cd3e40ef8be49a1/t/5ebab4cca375f52b541e8cdd/1589294292947/AustinP51+M3+Overview+Guide+-+Version+1.3.0.pdf. Accessed 8 May 2021.
23. About. Austin P51. https://www.p51ventilators.com/about. Accessed 8 May 2021.
24. How Are Brands Actually Making a Difference in the Age of COVID-19? Lemonade Blog. Published May 14, 2020. https://www.lemonade.com/blog/covid-brands-charity/. Accessed 9 May 2021.
25. Rice ventilator receives emergency FDA approval. George R. Brown School of Engineering | Rice University. https://engineering.rice.edu/news-events/rice-ventilator-receives-emergency-fda-approval. Accessed 8 May 2021.
26. LifeMech. https://lifemech.org/. Accessed 9 May 2021.
27. LifeMech · Machines Saving Lives, organized by Saurabh Gupta. gofundme.com. https://www.gofundme.com/f/efj4dc-lifemech-machines-saving-lives. Accessed 9 May 2021.

Part IV
Regulatory Factors and Device Testing

Chapter 17
Innovation and Regulation: The FDA's Response to the COVID-19 Pandemic

Rachel Fenberg, Emma McKinney, and Peter Kahn

Timeline of Initial SARS-CoV-2 Response

The World Health Organization first identified the SARS-CoV-2 virus in Wuhan, People's Republic of China, on December 31, 2019 [1]. Throughout the beginning of 2020, the SARS-CoV-2 virus spread throughout China as cases in Wuhan—the center of the outbreak—continued to spike.

By January 21, 2020, the United States reported its first confirmed case of coronavirus disease 2019 (COVID-19) [1]. On January 31, 2020, the United States Food and Drug Administration (FDA) declared a public health emergency under Section 319 of the Public Health Service Act [2]. Though this step was vital to provide protection against COVID-19-associated liability, it did not allow the FDA to issue Emergency Use Authorizations (EUA) [2]. On February 4, 2020, the United States had a total of 11 confirmed cases of COVID-19. On this date, the Secretary of the Department of Health and Human Services foresaw a significant threat to public health, and enacted Section 564 of the Federal Food, Drug, and Cosmetic Act (FD&C Act). With this in place, the FDA was able to issue EUAs [3].

Implementation of the Emergency Use Authorization

The general purpose of an EUA is to allow for rapid FDA authorization of devices, technologies, and other market products that could aid in the response to the COVID-19 pandemic. With a novel, deadly virus came the need for novel

R. Fenberg · E. McKinney
Albert Einstein College of Medicine, New York City, NY, USA
e-mail: Rachel.fenberg@einsteinmed.org; emma.mckinney@yale.edu

P. Kahn (✉)
Yale School of Medicine, Section of Pulmonary, Critical Care, and Sleep Medicine, New Haven, CT, USA
e-mail: peter.kahn@yale.edu

© The Author(s), under exclusive license to Springer Nature Switzerland AG 2022
A. A. Hakimi et al. (eds.), *Mechanical Ventilation Amid the COVID-19 Pandemic*,
https://doi.org/10.1007/978-3-030-87978-5_17

technology to match, and the umbrella EUAs issued by the FDA allowed entire categories of devices to be eligible for rapid authorization. Initially, there was a dire need for diagnostics, as cases of COVID-19 could not be definitively identified and tracked on a large scale. The first umbrella EUA authorized by the FDA addressed this concern and on February 4, 2020, an EUA for in vitro diagnostics for the detection and/or diagnosis of COVID-19 was issued [4].

Additionally, lack of personal protective equipment (PPE) for physicians and other healthcare workers became a growing crisis. Healthcare workers lacked essential gear such as gloves, gowns, and N95 respirators [5]. Recognizing this crisis, the FDA issued an umbrella EUA on March 2, 2020, for personal respiratory protective devices [4].

As the SARS-CoV-2 virus continued to spread, the challenges facing the medical field grew in tandem. The surge in COVID-19 cases caused great consternation regarding the inadequate number of ventilators to handle the flood of COVID-19 cases [6]. There was recognition by the FDA that novel devices could aid in the treatment of COVID-19 and therefore the FDA issued its final umbrella EUA on March 24, 2020, allowing for the authorization of emergency use of other medical devices, including alternative products to be used as medical devices [4].

The implementation of the umbrella EUAs was instrumental in the United States' response to the SARS-CoV-2 virus. A typical FDA application process for a medical device must provide evidence that the device is safe, effective, and potentially equivalent to another similar and legally marketed device. This process, from early product design to final FDA approval, can take anywhere from months to years [7].

The EUA process rapidly accelerated this cycle to match the urgency of the COVID-19 pandemic. While the FDA continued to require evidence regarding device safety and efficacy for *authorization*, it did not require the level of evidence necessary for full-fledged FDA *approval*. From the inventor's point of view, the EUA is critical as it allows for the rapid sale and deployment of novel technology with a significantly reduced market barrier to entry during a crisis. However, the EUA is only effective while the emergency declaration is in place. The EUA can be revoked or changed at any time, and the FDA regularly conducts reviews to determine which devices are still eligible. If the FDA decides to remove a device from the EUA category, the device can no longer be sold or used in an authorized manner [8].

Ventilator and Ventilator Accessory EUAs

One of the most important EUA categories developed was for ventilators and ventilator accessories. This EUA served two main purposes: it allowed for the rapid deployment of both novel devices and previously authorized devices in settings other than those for which they were initially approved. The FDA Appendix B lists authorized ventilators, ventilator tubing connectors, and ventilator accessories which were authorized in the umbrella EUA relating to the COVID-19 pandemic [9].

Ventilators

The ventilation devices authorized under the EUA could be further categorized as emergency resuscitators and ventilators. The category of ventilators includes critical care ventilators, emergency ventilators, continuous ventilators (non BiPAP/CPAP type), anesthesia ventilators, noncontinuous ventilators (non-BiPAP/CPAP type), and BiPAP/CPAP devices (Fig. 17.1). The EUA was largely a success, but there were authorized devices about which clinicians expressed concern regarding safety and efficacy [10].

Ventilators played a critical role during the pandemic for treatment of the most severe COVID-19 cases. Early on, there was concern that ventilators would have to be rationed; however, ventilator rationing was obviated due to the expanded supply in authorized devices under the umbrella EUA.

Ventilator Tubing Connectors

A novel category of devices, which allow for the splitting of ventilators, were authorized for use during the pandemic with a total of 13 devices authorized at one time (Fig. 17.2). The goal of these devices was to allow all patients access to a critical care-level ventilator. These devices could be further categorized into those that allowed for individual patient settings versus those that could not. There are also variations in these devices in the maximum number of patients that can be on one ventilator using one splitting device. None of these devices held prior FDA approval or were in use prior to the pandemic.

As the pandemic recedes any devices originally authorized under EUAs are now being removed from the Appendix B list, meaning that they are no longer FDA authorized for use. Challenges regarding ventilator-splitting devices include the need for paralysis and sedation, the lack of individual alarms, and the increased complexity of clinical decision-making. Certain ventilator-splitting devices also require the need to balance differences in respiratory mechanics of the co-vented patients, further compounding the difficulties of ventilator splitting. As a result of these challenges, and although there have been no adverse patient events due to the use of devices in this category, the FDA has recommended that these devices no longer be used in clinical practice [11] and has removed 9 of the 13 authorized ventilator-splitting devices [9]

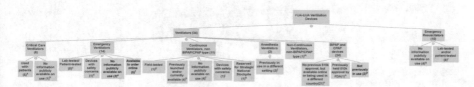

Fig. 17.1 Summary of ventilation devices

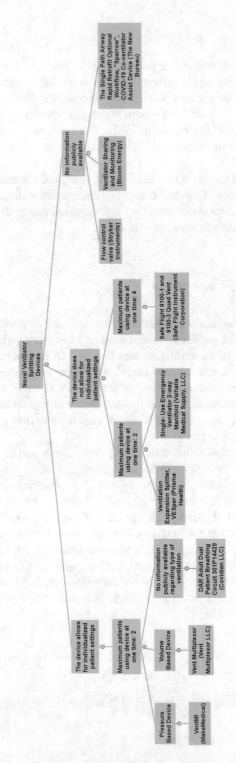

Fig. 17.2 Summary of novel ventilator-splitting devices

Challenges Associated with the FDA's Emergency Use Authorization

Availability of Information to Clinicians

While the design of devices was rapid, getting newly authorized devices into clinical use often posed a challenge. From the clinician's perspective, it was difficult to find the time to learn about new products available for use during an unprecedented pandemic. As a result, clinicians lacked the time and ability to investigate which devices were available and to learn how to properly deploy them. In addition, there was no simple method for inventors to get information to clinicians about these newly developed and authorized devices, with the FDA's Appendix B as the only consistent database of information. Despite this list being regularly updated, Appendix B did not contain sufficient information on how to best evaluate or deploy the devices on the list, limiting its utility. Further, there was no mutually effective way for inventors and clinicians to be in continuous contact, stunting inventors' efforts to share their developments with the proper people and help them deploy new treatments.

Lack of Data on Patient Use

While the FDA's Appendix B is a very valuable resource, it has many limitations. One of the most significant limitations of Appendix B is that it lacks any follow-up on device usage after approval or standard information that might be available for 510 k or de novo-approved products. It was therefore difficult for clinicians to know which devices had been safely used in patient setting.

Future Directions

The Future of the FDA Umbrella EUA

The FDA umbrella EUA has arguably been a very successful program. It has clearly demonstrated the FDA's ability to weigh risks and benefits and make decisions that are clinically safe yet accelerate the approval and deployment of new medical devices. Additionally, the direct interaction between the FDA and sponsors fosters an environment more conducive to rapid innovation.

Moving forward, the EUA can continue to serve an integral role in preparing for the next pandemic. Instead of reacting rapidly after a pandemic has already started to spread, having an existing EUA in place can encourage clinicians and inventors to prepare for future threats. With an EUA enacted, inventors are incentivized to create devices and get them authorized, even if they are only intended to be used at times when resources are scarce or during pandemic standards of care. This gives inventors the ability to continue creating devices that would mitigate the fear, uncertainty, and lack of preparedness that were seen in the early weeks of the COVID-19 pandemic.

The Response to Future Pandemics

The FDA's response to the SARS-CoV-2 pandemic helped strengthen the United States' hold on a virus that threatened to completely overwhelm the country and its medical system. Moving forward, it is critical that there be a better and more centralized database/usage record of these devices, so that both inventors and clinicians know which devices have had prior usage in which settings. Emphasizing the role of the EUA can strengthen our country's disaster response to future pandemics and can foster an innovative landscape for inventors.

Conflicts of Interest Dr. Kahn reports equity in Vent Multiplexor LLC and it is listed on the provisional patent for the Vent Multiplexor device.

Funding Information No funding was obtained.

References

1. Listings of WHO's response to COVID-19. World Health Organization; 2020, June 29. https://www.who.int/news/item/29-06-2020-covidtimeline
2. Emergency Use Authorization. FDA; 2021, March 24. https://www.fda.gov/emergency-preparedness-and-response/mcm-legal-regulatory-and-policy-framework/emergency-use-authorization
3. February 4 coronavirus news. CNN World; 2020, February 4. https://www.cnn.com/asia/live-news/coronavirus-outbreak-02-04-20/index.html
4. *Coronavirus* 2019 (COVID-19) Emergency Use Authorizations for Medical Devices. FDA; 2020, August 3. https://www.fda.gov/medical-devices/emergency-use-authorizations-medical-devices/coronavirus-disease-2019-covid-19-emergency-use-authorizations-medical-devices
5. Cohen J, Rodgers Y. Contributing factors to personal protective equipment shortages during the COVID-19 pandemic. Prev Med. 2020;141:106263. https://doi.org/10.1016/j.ypmed.2020.106263.
6. Neighmond P.. As The Pandemic Spreads, Will There Be Enough Ventilators? NPR; 2020, March 14. https://www.npr.org/sections/health-shots/2020/03/14/815675678/as-the-pandemic-spreads-will-there-be-enough-ventilators
7. Miller E.. FDA Approval Process. Drugwatch; 2021, March 15. https://www.drugwatch.com/fda/approval-process/
8. Understanding the Regulatory Terminology of Potential Preventions and Treatments for COVID-19. FDA; 2020, October 22. https://www.fda.gov/consumers/consumer-updates/understanding-regulatory-terminology-potential-preventions-and-treatments-covid-19
9. VentilatorsandVentilatorAccessoriesEUAs.FDA;2021,March22.https://www.fda.gov/medical-devices/coronavirus-disease-2019-covid-19-emergency-use-authorizations-medical-devices/ventilators-and-ventilator-accessories-euas
10. British doctors warn some Chinese Ventilators could kill if used in hospitals. NBC News; 2020, April 30. https://www.nbcnews.com/news/world/british-doctors-warn-chinese-ventilators-could-kill-if-used-hospitals-n1194046
11. Using Ventilator Splitters During the COVID-19 Pandemic- Letter to Health Care Providers. FDA; 2021, February 9. https://www.fda.gov/medical-devices/letters-health-care-providers/using-ventilator-splitters-during-covid-19-pandemic-letter-health-care-providers

Chapter 18
Regulatory Considerations for Bridge Ventilators

Elisa Maldonado-Holmertz and Sarah Mayes

Medical Devices 101

What Is a Medical Device?

The Food and Drug Administration (FDA) uses a somewhat antonymic definition to describe medical devices, primarily stating what is not a medical device (Section 201(h) of the FD&C Act). In plain speak, the FDA carves away (1) products not intended to diagnose, cure, or treat disease and (2) products that function via chemical actions or metabolic activity as *not* medical devices, leaving a vast landscape of products that are defined as medical devices. To further define devices within this broad scope, the FDA segregates devices into classes, based on risk. The higher the risk, the higher the class.

Mechanical ventilators may fall into almost any class of medical device (Fig. 18.1). Classification of a medical device is directly dependent on the indication for use and claims of the product. The indication for use statement is usually the inverse of the problem statement. Increasing complex clinical problems lead to higher risk indication for use statements which require more extensive testing to demonstrate safe and effective use of the device. In short, defining the problem statement(s) or clinical need(s) is the first and most critical step in medical device design.

A mechanical ventilator designed to simply actuate a bag-valve mask, with no claim to monitor or to support patient breathing, may be considered Class I. A

E. Maldonado-Holmertz (✉)
Obelix Biotech Solutions, Austin, TX, USA
e-mail: elisamh@obelixconsult.com

S. Mayes
Alafair Biosciences, Austin, TX, USA
e-mail: smayes@alafairbiosciences.com

© The Author(s), under exclusive license to Springer Nature Switzerland AG 2022
A. A. Hakimi et al. (eds.), *Mechanical Ventilation Amid the COVID-19 Pandemic*,
https://doi.org/10.1007/978-3-030-87978-5_18

Increasing:
- Claims
- Features
- Risks
- Testing

Product parts	Indication or claims	Class I	Class II	Class II Special Controls	Class III
Hammer-like appendage and means to hold an AMBU bag stationary	To squeeze an AMBU bag repeatedly (i.e. not intended to support patient breathing; a hammer hitting a bag; generic use)	✓			
AMBU bag and valve	To provide emergency respiratory support by means of a face mask or a tube inserted into a patient's airway (BTM Product Code)		✓		
Pneumatic logic and control system, breathing circuit, oscillator, airway pressure monitoring system, electronic controls and alarms, power supply	To mechanically control or assist patient breathing by delivering a predetermined percentage of oxygen in the breathing gas (MNT Product Code)			✓	
Pneumatic logic and control system, breathing circuit, oscillator (high frequency for pediatric population), airway pressure monitoring system, electronic controls and alarms, power supply	For ventilatory support and treatment of respiratory failure and barotrauma in neonates; for use in ventilatory support and treatment of selected pediatric patients who, in the opinion of their physician, are failing on conventional ventilation (LSZ Product Code)				✓

Fig. 18.1 Mechanical ventilator device classification and indication for use

mechanical ventilator designed to provide respiratory support via bag-valve mask actuation and monitoring of patient breathing may be considered a Class II device. A mechanical ventilator designed to mechanically control patient breathing may be considered a Class II or Class III device depending on the specific indication for use; for example, the narrowed indication for use to target pediatric patients increases the risk, and therefore device classification.

Medical Device Design

A mechanical ventilator is not intended to cure or heal the condition of the patient. While the intended use of the mechanical ventilator is slightly less lofty, to help a patient breathe, there are many ways the device can meet the goal of helping a patient breathe, with varying complexities. That complexity is directly related to the clinical need or clinical problem that the ventilator seeks to address. The indication of use of a mechanical ventilator may be consistent between two designs, but one design may include additional features intended to meet additional user needs. For instance, if the ventilator is intended to be used in senior living facilities, ease of transport and ease of turning knobs or pushing buttons may be a top priority. Alternatively, if the ventilator is intended for at-home use where child safety precaution is required, ensuring that knobs or buttons are less accessible or are difficult to manipulate (i.e., additional alarms) may be the top priority. Irrespective of the indication for use, each feature intended to meet a user need requires testing to ensure that the user need is met. The process of ensuring that design meets user needs is called design controls (Fig. 18.2).

Design controls begins with the clinical problem, or user needs. While the user needs guide the design and inform the design team *what* to build, the design controls process guides *how* to build the right design. The end user may be a physician, surgeon, surgical technician, nurse, or patient. User needs, also often referred to as customer requirements, may be identified in a myriad of ways. Surveys, labs, clinical case experience, market needs, and regulations may all guide identification of user needs. Counterintuitively, the user may not actually be able to articulate the exact needs/requirements they want. The job of the design team is to ask, listen, elicit, and interpret information into requirements. New or altered customer requirements may be identified throughout the design controls process. As described above,

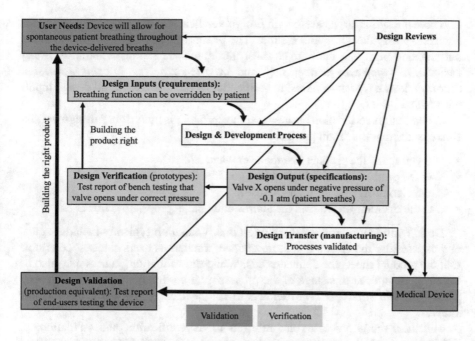

Fig. 18.2 Design controls waterfall process with mechanical ventilator example (Ref: https://www.fda.gov/media/116573/download)

the user needs may be related to the patient population (pediatric or geriatric) or location of device use (operating room, hospital room, patient home). The user needs of a mechanical ventilator depend on the target patient population and where, when, and how the ventilator will be used. User needs are translated into **design inputs**, or more plainly, the detailed requirements of what the device does.

Once customer requirements are identified and agreed upon, design inputs, such as specifications, are identified and prototypes are fabricated. Specifications include device size, flow rate, respiratory rate, controls, number of alarms, color, weight, etc. A customer requirement for pediatric-safe controls may lead to a design input of a protective cover over the device controls.

The completed list of design inputs describes the device requirements. **Design outputs** are the written drawings, specifications, and labeling that define the design inputs. The circuit diagram and power supply of the ventilator design are the design outputs that define the design input requiring 120 V of power

Once design inputs and outputs are defined and documented, prototypes are tested to determine the device functions as desired:

- Does the device perform as specified?
- Are the required flow rates and respiratory rates achieved?
- Do the displays show the proper information that maps to the actual device outputs?

These questions are answered via **design verification**: the process of testing the device to verify design inputs are met. The process of identifying inputs, creating outputs, and verifying the outputs meet the inputs via testing is iterative. *Many cycles of this loop may be necessary, and are often expected, to achieve a design that functions as intended.* Design verification is complete when all design inputs are verified.

While design verification ensures that the "product is built right," **design validation** ensures that the "right product is built."

• Did you make the product that the user wanted?
• Will the product address the problem you identified at the beginning?
• Are the controls safe for pediatric use?
• Can the operator understand the alarms and take appropriate action?

Design validation answers these questions. Validation typically includes actual end user testing the device in a representative manner as users can best determine that the product meets the defined needs. While the validation process may also be iterative, changes at this stage of the process may be timely and costly. *Correctly identifying the customer requirements at the beginning sets the project up for success.*

Together, these processes are referred to as verification and validation, or V&V. After V&V is complete the design process is finished. FDA regulatory clearance may be achieved at this stage. Obtaining FDA clearance may feel like the peak of the mountain, and while a celebration is often deserved, the final step of transferring the design to production remains. **Design transfer**, or transferring the design to production, can sometimes be the longest step. Repeatable scale-up manufacturing may present unforeseen challenges when compared to building prototypes in a lab setting and requires validation of processes not verified via inspection:

• Does each ventilator built meet the specifications that were verified and validated in the previous phase?

Design transfer ensures that the product sold meets the customer requirements defined, verified, and validated in earlier phases. Design or process changes implemented following design transfer must be evaluated and potentially verified or validated.

This description of design controls follows a traditional/ideal chronological process. While real-world projects may vary in execution, the fundamental principles remain. Sometimes the most difficult inflection point to identify is when to exit the design controls loop. No medical device is perfect. The design controls process is intended to be one of continuous improvement; therefore, it may be easy to be lured into new design changes developed in parallel to design transfer. While not inherently wrong, these types of late-stage changes can put significant constraints on product launch. Strong project management, effective design team, and well-documented goals including timeline and budget are imperative to product launch success.

Herding Cats (Creating the Team)

Mindset

The most important attribute of a design team is mindset. The successful mindset often referred to in medical device communities is a "quality mindset" and is in reference to a commonsense approach with great appreciation for the design process. The FDA takes a commonsense approach, so it behooves design teams to do the same. The design process of medical devices is truly a constantly flowing waterfall with previous decisions directly impacting and leading to future results. The selections made early in the process have profound impacts on the final product design. Keeping both the entire process and also each of its components in mind when designing a device ensures a system-level approach that greatly improves efficiency. At each step a quality mindset ponders what the next step is, how that step is connected to the current step, and if everything continues to make sense. In short, consider how the present task will affect the next and how that task meets the overall goals. And above all else, when in doubt, write things down. No matter how early you are in the design process, a quality mindset relentlessly documents decisions, tasks, and procedures.

Beyond the quality mindset, enthusiasm, focus, endurance, strong work ethic, initiative, and dedication are required for success. Medical device design is not for the faint-hearted; long hours and frequent failed results are bedfellows of design teams.

Team of Many Hats (Exploit Previous Experience)

Design teams often move together, as one, through the design process with individuals acting both independently and dependently. While individuals have a specific role, this role often requires wearing many "hats" to ensure that information is effectively transferred from one step to the next. Any single role impacts multiple others and yet is required to perform tasks independently to continue moving the ball forward.

As a team is worth exponentially more than the sum of its individuals, design teams are especially capable of high productivity and efficiency. Lean heavily on the previous experience that each team member brings to the table. For instance, a previous background in manufacturing inherently provides an understanding that small design changes significantly impact manufacturability. Include that expertise in design change decisions and documentation of those decisions to ensure that optimal decisions are made and that easily understood documentation is provided to the intended audience (i.e., design transfer to manufacturing).

Bells and Whistles: How Much Is Too Much for an Emergency Use Authorization (EUA) Device?

First and foremost, even in a pandemic or emergency-use situation, **market need and demand** must be considered. A mechanical ventilator with a simple design that is quickly approved by FDA is key. Typically, first approved FDA EUA medical devices have the lowest regulatory thresholds placed upon them. Additionally, a ventilator with a simple design would more quickly meet the needs of a pandemic market, whether due to high volume of ill patients creating healthcare pressures and/or supply-chain issues.

The smaller the existing gap between the pandemic market need and the developer's perception of the need translated into ventilator design, the clearer the ventilator **design inputs** will be. The **concept generation stage** is where the ventilator design takes shape and value-added features are created. Great importance is for designers to know the needs of the users, to define the ideal user experience (healthcare professional and patient), and to create a design that addresses those needs in the best and most streamlined way. Note that the usual time allocated for this stage will be sharply limited; therefore, expert users need to be part of the design team, and a strong project manager needs to be allocated to keep the design team on track, focused, and in adherence to the pressing demands of the pandemic.

Once agreement is reached on the ventilator **design concept**, then the actual **development** can proceed at full speed. At this point, stakeholders should commit to the development plan with as little design deviation as possible to deliver the agreed product on schedule and without design creep! The project then becomes the sole focus for the key members of the team responsible for driving the project forward to completion. Ideally, all team members should be solely focused on the ventilator development. If problems with development do occur, a dedicated sub-team committed to action plan development to resolve difficulties will keep the project moving forward. A dedicated and motivated team can achieve orders of magnitude more than a distracted or part-time team.

Once the design and development are in place, a ventilator **prototype** is the next step. A good approach to this stage is to conduct a risk management assessment. Identify the ways in which the ventilator might function incorrectly or fail. Patient care and safety are at the forefront of the process.

Awareness of FDA **regulatory requirements** and the EUA approval process is invaluable for a successful route to commercialization. Read FDA guidances, letters, and announcements carefully and fulfill their requests. Do not provide the FDA with partially completed documentation as a "gut check" or use communication with the FDA to answer questions they have already addressed in their published literature. The FDA is reasonable and understands the pandemic or emergency needs. For instance, in a non-pandemic, non-EUA environment the FDA requires adherence to critical care ventilators standard ISO 80601-2-121, or life-supporting homecare ventilators standard ISO 80601-2-722, or ventilatory support equipment standard ISO 80601-2-803. However, during an EUA scenario ventilator developers and manufacturers are not required to provide the same level of performance; the FDA makes requirements clear in published guidances. For instance, the FDA developed the **Emergency Use Resuscitator System Design Guidance** modeled on the MIT E-vent ventilator project where a machine was designed to replace a trained clinician by mechanically squeezing a user-powered resuscitator (e.g., "Ambu bag") as specified in ISO 10651-45. Ultimately, the need for speed allowed MIT to establish themselves as the new "gold standard" emergency resuscitator. The FDA then created an **Emergency Use Resuscitator System template** for EUA submissions. The requirements of this template are based on the following:

- AAMI CR503:2020 Emergency Use Resuscitator Systems Design Guidance

    - Note: AAMI CR503:2020 incorporates the requirements of IEC 60601-1 and parts of ISO 10651-4, and ISO 80601-2-80.

- AAMI CR504:2020 End User Disclosures for Emergency Use Resuscitator Systems
- Risk Management Process (IEC 60601-1 clause 4.2)
- Emergency Use Resuscitator Performance (IEC 60601-1 clause 4.3)
- Enclosure Protection rating per (IEC 60529)

    Should such an EUA environment occur again, refer to the **FDA Emergency Use Authorization webpage** [1] which includes:

- About Emergency Use Authorizations (EUAs)
- PREP Act
- EUA Guidance
- COVID-19 EUAs

    - Vaccines
    - Drug and Biological Therapeutic Products
    - Information About COVID-19 EUAs for Medical Devices

- Other Current EUAs
- Related Links

Performance and Analytical Testing to Support Bells and Whistles

Once a mechanical ventilator prototype is created, **design outputs** can be tested, including **design verification,** ensuring that design output conforms to design input. A **traceability matrix** links design inputs (requirements), design specifications, and testing requirements. The traceability matrix also provides a means of tying together identified hazards (risks) with the implementation and testing of mitigations.

During the **design validation** phase, the ventilator must meet the user needs and must satisfy its intended use. In design validation, the final design ventilator undergoes testing to confirm that performance is as stated. Testing should be conducted in a simulation of its expected environment.

Validation of a locked-down ventilator design for a non-EUA FDA submission is modified when compared to an EUA FDA submission. Standard, non-EUA **medical device testing** can include:

- Bench/analytical/in vitro testing (performance and use life)
- Animal testing (typically not required by FDA for an EUA submission)
- Usability testing (typically not required by FDA for an EUA submission)
- Clinical validation (typically not required by FDA for an EUA submission)
- Biocompatibility (typically not required by FDA for an EUA submission, though airway components must be biocompatible)
- Sterilization validation (if applicable)
- Electrical safety IEC 60601-1-1
- Electromagnetic conductivity (EMC) IEC 60601-1-2
- Software validation

This V shape (Fig. 18.3) demonstrates the relationships between each phase of the software development life cycle and its associated phase of testing, i.e., any phase in the development process begins only if the previous phase is complete.

Special emphasis should be placed on **Software Documentation Requirements** (Table 18.1), as software engineers may be unfamiliar with FDA requirements for software (SW) documentation.

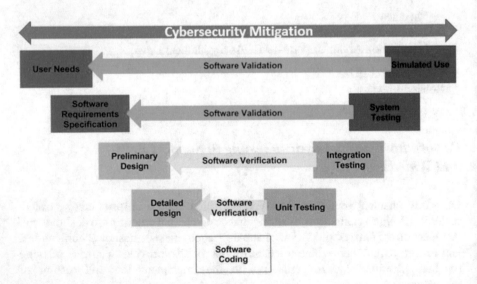

Fig. 18.3 The V-model: Validation and verification software development process (Ref: https://en.wikipedia.org/wiki/V-Model_(software_development))

Table 18.1 Software documentation

FDA SW Guidance Document: Major LOC	Documentation description
1. Level of concern (LOC)	Recommend that you clearly state which one of the three levels of concern is appropriate for your device and include documentation of the rationale for your decision.
2. Software description	A summary overview of the features and software operating environment.
3. Device hazard analysis	Tabular description of identified hardware and software hazards, including severity assessment and mitigations.
4. Software requirements specification (SRS)	The SRS documents the requirements for the software. This typically includes functional, performance, interface, design, developmental, and other requirements for the software. In effect, this document describes what the software device is supposed to do.
5. Architecture design chart	This document typically contains state diagrams and flowchart depicting the functional units and software modules, including relationships to hardware and to data flows such as networking.
6. Software design specification (SDS)	The SDS describes the implementation of the requirements for the software device. In terms of the relationship between the SRS and the SDS, the SRS describes what the software device will do and the SDS describes how the requirements in the SRS are implemented.
7. Traceability analysis	A traceability analysis links together your product design requirements, design specifications, identified hazards and mitigations, and verification and validation testing.
8. Software development environment description	Summary of the software life cycle development plan. Annotated list of the control documents generated during the software development process. Include the configuration management and maintenance plan documents.
9. Verification and validation documentation protocol and report	Description of V&V activities at the unit, integration, and system level. Unit-, integration-, and system-level test protocols, including pass/fail criteria, test report, summary, and tests results.
10. Revision-level history	Revision history log, including release version number and date.
11. Unresolved anomalies (bugs or defects)	List of remaining software anomalies, annotated with an explanation of the impact on safety or effectiveness, including operator usage and human factors.
12. Cybersecurity mitigation plan	Identification of cybersecurity risks and mitigations for each identified risk.

Ref: FDA Guidance for the Content of Premarket Submissions for Software Contained in Medical Devices (https://www.fda.gov/regulatory-information/search-fda-guidance-documents/guidance-content-premarket-submissions-software-contained-medical-devices)

Design transfer is to translate the ventilator design into production, distribution, and installation specifications. The **Design History File** (DHF) is a formal compilation of documents that contains all design documents from the earliest stages. Nearly every design control element contains activity that needs to be documented. All documentation is added to the DHF. By the time the product is shipped, an organized account of how that product came into existence must be documented for successful transfer to a medical device manufacturer.

Conclusion

A focused, commonsense, stepwise approach to the design and transfer of a mechanical ventilator will ensure delivery of the right device in a timely manner. Identifying user needs is the first step; user needs drive the design process and regulatory classification. Mechanical ventilators may fall into almost any class of medical device depending on the indication for use and product claims or features. Mechanical ventilator design, development, verification, validation, regulatory clearance/approval, and transfer to manufacturing can be arduous, depending on the product features selected. The more features the device has, the more complex problem the device seeks to solve, and thus the higher risk and classification. Each feature requires testing to satisfy regulatory requirements, which can be expensive and time consuming. Having a focused, experienced team with a quality mindset is critical to meeting the demands of the device design control process during a pandemic, or emergency, when speed is key. In short, limited bells and whistles create speed to FDA EUA approval. The first applicants have the lowest regulatory threshold as FDA demands and requirements increase over time. Moving quickly does not mean skipping steps required to ensure that the device meets its intended use; moving quickly means selecting a design that is the simplest path to meet the few, carefully selected user needs. A simple design that can more easily be validated will ensure that the device life cycle will fit within the timeframe of the pandemic.

Tips

- Select a team of experienced individuals with a quality mindset.
- Select a team lead who can make critical decisions, including a FDA regulatory expert.
- Document early and often; use templates from team member or community experience.
- Communicate frequently with team members for current and future steps (i.e., including manufacturing in all design meetings).
- Ensure that the lab that conducts testing is accredited.
- Ensure that testing equipment is calibrated.
- Ensure that documentation is created by the software engineers.
- Lock down the design early; do not change the design during transfer.
- Performance testing is to be conducted on the lockdown-designed mechanical ventilator.
- Assume that the FDA is reasonable; read all published literature carefully and adhere to their guidance.

Conflicts of Interest The authors declare no relevant conflicts of interest.

Funding Information None

Reference

1. FDAEmergencyUseAuthorization.https://www.fda.gov/emergency-preparedness-and-response/mcm-legal-regulatory-and-policy-framework/emergency-use-authorization.

Chapter 19
Human Factors Considerations in the User Interface Design of Bridge Ventilator Devices

Edmond W. Israelski

Introduction

Human factors engineering (HFE) is a discipline that originated in the World War II that includes in the design process data about human capabilities and limitations, as well as methods from the behavioral sciences, to make products and processes safe, effective, efficient, and usable for expected users, uses, and use environments.

The flowchart in Fig. 19.1 summarizes the core human factors processes that are systematic and scientific methods to design products. At its core HFE is a user-centered design, where from the beginning of the design, user considerations are included throughout. The HFE process starts with a very thorough understanding of the context of use, i.e., the task flows, the user profiles, and the use environment, through the use of contextual inquiry investigations informed by direct observations and interviews. The process proceeds to estimation of risk of harm to users and on to the setting of usability goals. A hallmark of HFE is to iterate the design using prototypes and simulations that are evaluated for usability using analytical techniques such as expert reviews and cognitive walk-throughs, together with empirical task-based usability testing. Usability testing is done one-on-one, where users' performance is observed and subjective opinions are recorded as they perform essential and critical tasks that are derived through contextual inquiry and use-related risk analysis. Formative usability testing is done early as the design is iterated and then at the end as a summative test to validate the design to satisfy that usability goals can be met and that risk is reduced as much as practicable.

Throughout the HFE process user task performance data is obtained to iterate both the design and the formal risk analysis, as appropriate. The result is a product that is effective, efficient, safe, and satisfying for its users, since they have been

E. W. Israelski (✉)
Human Factors Engineering AbbVie, Lake Barrington, IL, USA

© The Author(s), under exclusive license to Springer Nature Switzerland AG 2022
A. A. Hakimi et al. (eds.), *Mechanical Ventilation Amid the COVID-19 Pandemic*,
https://doi.org/10.1007/978-3-030-87978-5_19

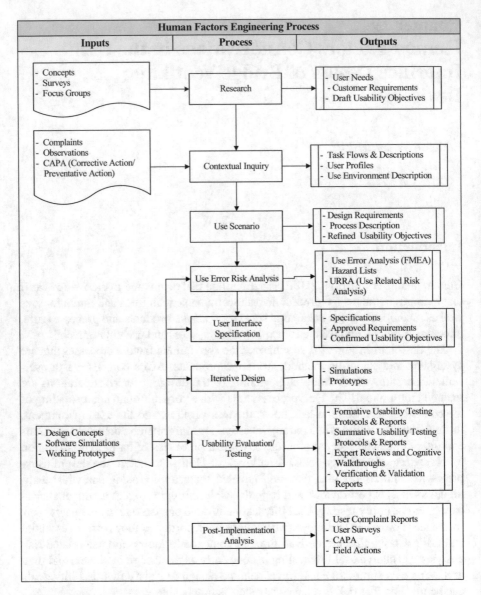

Fig. 19.1 Human factors engineering process

included during the entire design process. The following overview of human factors is adapted from Israelski [1].

The Human Factors Engineering (HFE) Process

In this chapter we describe the basic human factors process. Figure 19.1 is a flowchart depiction of the core methods of HFE in medical product development. This is the expected process for regulatory approvals such as 510 K clearance and premarket approval (PMA) in the USA and Conformité Europëenne (CE) mark in the European Union. In the remainder of the chapter, we give more detail on each of the core HFE methods. We point out that only a subset of these methods is expected in order to get a temporary Emergency Use Authorization (EUA) in a national emergency such as the COVID-19 pandemic that started in early 2020.

To better define the HFE process the following definitions are offered, followed by more detailed descriptions of how the core HFE methods are implemented (Table 19.1).

HFE Process Details

Design controls are required by the US Code of Federal Regulations for medical devices 21CFR820.30 [4] and also apply to combination products (drug-device combinations) for the device part of the product. Our focus in this book is on devices that are described as "bridge ventilators." Figure 19.2 depicts how the various HFE process steps fit into the overall flow of design controls.

Table 19.2 outlines the core process steps for HFE with a brief description of each step along with some commonly used names of HFE deliverables. Various development organizations use different names for these deliverables, but most are common terms.

To further explain some of the considerations in carrying out these HFE steps for combination products the following points should be considered.

User Research

The up-front user research is often done collaboratively with commercial or marketing research since both disciplines need to understand customer needs. The HFE focus is on the behavioral needs to support the ultimate design of the user's interaction with the product. The market research needs focus on user preferences, market segments, feature sets, and other important product considerations, such as willingness to pay.

Table 19.1 Definitions

Term	Definition
Contextual inquiry*	The process of observing and working with users in their normal environment to better understand the tasks they do and their workflow.
Critical task	A task where a use error can lead to serious harm (death or serious injury) including compromised medical care (e.g., extra therapy or hospitalization).
Effectiveness**	The accuracy and completeness with which users achieve specified goals.
Efficiency**	The resources expended in relation to the accuracy and completeness with which users achieve goals. Efficiency in the context of usability is related to "productivity" rather than to its meaning in the context of software efficiency.
Formative usability testing	Usability testing that is performed early with simulations or the earliest working prototypes and explores if usability goals are attainable, but does not have strict acceptance criteria.
Prototyping and iterative design	The design process that involves the rapid turnaround of user interface prototypes or simulations that are usability tested and improved in an iterative cycle until usability objectives are attainable.
Summative usability testing	Usability testing that is performed in the late stages of design. These tests include verification and validation. It is a recommended best practice to have formal acceptance criteria (e.g., qualitative for safety-related critical tasks and quantitative for usability objectives for human performance and satisfaction ratings that are non-safety related).
Task analysis*	Task analysis is a family of systematic methods that produce detailed descriptions of the sequential and simultaneous manual and intellectual activities of personnel who are operating, maintaining, or controlling devices or systems.
Usability inspection methods	Inspection methods involve analytical reviews and systematic walk-throughs of user interactions with simulated or working user interface designs looking to uncover usability problems.
Usability objectives*	Usability objectives (goals) are a desired quality of a user device interaction that may be expressed in written form, stipulating a particular usability attribute (e.g., task speed, first-time use completion rate, learning time) and performance criteria (e.g., number of seconds).
Usability testing*	Procedure for determining whether the usability goals have been achieved. Usability tests can be performed in a laboratory setting, in a simulated environment, or in the actual environment of intended use by observation and recording of users' task-based performance behavior.
User	A person who interacts with the device.
User interface	The hardware and software aspects of a device that can be seen (or heard or otherwise perceived) by the user, and the commands and mechanisms the user employs to control its operation and input data. It includes labeling, instructions for use, and training materials.
User group**	Subset of intended users who are differentiated from other intended users by factors such as age, culture, or expertise that are likely to influence usability (also described as a distinct user group).
Use environment*	The actual conditions and settings in which users interact with the device or system.

(continued)

Table 19.1 (continued)

Term	Definition
Use error	Use error is characterized by a repetitive pattern of failure that indicates that a failure mode is likely to occur with use and thus has a reasonable possibility of predictability of occurrence. Use error can be proactively identified through the use of techniques such as usability testing and hazard analysis. Use error can be addressed and minimized by the device designer. This term is preferred over user error because it is neutral about the cause of failure whereas user error implies that the user is to blame. Use error says that a use-related failure occurred and the root cause needs to be determined.
Use error risk analysis	Analysis focused on the use error component of fault and hazard analysis for medical devices.
User error	User error is characterized by an isolated pattern of failure that indicates a failure mode that is due to fundamental errors by humans and has no reasonable possibility of reliably being predicted. User error is not readily preventable and cannot easily be addressed by the device designer. As noted this term has been deprecated in favor of the neutral term use error, which does not imply blame on the user.
User profiles*	Summary of the mental, physical, and demographic traits of the end-user population as well as any special characteristics such as occupational skills and job requirements that may have a bearing on design decisions. (User groups are composed of groups with distinguishing user profiles based on use-related risk and task analysis.)

Note: Definitions marked by * are adapted from ANSI/AAMI HE-75:2009 Human factors engineering—Design of medical devices [2]. Those with ** are adapted from ISO 9241-210:2010, Ergonomics of human-system interaction [3]

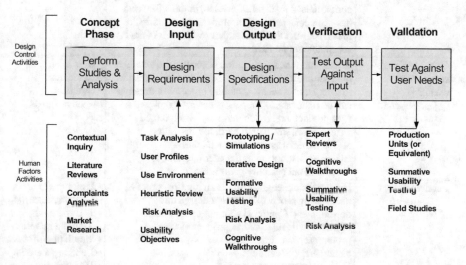

Fig. 19.2 Human factors engineering as part of the design control process

Table 19.2 HFE process steps and deliverables (with EUA considerations)

Process steps	Description (emergency use application EUA considerations)	Deliverables
System/product definition	A description of the specific system or product that is being evaluated for the purposes of the project. This would include a statement about intended use, which is also called a use specification EUA—Necessary to perform	• Documentation of User needs and customer requirements • Draft usability objectives/goals • Research data report • Product requirements document • Use specification
Contextual inquiry	An identification of the user profiles, use environment, and task(s) that will be performed with the system or product EUA—Necessary, even if done at a high level	• Contextual inquiry report • Customer Requirements
Use error risk analysis	The purpose of use error risk analysis is to identify use errors that may be potentially committed by users and determine the likelihood, hazard severity, and level of risk. In this step, risk control and mitigation strategies are established, and typically use error failure mode effect analysis (FMEA), use-related risk analysis (URRA), and hazard lists are generated EUA—Necessary. At a minimum to identify critical tasks that could lead to high-severity harm including compromised medical care. Also, to describe what has been done in the submitted design to mitigate these risks and a statement that residual risks are acceptable for an EUA	• Hazard lists • Use error risk analysis (FMEA) • Use-related risk analysis (URRA)
User interface specification/ usability objectives/goals	A user interface specification describes the details of the user interface including the critical tasks related to safety and efficacy. Usability objectives, or goals, can be established. They are a desired quality of a user-product interaction that may be expressed in written form, stipulating particular usability attributes and user performance criteria EUA—A description of the user interface is necessary, but usability goals are not	• User interface specification • Usability objectives/goals report
Iterative design	Human factors engineering is an iterative process used during process or product design and development. Continual changes should be implemented and tested as product models, prototypes, and simulations are subjected to usability testing and evaluation EUA—Not necessary, but if performed, it will be done with minimal iterations	• Prototype(s) – Labeling material – IFU material – Training material • Simulation(s) – Labeling material – IFU material – Training material

(continued)

Table 19.2 (continued)

Process steps	Description (emergency use application EUA considerations)	Deliverables
Usability testing	Usability testing is the formal method of systematically observing and recording representative users performing real tasks with real or simulated product. Evaluation of product usability will vary based on the stage of the design. Usability evaluation should be quantitative wherever possible • Formative usability testing (early stages—exploratory) • Summative usability testing (late stages) EUA—Not necessary, but can be beneficial in uncovering additional critical tasks that could lead to serious harm	• Formative test protocol • Screener document and consent form • Moderator guides • Formative test report • Verification report
Summative usability testing/ validation	Summative/validation usability testing takes place once the product or system has reached the final stages of development Following formative testing, summative usability testing is conducted for the purpose of determining how much progress has been made as a result of the formative testing and iterative designs and to validate the success of mitigations made to the user interface EUA—Not necessary, but would be required for eventual 510 K clearance or PMA approval	• Summative test protocol • Summative test report – Revised labeling, IFU, and training materials • HFE/UE summary report – Summarizes all HF work for the product
Post-implementation analysis	Post-implementation analysis provides a feedback loop for modification and improvement to products EUA—Necessary to collect and inform the future comprehensive work for 510 K clearance or PMA approval	• Post-market surveillance human factors report • Complaints report • Adverse events report • Recalls • Field actions

Contextual Inquiry

Contextual inquiry is all about understanding the context of use and is a foundational part of the design inputs for a device. It is related to ethnographic research and as noted earlier it is best gathered through observation and interviewing users.

The product user interface design should incorporate and match the following:

- The task flow for its relevant users
- User profiles for distinct user groups
- The characteristics of the use environment

The output of the contextual inquiry analysis answers three essential questions:

- What do users expect to do with the medical product?
- Who are the prime users of the product?
- In what environment or context of use will the product be used?

  This method may include the following techniques for data gathering:

- Observations (ethnographic studies)
- Follow-around studies (shadowing)
- Behavioral checklists
- Time slice sampling studies (of what they are doing at the time)
- Time and motion studies
- Usability studies repurposed to understand task behaviors via "talk aloud" protocols or pairs performing cooperative tasks
- Interviews and surveys (1:1 and focus groups)
- Review of job and task documentation
- Review of training materials, job descriptions, job evaluations
- User-kept diaries, activity logs, card sorting analyses

Use Scenarios

The use scenarios describe the user tasks or operational sequence of events. These use scenarios are most useful when they incorporate the findings of the contextual inquiry including the user profiles and the use environment descriptions. These scenarios are next examined through the lens of risk analysis.

Risk Analysis

The recommended steps for conducting a use error risk analysis in the form of a failure modes and effects analysis (FMEA) or its derivative (use-related usability analysis, URRA) are the same as traditional product design FMEA's with one addition, namely the need to initially perform a thorough task analysis. It is recommended that a group performing the use error risk analysis consist of individuals from the product development team with detailed knowledge of the product's user interface design. This group should include a human factors specialist as well as individuals from quality assurance, regulatory, product development, medical affairs, and marketing. For more detail on conducting risk analysis see Israelski and Muto [5, 6] and ANSI/AAMI HE-75:2009 section 5 [2]. Table 19.3 lists the basic steps to be taken during a use error risk analysis, which are also outlined in the ISO standard for Risk Management for Medical Devices in ISO 14971:2019 [8].

Table 19.3 Use error risk analysis steps

	Step	Description
1	Conduct a task analysis	A task analysis is usually done as part of the up-front user analysis (contextual inquiry) before or early in product development. The output of this analysis is a listing of all the tasks and related subtasks or steps that a user can perform with the product. These may be documented in a convenient form such as a task flow diagram or a table depicting each major step a user must take in interacting with a product. A draft user instructions manual is one source of user task descriptions since it is usually developed from a task analysis. Task analysis is a part of contextual inquiry.
2	Estimate the likelihood of use error (fault) occurrence for each major task leading to harm	This may also be called a frequency or probability estimate. Qualitative estimates can sometimes be informed by data where possible, such as use error frequencies observed in usability tests or from customer complaint data. The level of task detail should be sufficient to estimate what observable use errors might occur and does not need to be very microscopic in detail. All conceivable use errors that might be committed by a user or patient should be analyzed. • This analysis would include those use (human) errors that are common human mistakes, lapses of memory and attention that have previously been called user errors. Such errors would be in addition to use errors that may be design induced and that often follow predictable trends or patterns. • Each distinct user group should be considered in estimating the likelihood of use errors. • Each distinct use environment should be considered as different environments may lead to error-causing conditions. • Additional sources of use error data may come from predicate devices that have a history of use errors that may be catalogued in customer complaint data or medical device reports (MDRs). Another possible source of data would include computer modeling of human performance, but this is rarely done. • Consideration should be given to abnormal use. Technically, abnormal use including sabotage or reckless use is beyond a manufacturer's control, but if the likelihood is estimated to be high, then it is recommended to at least examine the possibility of risk mitigation, if technically feasible. • It should be strongly emphasized that the US FDA is highly skeptical of manufacturers' estimates of likelihood or probability of use error, because it is very difficult to make estimates of the rate at which humans make errors. Therefore, the FDA does not look favorably upon use-related FMEAs. They require a use-related risk analysis (URRA) to be used instead. A URRA example from the FDA [7] is shown in Table 19.4. It focuses solely on the severity of harm and ignores likelihood or probability of use error to determine critical tasks. • Estimations of likelihood of use error are often done by manufacturers to cover all user tasks (not just critical tasks) and because their quality systems are often based on traditional risk management methods which almost always include FMEAs. So, for FDA submission requirements manufacturers would extract a URRA from a use FMEA. The other use of likelihood estimates is to support statements of reducing as much as practicable residual risk which is usually done by reducing the likelihood of use error.

(continued)

Table 19.3 (continued)

	Step	Description
3	Estimate the severity of the resulting harms to users	The hazards and hazardous situations would be identified in a hazard analysis, which is the systematic method for enumerating all of the foreseeable hazardous situations and possible resulting harms that a product could inflict on a user. This step requires estimation of the severity of the resulting harm, which can range from catastrophic (death or serious injury) and moderate (serious reversible injury) to minor (a non-harmful nuisance). The FDA goes a further and includes compromised medical care as part of the estimation of harm severity. Compromised medical care can include additional therapy or medication or additional time in a clinic or hospital.
4	Determine the risk level or risk index	Determine the risk level or risk index by combining the estimates of use error leading to harm likelihood and hazard severity. This is usually done with a table or risk chart or if semiquantitative ratings are used, e.g., 1–5, then the risk index is the product of likelihood of harm times harm severity.
5	Determine what tasks need to be addressed	If the use error risk analysis is done early in the design cycle, as recommended, then the moderate and higher risk levels would indicate which tasks need to be addressed by mitigations or controls in the design of the user interface. If design mitigations are not feasible, then attention needs to be directed to product labeling, instructions for use, and possibly user training. It should be emphasized that the most effective design mitigations for use error will come from user interface design rather than relying on labeling, instructions, or training, especially for moderate and higher risk levels. Regulators expect to see a direct connection between risk analysis and critical tasks selected for summative usability testing.
6	Estimate the effectiveness of mitigation	The effectiveness of possible hazard mitigations can be estimated. If the analysis is done early in the design cycle, then the effectiveness of potential design controls will be more difficult to estimate with confidence, although formative usability testing and usability inspection methods will aid in these estimates. If done later in the development cycle, then data from summative validation usability testing will provide better estimates for the effectiveness of the mitigations.
7	Examine residual risk and determine the risk acceptability level	The US FDA has specific expectations for safety-critical tasks. The FDA ideal goal is for no task failures for safety-critical or hazard-related tasks, e.g., tasks that if not completed successfully could cause serious harm to patients or users, such as death or serious injury. All task failures are inevitably observed in a summative validation usability test, particularly for safety-critical tasks that should be rationalized for further risk control and mitigation to demonstrate the impact on product safety and effectiveness.

Usability Objectives or Goals

A usability objective is a measurable design objective for how usable a system needs to be. Usability objectives are a quality assurance metric that can serve as quantitative acceptance criteria for usability testing. The FDA does not accept the use of quantitative usability objectives for safety-critical tasks; for example, 95% of patients will be able to successfully inject themselves. The FDA expects qualitative criteria for judging if a submitted product is safe and effective for all users, uses, and

Table 19.4 Use-related risk analysis example format [7]

Task No.	Use task description	Description of potential use errors	Potential hazards/ harm and severity	Critical task (yes/no)	Risk mitigation measure for each use error	Evaluation method in HF validation study
4	Press green button and hold for 10 s	Button is held for less than 10 s	Full dose is not injected; leads to patient death	Yes	Redesign product to eliminate the need to hold for 10 s	Evaluated in HF validation study in use scenario 1: administration of drug, task 4

use environments. They require that each and every observed use error for safety-critical tasks that can lead to serious harm be investigated for root cause and whether further design mitigation is practicable. One optional use of quantitative usability objectives is to set the criteria for acceptance of business or marketing product claims or attributes, such as learning time or calibration time. Setting and confirming usability objectives should be done as early as possible in the product design process.

Usability objectives should be expressed as quantitative metrics of product usability. They may be specified as target human performance measures and optionally with additional user satisfaction measures. Usability objective measures may include:

- Human performance goals

  - Task completion time
  - Task success rate
  - Learning time
  - Accuracy (e.g., acceptable error rates)
  - Efficiency (e.g., number of missteps as a percentage of total steps)
  - Significant errors
  - Number of references to documentation
  - Number of calls to a helpline
  - Physical measures (e.g., fatigue, force, heart rate)

- User satisfaction (e.g., secondary and supplemental to observable human performance goals)

  - Rating scales (e.g., Likert, agree or disagree, or comparative ratings)
  - Rankings
  - Semantic differential (e.g., pick satisfaction rating between two opposite adjectives)

Iterative Design

One of the hallmarks of HFE is iterative design. The user-centered design process enables usability and safety improvements as the design is first tested using simulations and early prototypes. Modifications and improvements are made to the design as it is incremented in an iterative process. Rarely are first designs likely to meet usability goals and only through iteration can the design become progressively better and more usable and ultimately safer and more effective. The primary method to achieve improvement is through empirically based usability evaluations including usability testing.

Usability Evaluation and Testing

Usability evaluations are a critical component of the human factors engineering process. Usability testing is a key method of evaluation and typically involves representative users performing the core tasks, especially the most safety critical, under simulated use environment conditions. User's performance is observed and objectively measured without any method bias. Typically, a moderator directs the test participant (who is a representative user) to perform a use scenario under simulated but representative environmental conditions. This behavior is observed and recorded by the testing team. There are two main types of usability testing:

- Formative Testing
  Formative usability testing is performed early with simulations and first working prototypes and explores if usability goals are attainable but does not have strict acceptance criteria. These evaluations take place while the product design is being "formed." The purpose is to uncover design faults and correct them. Small sample size on the order of 5–8 per distinct user group is usually sufficient. Larger sample sizes might be required if a comparison between competing design alternatives is required, in which case a properly statistically powered test design is warranted.
- Summative Testing
  Summative or validation usability testing is performed in the final stage of design.

As noted previously, the US FDA has made summative testing a qualitative process without consideration of rigorous statistical acceptance criteria for safety-critical tasks; for example, 95% of patients will measure blood glucose level on their first attempt. But the FDA does want a measurable metric of critical task success; for example, the dose accuracy after patient preparation is within 10%. Sample sizes are larger for summative tests on the order of 15–25 per distinct user group or profile. The US FDA has recommended 15 as the minimum sample size per distinct user group. For non-safety-critical tasks (e.g., for business and marketing product claims) summative testing can be conducted using hypothesis testing using inferential statistics. Fortunately, statistically based usability testing using classical hypothesis testing also requires sample sizes in the range of 15–25 per distinct user group. For more detail on usability testing methodologies including sample size considerations see Israelski [9] and ANSI/AAMI HE-75:2009 section 9 [2].

Post-implementation Analysis

Regulators around the world expect a rigorous post-market surveillance process to record, trend, and monitor usability problems when the product is in use. In spite of the systematic and scientifically based user-centered design methods of human factors engineering not all usability problems will be caught during design. Only after use by large numbers of users in actual field conditions can some very-low-probability problems surface. That is why a carefully designed and executed post-market system is needed. Typical systems capture the following data post-product launch:

- Product complaints
- Product returns
- Field correction actions
- Medical device reports or other reports on adverse events
- Corrective action and preventative action (CAPA)
- Product recalls

Regulator Expectations

For medical devices and combination products the US FDA has been requesting manufacturers to submit the work on HFE in a specific summary report format. It is a logical and effective way to summarize HFE efforts and the author believes that it is a good model to follow for any medical product submission, regardless of the location in the world. As noted, the process is tailorable and the amount of HFE effort and resources is based on the product risk and complexity. There is also an international standard on HFE and usability engineering that is similar in its HFE requirements from IEC (2020) [10]. The FDA-recommended format, which was published in the HF guidance from CDRH, FDA (2016) [11], has eight sections, and they are presented in Table 19.5:

Table 19.5 US FDA Recommended Outline of HFE/UE Report

Sec.	Contents
1	Conclusion The <device> has been found to be safe and effective for the intended users, uses, and use environments • Brief summary of HFE/UE processes and results that support this conclusion • Discussion of residual use-related risk
2	Descriptions of intended device users, uses, use environments, and training • Intended user population(s) and meaningful differences in capabilities between multiple user populations that could affect user interactions with the device • Intended use and operational contexts of use • Use environments and conditions that could affect user interactions with the device • Training intended for users
3	Description of device user interface • Graphical representation of device and its user interface • Description of device user interface • Device labeling • Overview of operational sequence of device and expected user interactions with user interface
4	Summary of known use problems • Known use problems with previous models of the subject device • Known use problems with similar devices, predicate devices, or devices with similar user interface elements • Design modifications implemented in response to post-market use error problems
5	Analysis of hazards and risks associated with the use of the device • Potential use errors • Potential harm and severity of harm that could result from each use error • Risk management measures implemented to eliminate or reduce the risk • Evidence of effectiveness of each risk management measure
6	Summary of preliminary analyses and evaluations • Evaluation methods used • Key results and design modifications implemented in response • Key findings that informed the human factors validation test protocol
7	Description and categorization of critical tasks • Process used to identify critical tasks • List and descriptions of critical tasks • Categorization of critical tasks by severity of potential harm • Descriptions of use scenarios that include critical tasks

(continued)

Table 19.5 (continued)

Sec.	Contents
8	Details of human factors validation testing • Rationale for test type selected (i.e., simulated use, actual use, or clinical study) • Test environment and conditions of use • Number and type of test participants • Training provided to test participants and how it corresponded to real-world training levels • Critical tasks and use scenarios included in testing • Definition of successful performance of each test task • Description of data to be collected and methods for documenting observations and interview responses • Test results: Observations of task performance and occurrences of use errors, close calls, and use problems • Test results: Feedback from interviews with test participants regarding device use, critical tasks, use errors, and problems (as applicable) • Description and analysis of all use errors and difficulties that could cause harm, root causes of the problems, and implications for additional risk elimination or reduction

Conflicts of Interest   The author has no relevant conflicts of interest to disclose.

Funding   This work was not funded.

References

1. Israelski EW. Design inputs and associated design verification and validation —a primer on applying human factors engineering. In: Hornbeck L, editor. Combination products implementation of cGMP requirements. River Grove, IL: PDA- DHI Publishing; 2013.
2. ANSI/AAMI HE75: 2009, Human factors engineering—Design of medical devices.
3. ISO 9241-210:2010, Ergonomics of human-system interaction — Part 210: Human-centred design for interactive systems.
4. 21CFR820.30 PART 820 -- US Code of Federal Regulations Quality System Regulation Subpart C - Design Controls Sec. 820.30.
5. Israelski EW, Muto WH. Human factors risk management in medical devices. In: Carayon P, editor. Handbook of human factors and ergonomics in healthcare and patient safety. Mahwah, NJ: Lawrence Erlbaum; 2012.
6. Israelski EW, Muto WH. Risk management: human factors methods. Washington, DC: Human Factors and Ergonomics Society; 2021 in press
7. FDA. Contents of a complete submission for threshold analyses and human factors submissions to drug and biologic applications. Washington, DC: DRAFT, US Food and Drug Administration; 2018.
8. ISO 14971:2019 Medical devices — Application of risk management to medical devices.
9. Israelski EW. Testing and evaluation. In: Gardner-Bonneau D, Weinger MB, Wiklund M, editors. Handbook of human factors in medical device design. New York, NY: CRC Press; 2010.
10. IEC 62366-1:2015/AMD 1:2020 Medical devices – Part 1: Application of usability engineering to medical devices.
11. FDA. Applying human factors and usability engineering to medical devices. Washington, DC: US Food and Drug Administration; 2016.

Chapter 20
Preclinical Animal Testing of Emergency Resuscitator Breathing Devices

Aleksandra B. Gruslova, Nitesh Katta, Andrew G. Cabe, Scott F. Jenney, Jonathan W. Valvano, Tim B. Phillips, Austin B. McElroy, Van N. Truskett, Nishi Viswanathan, Marc D. Feldman, Thomas E. Milner, Richard Wettstein, and Stephen Derdak

Introduction

In vivo studies are important not only for evaluating prototype ventilation devices, but also to provide initial data for evaluation of device safety. Perfomance of a prototype ventilation device can be assessed in animal models so that investigators can better understand the interface with a live biological system.

This guide has been prepared to assist in designing ventilator device testing protocols and strategies and reporting the results of animal studies. Simulation experiments should test a device's ability to oxygenate and remove carbon dioxide in an animal model. Additionally, such experiments should assess the safety and efficacy of the test device in both a healthy lung (control) model and a diseased lung model (acute respiratory distress syndrome or ARDS). Simulating lung disease during

A. B. Gruslova · A. G. Cabe · M. D. Feldman
Department of Medicine, UT Health San Antonio, San Antonio, TX, USA
e-mail: gruslova@uthscsa.edu; cabe@uthscsa.edu; feldmanm@uthscsa.edu

N. Katta · T. E. Milner (✉)
Beckman Laser Institute, The University of California Irvine, Irvine, CA, USA

UT Austin Cockrell School of Engineering, The University of Texas, Austin, TX, USA
e-mail: nkatta@uci.edu; milnert@uci.edu

S. F. Jenney · J. W. Valvano · T. B. Phillips · A. B. McElroy · V. N. Truskett
UT Austin Cockrell School of Engineering, The University of Texas, Austin, TX, USA
e-mail: jonathan.valvano@engr.utexas.edu; vtruskett@utexas.edu

N. Viswanathan
Dell Medical School, UT Austin, Austin, TX, USA
e-mail: nishi.viswanathan@utexas.edu

R. Wettstein · S. Derdak
School of Health Professions, UT Health San Antonio, San Antonio, TX, USA
e-mail: wettstein@utscsa.edu

© The Author(s), under exclusive license to Springer Nature Switzerland AG 2022
A. A. Hakimi et al. (eds.), *Mechanical Ventilation Amid the COVID-19 Pandemic*,
https://doi.org/10.1007/978-3-030-87978-5_20

ventilator testing is especially important when considering test ventilation devices aimed to assist patients with viral infections like COVID-19. COVID-19 has been shown to cause an ARDS-like syndrome in some patients if the viral infection enters the lower respiratory tract [1].

Pigs are an excellent model for testing ventilator devices given their size and pulmonary gas exchange physiology similarity to that of humans and because there is an accepted research model of COVID-like ARDS for this species [2]. In addition, their relatively large size permits the use and testing of ventilator equipment that are designed for use in human adults.

Objectives of the Study

In this section, two primary objectives are outlined to test a ventilation device:

1. Assess ventilator test device function and efficacy to maintain appropriate O_2 and CO_2 blood concentrations in vivo during mechanical ventilation of healthy and injured lungs.
2. Assess test device function and animal model response to alteration of device parameters to include inspiratory time (T_I), positive end-expiratory pressure (PEEP), tidal volume (V_T), respiratory rate (RR), and oxygen flow rate.

Materials

A careful balance exists between generating valid scientific data to demonstrate reasonable safety and performance of the tested device while maintaining the ethical principles of reduction/replacement. The goal of ventilator testing using animal models should be to maximize data collection while using the minimum number of test animals. Any study design must be approved by the corresponding Institutional Animal Care and Use Committee (IACUC). Additionally, the care and handling of all animals should be in accordance with the National Institutes of Health guidelines for ethical animal research [3].

The following simulation methodology involved porcine animals weighing 50–80 kg. The procedure requires a suitable operating room including an operating table, ventilator, and equipment for invasive hemodynamic monitoring.

Animal Monitoring

The animal is placed on a surgical table with a heated pad in a prone position. For safe monitoring of the animal, the following instruments and protocols allow for conducting safe ventilation device testing:

- Invasive blood pressure monitoring lines for measurements of systemic blood pressure.

- Instrument with physiologic monitors: body temperature, electrocardiogram, end-tidal CO_2 ($P_{ET}CO_2$), in-line circuit FiO_2 analyzer, and pulse oximetry. Body temperature needs to be maintained in the normal range (38–39 °C).
- Peripheral arterial catheter to collect blood samples for arterial blood gas (ABG) analysis. After animal stabilization and collection of the baseline blood, ABG monitoring is required to assess the device's effectiveness in maintaining adequate oxygenation and ventilation.
- Syringes for drawing blood samples and a blood gas analyzer.

Anesthesia and Drugs

- Intramuscular injection syringe containing premedication to relax the animal before inducing anesthesia:

  – Premedication: telazol (4–8 mg/kg, IM), xylazine (1–2.2 mg/kg, IM)
- Anesthesia induction: propofol, 0.2–0.4 mg/kg/min
- Cuffed endotracheal tube of appropriate size for intubation
- Veterinary ventilator
- Isotonic saline (5–10 ml/kg, IV, continuous during the procedure)
- Neuromuscular paralysis: vecuronium, IV, 0.1–0.2 mg/kg
- Euthanasia: Euthasol, IV, 100 mg/kg

Study Protocol

Objective of the following method is to determine if the testing device can be used to maintain appropriate oxygenation (O_2) and carbon dioxide (CO_2) clearance under normal and injured lung (ARDS) conditions in a porcine model during general anesthesia. Both conditions occur sequentially in the same animal during a single event under anesthesia. The use of each animal for collection of multiple types of data (control and injured lung) also reduces the total number of animals required to complete the study.

Animals should be acclimatized in an appropriate facility close to the operating room and fasted overnight with free access to water. All equipment and monitoring systems should be prepared prior to inducing anesthesia.

Inducing and Maintaining Anesthesia

At a minimum the following protocol must be followed for inducing and maintaining anesthesia:

- Insert needle connected to a syringe containing premedication (telazol, 4–8 mg/kg) into the neck musculature and gently infuse. Wait until the animal dozes off.

- Insert a peripheral venous catheter into one of the ear veins and infuse drugs to induce anesthesia (propofol 0.2–0.4 mg/kg/min).
- Intubate the animal following visualization of vocal cords with a swine laryngoscope. Ensure proper position of endotracheal tube (ETT) by hand bagging and listening to breathing sounds with a stethoscope. Make sure that the ETT is fixed securely to the animal. Connect the ETT to a conventional veterinary ventilator with mainstream or sidestream end-tidal CO_2 monitor positioned at the circuit "Y".
- Adjust baseline conventional ventilator settings to achieve a tidal volume (V_T) of 6–8 ml/kg at a rate of 10–14 breaths per minute (BPM) with 21–50% oxygen (using a calibrated in-line FiO_2 analyzer) and a peak end-expiratory-pressure (PEEP) of 5 cm H_2O. Serial ABG analyses should be performed, ensuring pO_2 ≥12 kPa, 4.5 > pCO_2 > 6.5 kPa, and 7.35 > pH > 7.45.
- Maintain continuous anesthesia with 0.5–3% isoflurane in 100% O_2.
- Place the animal in supine position (dorsal recumbency) on a heated pad, fixed to the operating table. Body temperature must be kept between 38 °C and 39 °C.

Vascular Cutdown and Blood Pressure Catheter Placement

- Clip and clean the right or left medial thigh from gross dirt and debris.
- Make a 3–4 cm longitudinal skin incision lateral (left or right) to the femur. Use blunt and sharp dissection to expose and isolate the femoral artery.
- Place three vessel loops (silk ligatures) around the artery: two proximal and one distal to the catheter insertion site.
- Tie the distal loop and elevate the proximal loop to stop bleeding. Create a stab incision in the vessel and pass the blood pressure catheter (micromanometer) through the incision into the vessel. Advance the catheter until a clear blood pressure signal is obtained.
- Secure the catheter in place by tying the proximal ligatures. Close the skin using suture with the blood pressure catheter extending out through the incision site.

Healthy Lung Data Collection

- Place a catheter in a peripheral vessel for arterial blood samples. Collect the baseline arterial blood sample for immediate ABG analysis and synchronously record all data [fraction of inspired oxygen (FiO_2) analyzer, respirometer—tidal volume (V_T), respiratory rate, blood pressure, CO_2].
- Switch the animal to the test ventilator. This is done by connecting the test ventilator to the proximal end of the ETT via a 90° adapter plugged into the breath-

ing circuit (includes FiO_2 analyzer, respirometer, and mainstream or sidestream $ETCO_2$ analyzer).

- Data for all conditions is collected for physiological parameters including heart rate (HR), total respiratory rate (set ventilator rate plus spontaneous respiratory rate), oxygen saturation (SpO_2), end-tidal carbon dioxide ($P_{ET}CO_2$), mean arterial pressure (MAP), in-line FiO_2 analyzer, pH, partial pressure of carbon dioxide ($PaCO_2$), partial pressure of oxygen (PaO_2), SaO_2, and peak inspiratory pressure (PIP).
- Perform serial tests with various ventilation settings: tidal volume (V_T), respiratory rate (RR), and PEEP. Keep inspiratory time (T_I) and O_2 flow rate constant throughout the entire test.
- Confirm absence of ETT cuff leak and use an in-line flow meter or a manual Wright respirometer to measure delivered tidal volume, including tidal volume test and subsequent blood gas exchange measurement tests.

Tidal Volume Test

- Hypoventilation (V_T 200 mL, RR 10 BPM) to achieve $PaCO_2$ >60 mm Hg (use $P_{ET}CO_2$ to estimate when to do ABG).
- Set respiratory rate at 20 BPM, PEEP at 5 cm H_2O, T_I at 1 s, and oxygen flow rate at 5 L/min. Record FiO_2 with in-line FiO_2 analyzer. Measure animal response by decreasing V_T from 800 mL to 400 mL in 200 mL increments (i.e., 800 mL, 600 mL, 400 mL). Wait for 10 min after adjusting to the new setting before collecting data. Verify values on the testing device.
- Monitor physiological parameters of animal health to verify if the V_T in question can be supported.

Respiratory Rate Test (note: animal must be paralyzed during respiratory rate testing so that ventilator set rate = total respiratory rate):

- Hypoventilate (RR 10 BPM, V_T 200 mL) to achieve $PaCO_2$ >60 mm Hg (use $ETCO_2$ to estimate when to do ABG). ABG may be done when $P_{ET}CO_2$ and measured in-line FiO_2 have been stable for 5 min.
- Set V_T at 800 mL, PEEP at 5 cmH_2O, T_I at 1 s, and oxygen flow rate at 5 L/min. Measure the animal's physiological response at respiratory rates of 20, 30, and 40 BPM. Wait for 10 min after adjustment to each new setting and document the stability of $P_{ET}CO_2$ for 5 min before collecting physiological data. Verify values on the testing device.
- Monitor physiological parameters of animal health to verify if the respiratory rate in question can be supported.

Oxygen Flow Rate Test (note: animal must be paralyzed during O_2 flow rate and FiO_2 testing since spontaneous breathing will decrease delivered FiO_2 at any given O_2 flow rate):

- Set V_T at 800 mL, RR at 20 BPM, PEEP at 5 cmH$_2$O, and T_I at 1 s. Measure the animal's physiological response for oxygen flow rate at 5, 10, and 15 L/min. Record measured FiO$_2$ at each O$_2$ flow rate. Wait for 10 min after each adjustment before collecting physiological data. Verify values on the testing device.
- Monitor physiological parameters of animal health and confirm that FiO$_2$ >90% and SaO$_2$ >95% can be supported.

Acute Lung Injury by Saline Lavage (Porcine ARDS Lung Model)

To induce acute lung injury, surfactant deficiency may be induced by lung lavage with 30 mL/kg 37 °C normal saline. This technique induces a short-term injury with a PEEP-recruitable lung. Other methods of inducing more severe lung injury include smoke inhalation with thermal injury, oleic acid injection, and acid instillation, (ADD REFS) and may be considered depending on the application of the emergency resuscitator device being tested.

- Ensure that the animal is ventilated with an FiO$_2$ of 1.0 and set the PEEP to 2–4 cmH$_2$O for the lavage procedure. Disconnect the animal from the ventilator.
- Fill the lungs with warmed normal sterile saline (37 °C, 50 ml/kg body weight). For this, pre-fill a funnel and connect it to the ETT with a fitting elastic tube. Raise the funnel about 1 m above the animal and allow the saline to flow into the lungs as quickly as possible. The hydrostatic pressure will allocate the saline into all pulmonary sections.
- Stop filling when the MAP falls below 50 mm Hg.
- Lower the funnel manually to ground level, drain the lavage fluid passively, and reconnect the animal to the ventilator for oxygenation.
- Wait until the animal compensates (increase in MAP and SpO$_2$) and repeat the lavage as soon as possible. The time frame for successive lavages should not exceed 5 min.
- Take an ABG sample after the second or third lavage depending on the hemodynamic deterioration and compromise in SpO$_2$.
- Adjust the ventilator rate during the periods of lavage to maintain the arterial pH above 7.25. This will prevent hemodynamic decompensation.
- Start the experiment based on the surfactant washout model once the PaO$_2$ is persistently measured below 100 mmHg for at least 30 min.

Injured Lung Data Collection

- Collect baseline data at V_T of 400 mL, RR of 20 BPM, T_I of 1 s, oxygen flow rate of 5 L/min, and PEEP of 5 cmH$_2$O. Verify delivered FiO$_2$ with these values on the testing device.

ARDS Tidal Volume Test

- Hypoventilation/hypercapnia correction sequence (same sequence as normal lung hypoventilation (V_T 200 mL, RR 10 BPM, $PaCO_2$ >60 mm Hg)).
- Set RR at 20 BPM, PEEP at 5 cm H_2O, T_I at 1 s, and oxygen flow rate at 5 L/min. Confirm absence of spontaneous breathing. Measure the animal's physiological response by increasing V_T from 400 mL to 800 mL in 200 mL increments (400 mL, 600 mL, 800 mL). Wait for 10 min after adjusting to the new setting before collecting physiological data. Verify values on the testing device.
- Monitor physiological parameters of animal health to verify if the tidal volume can be supported. Desired $PaCO_2$ is <45 mm Hg.

Respiratory Rate Test

- Hypoventilation (RR 10 BPM, V_t 200 mL) to achieve $PaCO_2$ >60 mm Hg (use $ETCO_2$ to estimate when to do ABG).
- Set V_T at 400 mL, PEEP at 5 cmH_2O, T_I at 1 s, and oxygen flow rate at 5 L/min. Measure the animal's physiological response at RR of 20, 30, and 40 BPM. Wait for 10 min after adjusting to new settings before collecting physiological data. Verify values on the testing device.
- Monitor physiological parameters of animal health to verify if the RR can be supported. Desired $PaCO_2$ is <45 mm Hg.

ARDS PEEP Test

- Hypoxemia/PEEP recruitment sequence: Reduce O_2 flow rate from 15 L/min and PEEP from 10 (if needed) to obtain SpO_2 <85% mm Hg. Record FiO_2. Anticipate the need for IV fluids and pressors for hemodynamic support.
- Set V_T at 800 mL, RR at 20 BPM, T_I at 1 s, and oxygen flow rate at 5 L/min. Measure the animal's response by increasing PEEP of 5, 10, 15, and 20 cmH_2O. Wait for 10 min between each change in PEEP before collecting physiological data. Verify values on the testing device.
- Monitor physiological parameters of animal health to verify if PEEP can be supported. Target SpO_2 >95% (highest achievable). O_2 flow may be increased if SpO_2 is <95% at the highest PEEP. Record the highest FiO_2 achievable.

Euthanasia

Animals are euthanized (Euthasol, IV, 100 mg/kg) following completion of experiments (6–8 h) (Fig. 20.1).

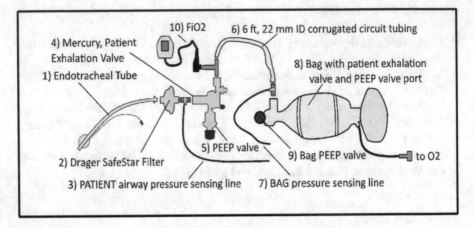

Fig. 20.1 Recommended breathing circuit for ventilator testing in a porcine model

Conflicts of Interest The authors declare no relevant conflicts of interest.

Funding Information UTHSCSA Clinical and Translational Science Award, Texas Innovation Center at the University of Texas at Austin

References

1. Jafari-Oori M, Ghasemifard F, Ebadi A, et al. Acute respiratory distress syndrome and COVID-19: a scoping review and meta-analysis. Adv Exp Med Biol. 2021;1321:211–28.
2. Russ M, Kronfeldt S, Boemke W, Busch T, Francis RCE, Pickerodt PA. Lavage-induced surfactant depletion in pig as a model of the acute respiratory distress syndrome (ARDS). J Vis Exp. 2016;(115):53610. https://doi.org/10.3791/53610.
3. Office of Science and Technology Policy, U.S. government principles for the utilization and care of vertebrate animals used in testing, research, and training. (Federal Register, May 20, 1985, Vol. 50, No. 97). https://olaw.nih.gov/policies-laws/gov-principles.htm.

Part V
Pandemic Innovations

Chapter 21
Multiplex Ventilation: Requirements and Feasibility of Ventilator Splitters

Pratyushya Yalamanchi, Peter Kahn, and Kyle VanKoevering

Introduction

Modern mechanical ventilators are complex devices that provide life-sustaining respiratory support. In keeping with the critical care adage to "fit the ventilator to the patient not the patient to the ventilator," each ventilator is traditionally adjusted to suit an individual patient's needs. While ventilators can provide lifesaving respiratory support, they significantly alter the respiratory physiology of the patient. Ventilators use positive pressure to drive airflow into a patient's lungs while relying on pulmonary recoil to allow exhalation as the pressure is reduced. Although the system's pressure is reduced to allow for exhalation, it is typically still maintained above atmospheric pressure to maintain alveolar recruitment, and is referred to as positive end-expiratory pressure (PEEP). Modern ventilators utilize two primary mechanisms to cycle each breath: volume-limited and pressure-limited ventilation [1–5]. In volume-limited ventilation, the volume of air delivered at each respiratory cycle (tidal volume) is defined by the user along with the flow dynamics. In pressure-limited ventilation, the target inspiratory and PEEP pressures are set by the user to define the ventilation, with the tidal volume dependent on lung compliance. A

P. Yalamanchi
Department of Otolaryngology-Head and Neck Surgery, University of Michigan, Ann Arbor, MI, USA
e-mail: ypratyus@med.umich.edu

P. Kahn
Department of Internal Medicine, Yale School of Medicine, Hartford, CT, USA
e-mail: peter.kahn@yale.edu

K. VanKoevering (✉)
Department of Otolaryngology-Head and Neck Surgery, Ohio State University, Columbus, OH, USA
e-mail: kyle.vankoevering@osumc.edu

© The Author(s), under exclusive license to Springer Nature Switzerland AG 2022
A. A. Hakimi et al. (eds.), *Mechanical Ventilation Amid the COVID-19 Pandemic*,
https://doi.org/10.1007/978-3-030-87978-5_21

number of parameters can be adjusted within each of these primary ventilation strategies, including respiratory rate, fraction of inspired oxygen, and various techniques to synchronize breathing with the patient's efforts.

The ability to customize ventilation to each patient's specific physiologic needs is critical. However, the worldwide COVID-19 pandemic has highlighted a global respiratory crisis where available ventilator supply may be insufficient to meet the demand of a large number of patients in respiratory failure. With the rising pandemic, vigorous manufacturing efforts were undertaken to create new ventilators. However, given the supply-chain constraints of this just-in-time ventilator production, there has been increasing interest in expanding ventilator capacity through "vent splitting" or multiple-patient ventilation, in which more than one individual is simultaneously provided respiratory support by a single ventilator [6–10]. Here we review the purpose of ventilator splitters, mechanics of split ventilation, design strategies, and advantages and limitations in implementation.

Purpose of Ventilatory Splitters

The purpose of ventilatory splitters is to expand respiratory support capacity. Ideally, vent splitting facilitates appropriate lung-protective ventilation of multiple patients with a single ventilator. The use of split ventilation is particularly attractive in resource-constrained environments, such as respiratory pandemics, disaster relief environments, and field hospital settings, to avoid rationing of limited ventilator capacity. A guiding principle of multiple-patient ventilation is that each patient should have no effect on the ventilation of other patients attached to the ventilator. Ideally, the ventilator-splitting system facilitates adaptation to a range of clinical scenarios including varying patient physiologies, procedural insults, coughing, disconnection, and movement.

Mechanisms of Split Ventilation

Simple Shared Ventilation Strategy

Initial descriptions of ventilator splitting utilized "simple" tube-splitting techniques to connect multiple circuits to the ventilator [1, 4]. Pressure-controlled and volume-controlled modes may be used to maintain control over each patient's pressures and volumes in an effort to facilitate lung-protective ventilation [4]. Traditional approaches often utilized a high PEEP and a low driving pressure or smaller tidal volumes to achieve lung protection. To prevent patients from triggering breaths and affecting other patients, the ventilator trigger is locked out. Patients often require deep sedation to prevent coughing and ensure that they are passive on the ventilator.

An end-tidal CO_2 monitor placed in-line with each patient's endotracheal tube can be used to monitor ventilator efficacy. Permissive hypercapnia must often be expected and managed as tidal volumes may be challenging to track for each patient. It is important to consider that y-site connections and tubing length increase dead space and ultimately affect carbon dioxide clearance [5].

While this approach expands ventilator capacity, there are several challenges with this simplified approach as each circuit is identical. This requires that patients sharing a ventilator be "matched" in ventilator requirements, with comparable lung volumes and compliance (degree of lung injury), with similar ventilation settings [1]. These systems have previously been thought to result in cross-contamination, provide limited control over ventilatory parameters, and have historically been challenging to implement in practice, particularly in resource-constrained environments. However, in the absence of alternative ventilation support strategies, clinicians were forced to ration, triage, or split ventilation. A formalized protocol for ventilator sharing was developed by Bietler et al. at New York-Presbyterian Hospital as the pandemic was peaking [10]. This protocol requires appropriate patient selection, optimization of ventilatory settings, deep sedation and/or paralysis, and tolerating hypercapnia. Specifically, patients with similar compliance and comparable PEEP and FiO_2 requirements are chosen. Of note, while patients are ideally of similar size or BMI, larger patients typically have greater compliance and will therefore receive larger breaths so patient size difference could be tolerated [3].

While this protocol attempted to manage some of the challenges of simple split ventilation, there were several potential safety concerns raised. In fact, the use of "simple" ventilator splitting was specifically condemned in a joint statement from the Anesthesia Patient Safety Foundation (ASPF), Society of Critical Care Medicine (SCCM), American Association for Respiratory Care (AARC), American Society of Anesthesiologists (ASA), American Association of Critical-Care Nurses (AACN), and American College of Chest Physicians (CHEST) due to these concerns [2].

Ultimately, this simple shared ventilation strategy offers less control of precise tidal volumes and relies on acceptance of permissive hypercapnia with a risk of suboptimal ventilation for each individual patient. This joint statement highlighted several major concerns that revolved around the lack of individualization in split ventilation which ultimately led to ventilator-associated lung injury in patients as well as concerns for cross-contamination. These concerns, in turn, drove innovative new strategies for individualized ventilator splitting, to allow each patient to receive unique, tailored ventilation in both volume- and pressure-limited ventilation modes, from a single source of mechanical ventilation.

Individualized Shared Ventilation Strategies

Due to requirements for matched patient settings, risks of cross-contamination, harmful interference between patients, and inability to individualize ventilator support parameters, split ventilation has had limited adoption in resource-limited settings. Recent research has sought to circumvent these limitations. However, novel strategies and devices have helped circumvent several key limitations in shared ventilation by effectively creating completely separate circuits on the same ventilator. These strategies allow for customization of each circuit, which can be adapted to best accommodate each patient's needs. One-way valves separate each circuit to allow differential ventilation to each patient. These solutions have been developed for both pressure-limited and volume-limited ventilation strategies, and are reviewed here.

Pressure-Mode Individualized Ventilation Devices

Pressure-mode devices seek to allow a single ventilator to support multiple patients with individualized pressure control settings.

One such delivery system, VentMI, has been developed to allow individualized peak inspiratory pressure settings and PEEP using a pressure regulatory valve, developed de novo, and an in-line PEEP "booster." One-way valves, filters, monitoring ports, and wye splitters were assembled in-line to complete the system. VentMI was then investigated in mechanical and animal trials (with a pig and sheep concurrently ventilated from the same ventilator) and demonstrated the ability to provide ventilation across clinically relevant scenarios including circuit occlusion, unmatched physiology, and a surgical procedure while allowing significantly different pressures to be safely delivered to each animal for individualized support [6]. This system received emergency use authorization from the United States Food and Drug Association (FDA) for use during the COVID-19 pandemic.

The core of the design utilizes an inspiratory pressure regulator that downregulates the inspiratory pressure in one circuit, while the ventilator sets the higher inspiratory pressure in the second circuit. Additionally, PEEP can be differentially modulated by placing a "PEEP booster" on whichever circuit that requires higher PEEP. The pressure regulators are paired with one-way flow valves to ensure that pressures do not equilibrate across the circuits and viral/bacterial filters to limit risks of cross-contamination. A schematic diagram of the VentMI system in use is shown in Fig. 21.1.

A number of other pressure-controlled systems have been described. The Mount Sinai HELPS Innovate Group described the use of a single ventilator in pressure-control mode with flow-control valves to simultaneously ventilate two patients with different lung compliances. A 3D printed inspiratory flow-control valve was designed to allow individualized settings of tidal volume and airway pressure and

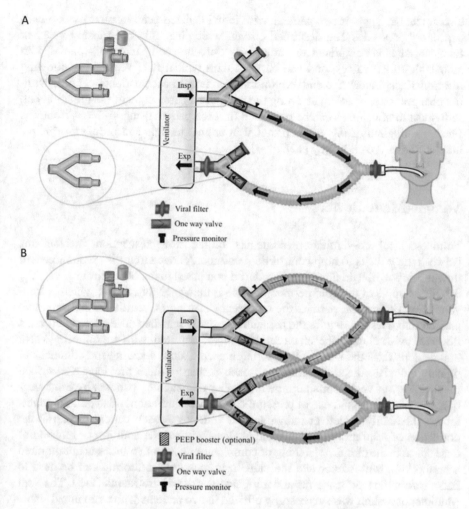

Fig. 21.1 Schematic diagram of VentMI system. (**a**) A single patient is connected to the VentMI system in "standby" mode, awaiting a second patient, and (**b**) both patients are connected to VentMI with one patient having inspiratory pressure downregulated by the regulator and the second controlled by the ventilator. Reproduced from VanKoevering et al. PLoS One, 15(12), e0243601

evaluated first using simulator mannequins with similar or different lung compliance and it was found to deliver stable tidal volumes to each mannequin. The custom-designed flow-control valve system was then tested in two pairs of volunteer COVID-19 patients with acute respiratory failure and found to enable delivery of stable tidal volume and peak airway pressure similar to those provided by individual ventilators for 1 h [11].

Similarly, the Pressure-Regulated Ventilator Splitting (PReVentS) Yale University protocol describes the use of pressure-controlled ventilator mode for a ventilator circuit that can support two patients with individualized peak inspiratory and end-expiratory pressures. The described circuit, which has only been tested in mock lungs to date, is comprised of exclusively "off-the-shelf" materials paired with adjustable PEEP valves, and can be used with typical ICU ventilators, allowing titration of inspiratory and end-expiratory pressures for each patient over time without changes for one patient affecting the ventilation parameters of the other patient. Individual tidal volumes can be measured for each patient using in-line spirometry. Further validation of this novel protocol in animal models and proof-of-principle human studies are underway [12].

Volume-Mode Devices

Volume-control co-ventilation strategies utilize flow restriction mechanisms between the circuits to help control tidal volume. As one circuit is given increased flow restriction, the tidal volume is reduced compared to the other circuit.

One example of the volume-mode device is the Vent Multiplexor, which is a co-ventilation device that permits the emergency sharing of ventilators between two patients and does not require the patients be equally matched. The system utilizes a flow restriction clamp on each circuit that can be adjusted, with a monitoring valve that demonstrates the relative flow through each circuit, allowing the clinicians to quickly calculate the tidal volume to each patient. Unlike previously described methodology of ventilator sharing which relies on matching patients by exact ventilator requirements and use of pressure-controlled ventilation, this ventilator splitter has the ability to deliver individualized volumes to each patient to permit the correction of respiratory alkalosis and acidosis without the addition or removal of dead space to the circuit. Matching of compliance and tidal volumes is not required with the Vent Multiplexor and individualized pressure monitoring can be used to better inform flow adjustments and mitigate the risk of barotrauma [8, 9]. The Vent Multiplexor system was successfully utilized in two patients who maintained stable ventilation throughout the trail and received emergency use authorization.

Another volume-control co-ventilation system is the individualized system for augmenting ventilator efficacy (iSAVE), which was designed as a rapidly deployable platform that enables individual-specific volume and pressure control in response to improvement or deterioration in an individual's respiratory status. The iSAVE similarly incorporates a series of valves and flow regulators in parallel limbs to effectively maintain the desired tidal volume and positive end-expiratory pressure for each patient under volume-control mode. The iSAVE was shown to temporarily ventilate two pigs on one ventilator as effectively as each pig on its own ventilator while mitigating cross-contamination and backflow [7].

Other Ventilator Splitter Designs

Compact delivery systems capable of enabling mechanical ventilation for multiple patients from a single ventilator offer timely solutions to acute shortages of ventilators. This initial development of split ventilation used in pair-matched patients, use of one-way valves, filters, and flow restrictors were all considered and tested in the COVID-19 pandemic with basic splitting devices without the ability to regulate individual ventilator settings [7]. Various designs involving a two-way ventilator split mechanism versus three- or four-way split have also been suggested, but lack of robust testing leads to limited applicability.

Implementation

Ultimately, supporting multiple patients with a single ventilator is not considered standard of care and poses unique ethical considerations, as long as adequate ventilator resources are available [2, 3]. However, in the setting of large-scale crises such as the COVID-19 pandemic, natural disaster, or other conditions in which the number of patients requiring urgent ventilatory support exceeds ventilator supply necessary for single-patient ventilation, ventilator splitter technology can be used to support patients for whom invasive ventilation has a reasonable probability of being lifesaving. Patient selection is carefully considered, and a supply of ventilators should be reserved for patients who need individualized support or are ready to wean. During the COVID-19 pandemic, hospital protocols in which ventilator sharing was considered often required that at least one rescue ventilator to be placed near each cluster of patients that are supported by dual-patient ventilation to facilitate rescue of a patient undergoing dual-patient ventilation who needs to be urgently placed back on a single ventilator [9]. Furthermore, any extended period of co-ventilation would require dedicated monitoring of patients, well-trained nursing and respiratory technician staff, and an experienced clinical team. The personnel requirements can also be a limiting resource in such emergency environments. Most experts agree that the use of multi-patient ventilation should be discontinued as soon as a sufficient supply of ventilators to support single-patient ventilation is available.

Recent FDA guidance in February 2021 recommended the use of noninvasive ventilation such as high-flow nasal oxygen or noninvasive positive-pressure ventilation as the first option prior to using an authorized ventilator splitter. If invasive ventilation using an authorized ventilator splitter is required due to lack of available individual ventilator supply, the FDA advises careful patient selection with limited sharing of ventilation to two patients with similar ventilatory requirements and to limit the duration of sharing ventilation to 48 h. The FDA also recommends that a single-patient ventilator should be reserved and available for emergencies or to wean a patient off ventilation support as needed. Ideally, utilized ventilator splitters incorporate one-way valves in the breathing circuit, flow restrictors or pressure regulators at each inspiratory limb of the circuit, individual positive end-expiratory pressure (PEEP) valves, and inspiratory and expiratory tidal volume and pressure sensors to minimize risks of shared ventilation [13].

Advantages

Novel ventilator splitter technologies such as VentMI, HELPS, iSAVE, and Vent Multiplexor address many historical concerns regarding ventilator splitting such as managing differential compliance and PEEP requirements, personalized monitoring with alarm capacity, ability to simply cap a disconnected circuit if needed, and precluding circuit occlusion from significantly affecting ventilation to the co-ventilated patient. A standard arterial line pressure transducer and monitor can be used to individually monitor each patient's ventilation pressures in real time remotely. These systems are light, portable, and available at a fraction of the cost that would

Table 21.1 Multiplex ventilation: advantages and limitations of ventilatory splitters

Multiplex Ventilation: Advantages and Limitations of Ventilatory Splitters	
Advantages of Available Splitter Systems	**Limitations**
✓ Expanded Ventilator Capacity	✓ Limited data regarding long-term reliability
✓ Light, portable, and easily reproducible facilitating deployment during crises	✓ Risk of cross contamination
✓ Significantly reduced cost compared to full size ventilator alternative	✓ Difficult to individualize FiO2 and respiratory rate
✓ Extended monitoring capacity to evaluate individual tidal volumes and pressures	✓ Increased personnel and experience may be required
✓ Adjustable to each patient's specific ventilation requirements	✓ Deep sedation and paralysis requirements to prevent asynchrony

be required for comparably capable, full-size ventilators, thus facilitating rapid deployment during crises. Advantages and limitations of the novel, individualized ventilation-splitting systems are summarized in Table 21.1.

Limitations

During the COVID-19 pandemic, clinicians have increasingly gained real-world experience with shared ventilators and continue to improve our understanding of the known and potential risks and benefits of ventilator splitters. Reported limitations include (1) the constant need to balance differences in respiratory mechanics of co-ventilated patients to prevent barotrauma and (2) deep sedation and paralysis requirements to prevent asynchrony. Many have highlighted a lack of individual ventilator alarms as another concern, though this has been addressed in some systems. There are several additional limitations to ventilator splitters such as VentMI. These include the inability to deliver variable respiratory rates or differential FiO_2.

Conclusions

The COVID-19 pandemic created a global respiratory crisis which motivated innovative solutions to improve ventilator support. One significant advantage was the development of several split-ventilation systems utilizing both pressure- and volume-controlled ventilation. These systems have been vigorously tested in laboratory simulations and short animal and human trials, and have demonstrated remarkable capacity to support multiple patients safely. Ventilator splitting with systems that allow for individualized ventilation improves safety. As discussed, split ventilation should *only* be utilized when conventional ventilator resources have been exhausted. Nevertheless, split ventilation can provide a reliable alternative to triage and rationing when faced with limited respiratory resources in emergency settings and is a promising strategy in disaster relief medicine or future respiratory pandemics.

Conflicts of Interest Author PK was a developer of Vent Multiplexor Author KV was a developer of VentMI. Both devices received FDA Emergency Use Authorization for use and sale in the United States during the COVID-19 pandemic.

Funding Information None.

References

1. Greg N, Irvin CB. A single ventilator for multiple simulated patients to meet disaster surge. Acad Emerg Med. 2006;13(11):1246–9.
2. Anesthesia Patient Safety Foundation. Joint statement on multiple patients per ventilator. 2020. https://www.apsf.org/news-updates/joint-statement-on-multiple-patients-per-ventilator. Accessed 03 Jan 2021.
3. Hess DR, Kallet RH, Beitler JR. Ventilator sharing: the good, the bad, and the ugly. Respir Care. 2020;65:1059–62.
4. Amato M, Meade M, Slutsky A, et al. Driving pressure and survival in the acute respiratory distress syndrome. N Engl J Med. 2015;372(8):747–55. https://doi.org/10.1056/NEJMsa1410639.
5. Paladino L, Silverberg M, Charchaflieh J, et al. Increasing ventilator surge capacity in disasters: ventilation of four adult-human-sized sheep on a single ventilator with a modified circuit. Resuscitation. 2008;77(1):121–6. https://doi.org/10.1016/j.resuscitation.2007.10.016.
6. VanKoevering KK, Yalamanchi P, Haring CT, et al. Delivery system can vary ventilatory parameters across multiple patients from a single source of mechanical ventilation. PLoS One. 2020;15(12):e0243601.
7. Srinivasan S, Ramadi KB, Vicario F, Gwynne D, Hayward A, Lagier D, et al. A rapidly deployable individualized system for augmenting ventilator capacity. Sci Transl Med. 2020; https://doi.org/10.1126/scitranslmed.abb9401.
8. Milner A, Siner JM, Balcezak T, Fajardo E. Ventilator sharing using volume-controlled ventilation during the COVID-19 pandemic. Am J Respir Crit Care Med. 2020;202(9):1317–9.
9. Beitler JR, Mittel AM, Kallet R, Kacmarek R, Hess D, Branson R, Olson M, Garcia I, Powell B, Wang DS, Hastie J. Ventilator sharing during an acute shortage caused by the COVID-19 pandemic. Am J Respir Crit Care Med. 2020;202(4):600–4.
10. Beitler JR, Kallet R, Kacmarek R, Branson R, Brodie D, Mittel AM, Olson M, Hill LL, Hess D, Thompson BT. Ventilator sharing protocol: dual-patient ventilation with a single mechanical ventilator for use during critical ventilator shortages. Last accessed 2020 Mar 24. pp. 09–17.
11. Levin MA, et al. Differential ventilation using flow control valves as a potential bridge to full ventilatory support during the COVID-19 crisis from bench to bedside. Anesthesiology. 2020;133(4):892–904.
12. Raredon MSB, et al. Pressure-regulated ventilator splitting (PreVentS): a COVID-19 response paradigm from Yale University. medRxiv. 2020.
13. "Using Ventilator Splitters During the COVID-19 Pandemic - Letter to Health Care Providers." https://www.fda.gov/medical-devices/letters-health-care-providers/using-ventilator-splitters-during-covid-19-pandemic-letter-health-care-providers. Accessed 5 May 2021.

Chapter 22
CPAP-to-Ventilator: Open-Source Documentation, UC Irvine

Cody E. Dunn, Christian Crouzet, Mark T. Keating, Thinh Phan, Matthew Brenner, Elliot L. Botvinick, and Bernard Choi

Project Overview

We set out to develop a ventilator based on a continuous positive airway pressure (CPAP) device. CPAP devices generally have a maximum pressure output of approximately 20 cm H_2O. However, for ventilators in the hospital setting, the peak inspiratory pressure (PIP) can sometimes reach 40 cm H_2O. To this end, we modified an existing CPAP device to allow for a maximum PIP of approximately 40 cm H_2O using an electronic speed controller (ESC). An ESC is oftentimes used to control the motor of remote-controlled vehicles. The documentation presented here describes the components, general schematic, wiring diagram, code, limitations,

---

C. E. Dunn · T. Phan
Beckman Laser Institute and Medical Clinic, University of California, Irvine, CA, USA

Department of Biomedical Engineering, University of California, Irvine, CA, USA
e-mail: cedunn@uci.edu; thinhqp@uci.edu

C. Crouzet · M. T. Keating
Beckman Laser Institute and Medical Clinic, University of California, Irvine, CA, USA
e-mail: ccrouzet@uci.edu; keatingm@uci.edu

M. Brenner
Beckman Laser Institute and Medical Clinic, University of California, Irvine, CA, USA

Department of Medicine, University of California, Irvine, CA, USA
e-mail: mbrenner@hs.uci.edu

E. L. Botvinick (✉) · B. Choi (✉)
Beckman Laser Institute and Medical Clinic, University of California, Irvine, CA, USA

Department of Biomedical Engineering, University of California, Irvine, CA, USA

Department of Surgery, University of California, Irvine, CA, USA

Edwards Lifesciences Center for Advanced Cardiovascular Technology, Irvine, CA, USA
e-mail: Elliot.botvinick@uci.edu; choib@uci.edu

© The Author(s), under exclusive license to Springer Nature Switzerland AG 2022
A. A. Hakimi et al. (eds.), *Mechanical Ventilation Amid the COVID-19 Pandemic*,
https://doi.org/10.1007/978-3-030-87978-5_22

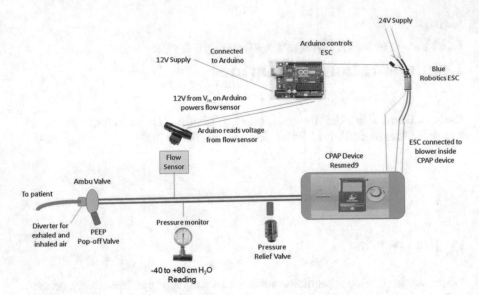

Fig. 22.1 CPAP-to-ventilator global layout schematic

and potential improvements to be made. A layout schematic is shown in Fig. 22.1.
A video showing the functionality is available on our website www.bli.uci.edu/bvc.

Components List

- ResMed S9 AutoSet™ CPAP Machine

    - Supplier: cpap.com
    - Part number: 36005
    - Link: https://www.cpap.com/productpage/resmed-s9-autoset-cpap-machine

- Blue Robotics Basic ESC

    - Supplier: Blue Robotics
    - Part number: BESC30-R3
    - Link: https://bluerobotics.com/store/thrusters/speed-controllers/besc30-r3/

- Analog Manometer

    - Supplier: Parts Source
    - Description: MANOMETER, PRESSURE, −40 TO +80 CMH2O W/ 22MMF
      X 22MMM/15MMF TEE
    - Part number: 00-266-G
    - Link: https://www.partssource.com/parts/anesthesia-associates/00266G/
      ps83fcjwxar

- Flow Meter

  - Supplier: Honeywell
  - Description: AWM700 Series airflow sensor, amplified, flow/pressure range: 200 SLPM; port style: tapered, 22 mm
  - Part number: AWM720P1
  - Link: https://sensing.honeywell.com/awm720p1-amplified-airflow-sensors2

- Arduino-Uno

  - Supplier: Arduino
  - Part number: A000066
  - Link: https://store.arduino.cc/usa/arduino-uno-rev3

- Three linear potentiometers

  - Potentiometer 1: peak inspiratory pressure
  - Potentiometer 2: minimum constant pressure
  - Potentiometer 3: respiratory rate

- Pressure-relief valve (not in description video)

  - Supplier: Parts Source
  - Description: VALVE, PRESSURE RELIEF, 0–55 cmH$_2$O TRUE APL, 1/2-20, CHROME BRASS
  - Part number: 00-273
  - Link: https://www.partssource.com/parts/anesthesia-associates/00273/ ps76frqejah

- PC with USB port
- 12 V/2 A Power Supply connected to Arduino to power the flow meter
- 24 V/2 A Power Supply for ESC

Modifying a CPAP Device to Gain Access to Blower and Connecting ESC

Modifying the CPAP device is a fairly simple process. First, the user needs to gain access to the blower inside the CPAP. To do this, the cover for the CPAP device can be pulled off. Second, the user needs to find the connector that gives power to the blower inside the CPAP and disconnect it (Fig. 22.2).

Fig. 22.2 Access connector that gives power to blower inside CPAP device

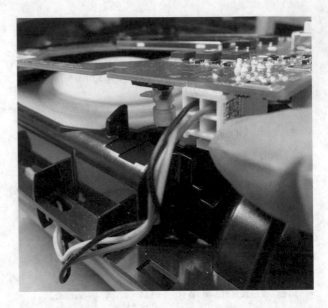

Next, connect the three motor wires from the ESC to the blower (Fig. 22.3). Power the ESC with the 24 V power supply and connect the signal of the ESC to the PWM pin 9. See wiring diagram for circuit connections (Fig. 22.4).

Note: Test to make sure that the airflow from the blower is in the outward direction. If the flow from the blower is inward, switch any two of the three motor wires to have the flow from the blower be in the outward direction.

CPAP-to-Ventilator Wiring Diagram

Arduino Code

The Arduino code to control the CPAP-to-ventilator design can be found starting on page 238.

Fig. 22.3 Connect three motor wires from ESC to blower of CPAP

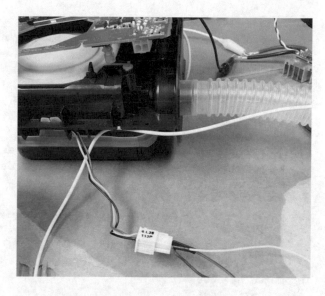

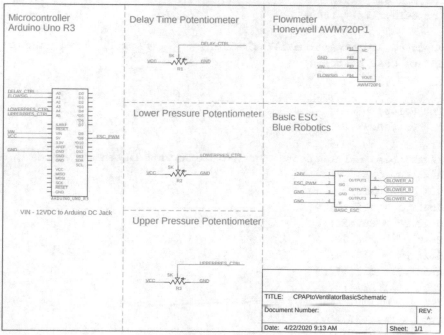

Fig. 22.4 CPAP-to-ventilator wiring diagram

```
// Authors: Mark Keating and Cody Dunn, 04/23/2020
// Example code for CPAP control and reading flow sensor

int pot = A0; // potentiometer input
int flowmeter = A1; // flowmeter input
int uppressure = A5; // inspiratory pressure
int lowpressure = A4; // expiratory pressure

// analog reading max and min (note this is across all pots)
int maxValue = 1023; // 10 bit default on arduino uno
int minValue = 0;


int cpapon = 2; //Determine whether CPAP inspiratory or expiratory


// max and min delay times in milliseconds
int maxDelay=5000;
int minDelay=100;
int delayTime = 1000;

unsigned long previousMillis = 0;              // will store time to
update CPAP status


int value;
int valueflow;

//variables and constants to calculate flowrate in LPM and volume in L
float flowrate;
float flowscale;
float p1 = 5.6356;
float p2 = 58.498;
float p3 = 216.06;
float p4 = 313.94;
float p5 = 151.17;
float volInhale;

int potValue3;
int potValue4;

#include <Servo.h>
Servo ESC;       // create servo object to control the ESC
int potValue;   // value from the analog pin
int potValue2;   // value from the analog pin
```

```
void setup() {
  // Attach the ESC on pin 9
  ESC.attach(9, 1000, 2000); // (pin, min pulse width, max pulse
width in microseconds)
  ESC.writeMicroseconds(1500); // send "stop" signal to ESC. Also
necessary to arm the ESC.
  delay(1000);
  Serial.begin(9600);
  pinMode(pot, INPUT);
  pinMode(flowmeter, INPUT);
  pinMode(uppressure, INPUT);
  pinMode(lowpressure, INPUT);
}


void loop() {
  // read trimpot value
  value = analogRead(pot);
  valueflow = analogRead(flowmeter);
  // scale to max and min delay
  delayTime = map(value, minValue, maxValue, minDelay, maxDelay);
  potValue = analogRead(uppressure);    // reads the value of the
potentiometer (value between 0 and 1023)

  //Inspiratory ESC value
  potValue3 = map(potValue, minValue, maxValue, 1685, 1850);   //
scale it to use it with the servo library

  potValue2 = analogRead(lowpressure);   // reads the value of the
potentiometer (value between 0 and 1023)
  //Expiratory ESC value
  potValue4 = map(potValue2, minValue, maxValue, 1500, 1600);   //
scale it to use it with the servo library

  //Estimate flowrate and volume continuously
  flowscale = 5 * valueflow / maxValue;
  flowrate = abs((p1 * (pow(flowscale, 4)) - (p2 * pow(flowscale, 3))
+ (p3 * pow(flowscale, 2)) - (p4 * (flowscale)) + p5));
  volInhale = flowrate * delayTime * 0.001 * 0.0167;
  //Print values to serial monitor
  Serial.print("Delay Time (ms): ");
  Serial.println(delayTime);
  Serial.print("Flow Rate (LPM): ");
  Serial.println(flowrate);
  Serial.print("Volume (L): ");
  Serial.println(volInhale);
```

```
  delay(10);


  //Determine when to switch from inhalation to exhalation pressure
and vice versa
  if ((unsigned long)(millis() - previousMillis) > delayTime) {
  previousMillis = millis();
    // cycle START;
    if (cpapon > 1) {
        ESC.writeMicroseconds(potValue3);        // Send the signal
to the ESC
      cpapon = 0;
    }
    else {
        ESC.writeMicroseconds(potValue4);        // Send the signal
to the ESC
      cpapon = 2;
    }
  }
  // cycle END
}
```

Limitations and Areas for Improvement

Although our design is simple and requires few modifications to a CPAP device for ventilator-like capabilities, it has several limitations. Some of the limitations are as follows:

1. Our design does not contain any alarms.
2. We did not perform stress tests.

   (a) We do not know how long the device can run continuously or which components would fail first.
   (b) We have not performed in vivo testing.

3. Our design does not have oxygen-mixing capabilities to change the FiO_2. An oxygen-mixing device can be coupled into the system to change the FiO_2 per provider's need.
4. We have not incorporated a filter to capture exhaled air. A filtration system can be integrated on the expiration end to prevent aerosolized viral particles.
5. Our device uses an inexpensive Arduino to serve as the main controller. Other microcontrollers may be better suited in terms of stability and reliability.
6. Currently, the constructed device does not have a pressure-relief valve. We plan to add the relief valve.

7. We only tested our design with the Resmed 9 CPAP device. Modifications may be necessary with alternative CPAP devices.
8. The conversion from the flow meter analog Arduino input to flow/volume involved a crude fitting that leaves room for improvement.
9. Presently, the inhalation pressure can only be set between approximately 10 and 40 cm H_2O. The exhalation pressure can only be set between approximately 0 and 10 cm H_2O.
10. The CPAP was powered with a 24 V supply and the flow meter was powered with a separate 12 V supply. Constructing a buck converter would reduce the need for two supplies.
11. The addition of a small display would remove the need for a computer after loading the code onto the Arduino.

Disclaimer

THE CPAP-TO-VENTILATOR INFORMATION IS PROVIDED "AS-IS, WHERE-IS," WITHOUT REPRESENTATIONS, CONDITIONS, OR WARRANTIES OF ANY KIND, WHETHER EXPRESS OR IMPLIED, INCLUDING, BUT NOT LIMITED TO, WARRANTIES OF MERCHANTABILITY OR FITNESS FOR A PARTICULAR PURPOSE, OR THAT THE USE OF THE CPAP-TO-VENTILATOR INFORMATION WILL NOT INFRINGE ANY PATENT, COPYRIGHT, TRADEMARK, OR OTHER PROPRIETARY RIGHTS. THE RECIPIENT IS SOLELY RESPONSIBLE FOR DETERMINING THE APPROPRIATENESS OF USING, REPLICATING, OR REDISTRIBUTING THE UNIVERSITY OF CALIFORNIA, IRVINE, INFORMATION AND DESIGN. IN THIS REGARD, THE RECIPIENT ASSUMES ALL LIABILITY FOR DAMAGES, OF WHATEVER NATURE AND DESCRIPTION, WHETHER IN CONTRACT OR IN TORT, WHICH MAY ARISE FROM THE USE OF THE CPAP-TO-VENTILATOR INFORMATION AND DESIGN. THE UNIVERSITY OF CALIFORNIA, IRVINE, INCLUDING ITS EMPLOYEES AND AGENTS, WILL NOT BE LIABLE TO THE RECIPIENT OR TO ANY THIRD PARTY FOR ANY LOSS, CLAIM, OR DEMAND MADE BY THE RECIPIENT, OR ANY LOSS, CLAIM, DEMAND, OR JUDGMENT AGAINST THE RECIPIENT BY ANY OTHER PARTY, DUE TO OR ARISING FROM THE USE OF THE VENTILATOR INFORMATION AND DESIGN BY THE RECIPIENT.

Conflicts of Interest The authors declare no relevant conflicts of interest.

Funding Information Institutional support from the Arnold and Mabel Beckman Foundation

Chapter 23
Alternatives to Conventional Noninvasive Positive-Pressure Ventilation Devices

Pauline Yasmeh, Annie Chen, Alexis Ha, Riley Oh, and Grant Oh

Standard Noninvasive Ventilation

During the COVID-19 pandemic, the recommendation to use noninvasive positive-pressure ventilation (NIPPV) was split amongst medical societies. Namely, the National Institutes of Health [1], the Society of Critical Care Medicine/European Society of Intensive Care Medicine Surviving Sepsis Campaign [2], the English National Health Service [3], the Italian Thoracic Society, and the Italian Respiratory Society [4], as well as the World Health Organization [5], support the use of NIPPV in patients with COVID-19 and acute hypoxic respiratory failure, at least in certain circumstances. Meanwhile, the Australian and New Zealand Intensive Care Society [6] recommend against the use of NIPPV in patients with COVID-19 in favor of early intubation.

The most common standard, preexisting, noninvasive oxygen delivery devices include oxygen via nasal cannula or prongs, simple face mask, non-rebreather masks, high-flow nasal cannula (HFNC), and NIPPV via continuous positive airway pressure (CPAP) and bi-level positive airway pressure (BiPAP). Each of these mechanisms has certain benefits and disadvantages to their use in COVID-19.

Nasal cannula, simple face mask, and non-rebreather masks are the simplest of the oxygen delivery devices as they do not require a respiratory therapist or specialist nursing competency and can be applied and managed by any member of the healthcare team. These devices are widely available in most hospitals and are effective especially for patients with do-not-intubate orders. Disadvantages of these devices, however, are that they would not serve patients who are severely hypoxic,

P. Yasmeh (✉) · A. Chen
David Geffen School of Medicine at UCLA, Olive View-UCLA Medical Center, Sylmar, CA, USA

A. Ha · R. Oh · G. Oh
Beckman Laser Institute and Medical Clinic, Irvine, CA, USA
e-mail: riley.oh@students.lhsoc.org

© The Author(s), under exclusive license to Springer Nature Switzerland AG 2022
A. A. Hakimi et al. (eds.), *Mechanical Ventilation Amid the COVID-19 Pandemic*,
https://doi.org/10.1007/978-3-030-87978-5_23

they are less effective at reducing the work of breathing and dyspnea in patients who are more severely ill as compared to high-flow nasal cannula or NIPPV devices, and they generate aerosol distribution at higher flow rates.

High-flow nasal cannula may be more beneficial than nasal cannula, simple face masks, and non-rebreather masks for its ability to deliver oxygen at higher flow rates while providing a degree of positive end-expiratory pressure. Its ability to deliver sufficient levels of oxygen to relieve the work of breathing and ability to provide positive end-expiratory pressure can promote ventilation by allowing for more effective gas exchange, thereby allowing it to treat hypercapnia in addition to hypoxemia. HFNC is typically well tolerated by patients because it allows them to eat, drink, and speak comfortably while relieving some work of breathing and dyspnea. HFNC can also deliver humidified air for added comfort to avoid epistaxis and dry nasal passages. HFNC is also a compatible mechanism for patients with do-not-intubate orders. While typically HFNC can be used in standard patient rooms, outside of the intensive care unit, a possible disadvantage is that some hospitals and centers require specialized nursing competency, or respiratory therapy, to manage the device. Similar to nasal cannula, simple face mask, and non-rebreather masks, HFNC has a high propensity for aerosol production given its high flow rate and can increase transmission to those in proximity to the affected patient.

NIPPV including CPAP and BiPAP are more advanced devices for oxygenation and ventilation but are less invasive than intubation. Benefits of NIPPV are that it may better alleviate dyspnea and work of breathing compared to the above oxygen therapies and it is still compatible with patients with do-not-intubate orders. These devices also avoid sedation and can be used outside of the intensive care unit in most facilities. However, these devices require specialist nursing competency and/or respiratory therapy to apply and titrate settings. Further disadvantages are that these devices may become uncomfortable due to the nature of using a tight-fitting mask and limit the patient's ability to communicate over the mask. These devices also prohibit patients from eating during oxygen delivery and can increase the risk of aspiration if applied too soon after eating. Similar to the devices mentioned above, NIPPV devices carry a high propensity for aerosol production and can increase transmission of the infection to those in proximity to the affected patient.

Innovative Noninvasive Ventilation Devices

The COVID-19 pandemic imposed a tremendous burden on medical resources, creating a drastic shortage on respiratory devices and masks with medical supply manufacturers unable to keep up with the level of demand, and limiting access to ventilators and other oxygen therapies. This spawned a worldwide initiative to create innovative devices and adjuncts to combat the shortage. Individuals, manufacturers, and various institutions collaborated to produce alternative respiratory equipment, whether it was by modifying existing equipment or by using additive manufacturing (3D printing) to construct new devices.

Snorkel Masks

One effort to address the shortage in respiratory supplies was made by adapting snorkel masks to be compatible with NIPPV machines (Fig. 23.1). In one of the most prominent examples, ISINNOVA, an Italian engineering startup, created a 3D printed adaptor called the Charlotte valve fitted to the Decathlon Easybreath snorkel mask in response to the urgent shortage of respiratory masks and Venturi valves [8, 9]. The same concept was subsequently expanded by other groups, leading to the production of adaptors and connector pieces compatible with alternative snorkel mask manufacturers. Distinctions between the various brands of snorkel masks, as well as different adaptor designs, will not be addressed in this chapter.

Advantages

Use of the modified snorkel mask and adaptor is first and foremost advantageous in its adaptability, utilization of readily available materials, as well as accessibility (Fig. 23.2). 3D printing is relatively low cost and allows for rapid prototyping and production times [10, 11]. The Charlotte valve's digital design files are open access and available for download online and roughly cost $2 to $3 to print [12].

In a comparative bench study by Ferrone et al. comparing variables of patient-ventilator interaction between the modified snorkel mask and the standard

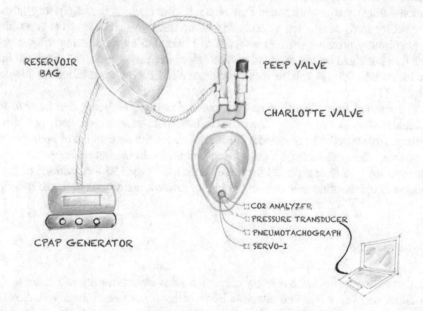

Fig. 23.1 Diagram of a modified snorkel mask as a NIPPV device. *Image courtesy of Noto* et al. [7]

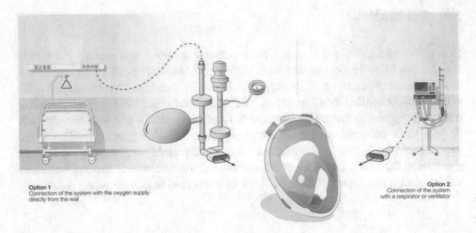

Fig. 23.2 Adaptability of the snorkel mask configuration depending on connection requirements. *Image courtesy of Profili* et al. [10]

noninvasive CPAP full-face mask, the snorkel mask was found to perform as well as or better than the full-face mask [13]. Specifically, the snorkel mask demonstrated significantly shorter pressurization time (defined as the time necessary to achieve the preset level of pressure support from the baseline value), significantly shorter expiratory trigger delay (defined as the delay between the end of the inspiratory effort and the end of the mechanical insufflations), as well as significantly longer pressure time product at 200, 300, and 500 ms indicating a higher capacity to maintain the pressurization during the aforementioned time intervals after opening the inspiratory valve.

Another study conducted air leakage tests on three volunteer subjects at positive end-expiratory pressure (PEEP) levels of 5–12 cmH$_2$O by monitoring the gas volume loss indicated on the mechanical ventilator interface screen. The results of this test indicated a 0% gas volume loss throughout all PEEP intervals tested for all three subjects [11].

The snorkel mask interface has also been described as being comfortable for patients to wear. A descriptive case series following 25 patients reported good initial tolerance in 92% of their enrolled subjects, defined as the percentage of patients able to maintain their masks for 1 h [14]. Furthermore, the immediate oxygen saturation after therapy initiation reported for these patients averaged 95.8%, with 21 of these patients demonstrating a three-point or higher improvement in oxygen saturation.

Disadvantages

As there have been relatively few clinical studies evaluating these products, the modified snorkel masks and adaptors by large have not been clinically validated. There are few case studies in the existing literature to support their use, and the existing studies all report small sample sizes, limiting the validity and generalizability of their results.

There are also limitations in using 3D printing to produce the adaptor valves. As 3D printers have become more accessible, there are many who own 3D printers and are able to download online digital design files for respiratory device parts and produce them from home. However, this introduces problems in quality control and reproducibility due to inherent differences in machine calibration and software, resulting in production errors [11, 14].

Additionally, while good initial tolerance with the modified snorkel mask has been reported, prolonged use appears to be poorly tolerated. In the aforementioned study by Bibiano et al., only 52% of their enrolled patients were able to tolerate the therapy for 24 h and the main overall cause of cessation was reported to be due to physical intolerance [14]. Furthermore, it may be poorly tolerated with patient proning, a valuable therapy in managing COVID-19 patients. A case report detailing the course of a COVID-19 patient being oxygenated with the modified snorkel mask while prone reported patient complaints of cervical pain and difficulty sleeping after 2 days of use, requiring pharmacologic relief as well as massage therapy [15].

Rebreathing of expired carbon dioxide (CO_2) is also a concern with use of the modified snorkel mask. High rates of CO_2 rebreathing have been observed with the use of such devices in healthy adult volunteers, as well as worsening of CO_2 levels with higher respiratory rates up to 30 breaths/min [7, 16]. This is thought to be due to the wide dead space (800–900 mL) associated with the mask along with a fixed production of CO_2 by the patient [7]. As a result, high flow rates are required to wash out the high levels of CO_2. One study suggested that a flow rate of at least 80 L is required to achieve this, while another reported that at least 50 L was needed [7, 17].

There is also concern that the modified snorkel mask is unable to maintain targeted CPAP levels. Noto et al. evaluated the snorkel mask's stability of pressure generated at PEEP levels of 5, 10, and 15 with a high-flow system generator set at 40, 80, and 120 L of flow. At 40 L of flow, the system was unable to achieve pressures higher than 5 cmH_2O, while 80 L of flow demonstrated inconsistent performance, at times under the targeted pressure while at other times over the targeted pressure. While 120 L of flow was able to meet the goal CPAP level at each interval, it frequently exceeded the target and delivered more pressure than desired [7]. Another study likewise demonstrated plateauing mask pressure measurements beyond 14 cmH_2O despite increasing CPAP settings [16].

While the absence of air leakage was suggested in an aforementioned study for lower levels of PEEP, this has not been redemonstrated with higher pressures. Landry et al. compared the modified snorkel mask with a standard oronasal CPAP mask in high-flow oxygen delivery performance. Both interfaces demonstrated dilution of oxygen delivery upon application of positive pressure. However, while the standard CPAP mask exhibited a small linear decline in measured FiO_2 (0.8%/cmH_2O), this was far more pronounced in the snorkel mask, which responded with a steep decline in FiO_2 that accelerated when PEEP was increased beyond 12 cmH_2O [16]. This was similarly reported in the study by Ferrone et al. in which significant air leaks were felt to contribute to asynchrony as well as double triggering of breaths by the patient after PEEP was increased beyond 18 cmH_2O [13]. Collectively, these findings are concerning for an inadequate face seal with the snorkel mask interface at higher pressures, posing a risk for exposure and aerosolization of viral particles, which, in the context of the COVID-19 pandemic, may prove highly problematic.

Helmets

Another solution to oxygen delivery for patients with respiratory distress or hypoxemic respiratory failure in COVID-19 was the use of helmet noninvasive ventilation. The helmet is used as an alternative to standard mask CPAP machines. A popular helmet design is one made of a clear plastic hood on a hard-plastic ring with an adjustable collar that is suitable for various neck dimensions [18]. During the COVID-19 pandemic, helmet CPAP machines were studied as they delivered continuous treatment with PEEP of 10–12 cmH_2O and pressure support of 10–12 cmH_2O [19].

Advantages

In a multicenter randomized clinical trial conducted by Grieco et al. across four intensive care units in Italy with 109 COVID-19 patients, those who received helmet therapy showed to have a significantly lower rate of endotracheal intubation than patients who received therapy with HFNC, 30% and 51%, respectively ($p = 0.03$). Furthermore, the median number of days free of invasive respiratory support was significantly higher in patients using a helmeted device compared to those using HFNC, 28 and 25 days, respectively ($p = 0.04$) [19]. Helmets also carry the advantage of decreased aerosolization and increased comfort for the patient as compared to masks and other standard oxygen delivery mechanisms [18, 20].

Disadvantages

In their same aforementioned study, Grieco et al. did not find a statistically significant difference in the median days free of respiratory support, 20 and 18 days, respectively ($p = 0.26$) [19]. Furthermore, helmets can generate loud noises that can be disturbing to the patient and would restrict the patient's ability to eat given the need for a tight seal at the neck to promote proper gas exchange while limiting aerosolization. In prior studies of helmet devices, namely in patients with chronic obstructive pulmonary disease, the helmet was less effective than a face mask at decreasing patient's inspiratory effort and significantly worsened patient-ventilator synchrony demonstrated by longer delays between inspiratory effort and oxygen support delivery [21].

Discussion

Due to a shortage of ventilatory systems, products such as masks and helmets have been refashioned to serve as noninvasive ventilatory support for patients during the COVID-19 pandemic as described in this chapter. The overarching benefits of these devices include their use of often readily available materials and their ability to deliver oxygen to patients in respiratory distress without invasive measures. This includes the avoidance of sedation, inability to communicate, and decreased potential for delirium. Additionally, noninvasive measures serve as an option for enhanced oxygen delivery in patients who otherwise have opted for "do-not-intubate" measures.

Snorkel masks serve as an inexpensive and simple-to-recreate design via 3D printing and have demonstrated both comfort and efficiency in delivering oxygen to patients. However, given inter-user variability in production, which limits quality control, and its relatively recent creation, its use is yet to be validated in clinical trials. Furthermore, its use is also impeded by patient discomfort over prolonged periods of time and its inability to consistently deliver goal pressure levels.

Helmet CPAP machines were found to be advantageous as they operate like a standard CPAP device; however, the helmet design as opposed to a facial mask was found to be less tolerable for patients. Studies also found that, when compared to HFNC, helmets demonstrated significantly decreased intubation rates as compared to HFNC. However, overall, the helmet did not produce a significant change in median days free of respiratory support for patients with COVID-19 and was less efficacious than the mask at relieving patient's inspiratory effort.

Conclusion

The use of modified snorkel masks in conjunction with 3D printed adaptors and helmet devices to deliver NIPPV therapy, while presenting an innovative solution in a massive shortage of resources, does not replace standard ventilating options. While these devices may have a role in limited settings, their clinical value in patients with higher ventilation requirements and the potential for design modifications would benefit from further clinical evaluation.

Conflicts of Interest The authors declare no relevant conflicts of interest.

Funding This work was not funded.

References

1. National Institutes of Health (NIH) COVID-19 Treatment Guidelines. Oxygenation and ventilation. https://covid19treatmentguidelines.nih.gov/critical-care/oxygenation-and-ventilation/
2. Alhazzani W, Møller MH, Arabi YM, et al. Surviving sepsis campaign: guidelines on the management of critically ill adults with coronavirus disease 2019 (COVID-19). Crit Care Med. 2020;48(6):e440–69. https://doi.org/10.1097/CCM.0000000000004363.
3. National Health Service (NHS) Guidance for the role and use of non-invasive respiratory support in adult patients with COVID-19 (confirmed or suspected). 6 April 2020, Version 3.
4. Italian Thoracic Society (AIPO/ITS) and Italian Respiratory Society (SIP/IRS). Managing the Respiratory care of patients with COVID-19. https://ers.app.box.com/s/j09ysr2kdhmkcu1ulm8y8dxnosm6yi0h

5. World Health Organization Clinical management of severe acute respiratory infection (SARI) when COVID-19 disease is suspected. Interim guidance. 13 March 2020. https://www.who.int/publications/i/item/clinical-management-of-covid-19

6. Australian and New Zealand Intensive Care Society. ANZICS COVID-19 Guidelines. Melbourne: ANZICS; 2020. https://www.anzics.com.au/wp-content/uploads/2020/04/ANZI_3367_Guidelines_V2.pdf

7. Noto A, Crimi C, Cortegiani A, et al. Performance of EasyBreath Decathlon Snorkeling mask for delivering continuous positive airway pressure. Sci Rep. 2021;11(1):5559. https://doi.org/10.1038/s41598-021-85093-w. Published 2021 Mar 10.

8. Charlotte Valve - Easy Covid-19. isinnova.it. https://isinnova.it/archivio-progetti/easy-covid-19/. Published April 27, 2021. Accessed 26 June 2021.

9. Decathlon Easybreath Mask & COVID-19. Decathlon. https://www.decathlon.com/blogs/inside-decathlon/decathlon-easybreath-mask-covid-19. Accessed 26 June 2021.

10. Profili J, Dubois EL, Karakitsos D, Hof LA. Overview of the user experience for snorkeling mask designs during the COVID-19 pandemic. Healthcare (Basel). 2021;9(2):204. https://doi.org/10.3390/healthcare9020204. Published 2021 Feb 14

11. Longhitano GA, Candido G, Ribeiro Machado LM, et al. 3D-printed valves to assist noninvasive ventilation procedures during the COVID-19 pandemic: a case study. J 3D Print Med. 2020; https://doi.org/10.2217/3dp-2020-0017.

12. Feldman A. Meet The Italian Engineers 3D-Printing Respirator Parts For Free To Help Keep Coronavirus Patients Alive. Forbes. https://www.forbes.com/sites/amyfeldman/2020/03/19/talking-with-the-italian-engineers-who-3d-printed-respirator-parts-for-hospitals-with-coronavirus-patients-for-free/. Published March 19, 2020. Accessed 26 June 2021.

13. Ferrone G, Spinazzola G, Costa R, et al. Comparative bench study evaluation of a modified snorkeling mask used during COVID-19 pandemic and standard interfaces for non-invasive ventilation. Pulmonology. 2021; https://doi.org/10.1016/j.pulmoe.2021.05.009. [published online ahead of print, 2021 Jun 8]

14. Bibiano-Guillen C, Arias-Arcos B, Collado-Escudero C, et al. Adapted Diving Mask (ADM) device as respiratory support with oxygen output during COVID-19 pandemic. Am J Emerg Med. 2021;39:42–7. https://doi.org/10.1016/j.ajem.2020.10.043.

15. Wagner LE, Basegio KG, Dornelles CFD, et al. Diving mask adapted for non-invasive ventilation and prone position in a patient with severe Covid-19: case report. Rev Epidemiol Control Infecç. 2020;10(3) https://doi.org/10.17058/reci.v10i3.15402.

16. Landry SA, Mann DL, Djumas L, et al. Laboratory performance of oronasal CPAP and adapted snorkel masks to entrain oxygen and CPAP. Respirology. 2020;25(12):1309–12. https://doi.org/10.1111/resp.13922.

17. Montalvo R, Castro E, Chavez A. Alternative to traditional noninvasive ventilation using a modified snorkel mask in a patient with SARS-CoV-2: A case report. Can J Respir Ther. 2021;57:18–21. https://doi.org/10.29390/cjrt-2020-039. Published 2021 Feb 9

18. Lucchini A, Giani M, Isgrò S, Rona R, Foti G. The "helmet bundle" in COVID-19 patients undergoing noninvasive ventilation. Intensive Crit Care Nurs. 2020;58:102859. https://doi.org/10.1016/j.iccn.2020.102859.

19. Grieco DL, Menga LS, Cesarano M, et al. COVID-ICU Gemelli Study Group. Effect of Helmet Noninvasive Ventilation vs High-Flow Nasal Oxygen on Days Free of Respiratory Support in Patients With COVID-19 and Moderate to Severe Hypoxemic Respiratory Failure: The HENIVOT Randomized Clinical Trial. JAMA. 2021; https://doi.org/10.1001/jama.2021.4682.

20. Cabrini L, Landoni G, Zangrillo A. Minimise nosocomial spread of 2019-nCoV when treating acute respiratory failure. Lancet. 2020;395(10225):685. https://doi.org/10.1016/S0140-6736(20)30359-7.

21. Navalesi P, Costa R, Ceriana P, et al. Non-invasive ventilation in chronic obstructive pulmonary disease patients: helmet versus facial mask. Intensive Care Med. 2007;33(1):74–81. https://doi.org/10.1007/s00134-006-0391-3.

Chapter 24
Development of an Inexpensive Noninvasive Ventilation Hood

Ellen Hong, Amir A. Hakimi, and Brian J.-F. Wong

Introduction

The novel COVID-19 virus can affect the respiratory system through complications such as pneumonia and acute respiratory distress syndrome (ARDS) [1]. Both complications can cause difficulty breathing in patients and require ventilation to treat. However, at the height of the COVID-19 pandemic, patients requiring ventilation outpaced the availability of conventional ventilators. Noninvasive ventilation (NIV) methods, such as continuous positive airway pressure (CPAP), were examined as an available alternative. However, CPAP masks can aerosolize the SARS-CoV-2 virus, necessitating further containment methods. This chapter describes the use of household items to create a low-cost, available CPAP hood that provides enhanced aerosol containment.

E. Hong (✉)
Beckman Laser Institute and Medical Clinic, University of California - Irvine, Irvine, CA, USA

A. A. Hakimi
Beckman Laser Institute and Medical Clinic, University of California - Irvine, Irvine, CA, USA

Department of Otolaryngology – Head and Neck Surgery, Medstar Georgetown University Hospital, Washington, DC, USA
e-mail: amir.a.hakimi@medstar.net

B. J.-F. Wong
Beckman Laser Institute and Medical Clinic, University of California - Irvine, Irvine, CA, USA

Department of Biomedical Engineering, Samueli School of Engineering, University of California - Irvine, Irvine, CA, USA

Department of Otolaryngology, Head and Neck Surgery, University of California - Irvine, Orange, CA, USA
e-mail: bjwong@uci.edu

© The Author(s), under exclusive license to Springer Nature Switzerland AG 2022
A. A. Hakimi et al. (eds.), *Mechanical Ventilation Amid the COVID-19 Pandemic*,
https://doi.org/10.1007/978-3-030-87978-5_24

Methods

To build the hood, the following items were sourced. A luggage compression bag (Accenter; Amazon.com Inc., Seattle, WA) was used as the containment "helmet." Each bag is inherently outfitted with a vacuum port containing a triple-seal valve. The screw tops of two water bottles were cut and used as additional ports for access to the patient's face if necessary. Every connection point in the bag, including the openings for the neck and vacuum ports, was sealed with hydrocolloid dressings (Fig. 24.1).

Hydrocolloid dressings are occlusive bandages made of a polymerized resin on a polyurethane film. The resin actively absorbs moisture, holding it within the adhesive. This prevents moisture retention in the underlying skin with prolonged bandage application [2]. The polyurethane film is impermeable to water, gases, and microorganisms and can reduce external friction and shear [3, 4]. No additional fixatives are necessary to adhere hydrocolloid dressings onto skin. They are commonly used for treating superficial wounds and preventing pressure damage to the skin [3, 5]. Also, due to the aforementioned properties, hydrocolloid dressings have become the material of choice for long-term wounds that can require frequent removal and reapplication, such as stoma care [2]. These qualities were highlighted in the decision for their use in adhering the hood to skin and creating a seal. With supervision, the hood was tested on a human volunteer. A commercial, at-home CPAP (ResMed, San Diego, CA) fit into the vacuum port of the luggage compression bag (Fig. 24.2). The volunteer used the hood for one hour (h).

Fig. 24.1 The luggage compression bag was sealed around the subject using hydrocolloid dressings

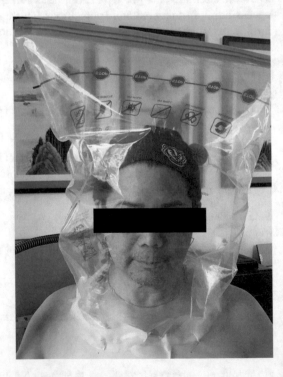

Fig. 24.2 An at-home
CPAP fit into the vacuum
port of the luggage
compression bag

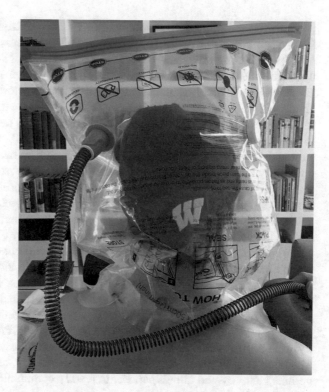

Results

The low-cost hood provided positive pressure in an environment that contained
aerosolized particles. The volunteer was comfortable and noted minimal increase in
pressure. The material cost for the hood is under $5, not including the cost of the
hydrocolloid dressing.

Discussion

This chapter describes the feasibility of using common household items to create a
low-cost yet functional aerosol containment helmet for noninvasive ventilation.

To alleviate the need for ventilators, NIV methods such as CPAP were assessed
as alternatives for early intubation. CPAP use in lieu of ventilators in early treatment
of COVID-19 was found to be effective with careful monitoring [6–9]. Because
careful CPAP titration can successfully ventilate the lungs and improve hypoxemia,
these outcomes demonstrate the utility of CPAP to potentially delay or prevent intubation or as supportive treatment.

However, the implementation of CPAP was scrutinized and criticized particularly when used with COVID-19 patients. NIV, including CPAP, are high-risk, aerosol-generating procedures [10–12]. Aerosolized SARS-CoV-2 is found to have a half-life of 1.1 h in the air, increasing the risk of exposure to healthcare providers. To prevent the spread of aerosolized particles, careful use of personal protective equipment (PPE) is critical. Nightingale et al. reported the use of a negative-pressure room and extra training in PPE usage to account for this risk [8]. While this proved to be effective, as they reported no cases of COVID-19 in the nursing staff that treated the CPAP cohort, this is still an extra burden on healthcare systems that are potentially lacking in resources and space to dedicate to isolation wards.

The proposed CPAP hood answers the call for both protection and accessibility. It follows the model of previously established CPAP helmets: high-flow oxygen enters from one side and an expiratory port is on the other, and the device is sealed around the patient's head using medical-grade dressing. CPAP helmets performed comparably to traditional masks [13]. Furthermore, helmets with an airtight seal around the neck and attachment ports have negligible air dispersion, minimizing room-air contamination [14]. However, previous helmets, with manufacturing variations, were made of latex-free polyvinylchloride attached to a soft polyvinylchloride collar by a metal or plastic ring [13]. Such materials grew in high demand, limiting the availability of such helmets. Our proposed CPAP hood is made of readily available materials: vacuum storage bags, water bottles, and hydrocolloid sheets. The hood is easily removable via scissors if necessary, and the clear, pliable bag permits visibility and allows patients to readily communicate with providers. At a time when demand outpaces traditional resources, the CPAP hood accessibly provides protection to healthcare workers and comfort for patients.

The trial of the CPAP hood was limited in execution, necessitating future rigorous testing. Similar to previous helmets, the hood could be outfitted with a pliable yet sturdy frame, such as hoop skirt boning, to help prevent collapse in case of CPAP failure. Additionally, the proposed hood was only used for 1 h, and prolonged testing would be necessary before clinical application. The initial iteration of the hood did not include a filter at its expiratory port, but an attachment with a HEPA filter to prevent aerosolization spread could be easily added. Considerations for how often the hood would need to be replaced are also needed. Further development of the seal is possible: while strips of hydrocolloid bandages were used in the current trial, production of ring-shaped bandages is easily feasible on a manufacturing scale. Ostomy paste is an alternative that could also be explored.

Conclusion

With the build method proposed in this study, it is possible to provide noninvasive ventilation to COVID patients with aerosol containment at minimal cost. The common materials used are readily available and do not place a burden on existing resources. While there are improvements to be made on the model, this study provides a preliminary guide for the development of an inexpensive NIV device that may be considered in resource-limited emergency situations.

Conflicts of Interest The authors declare no relevant conflicts of interest.

Funding No funding was received for this work.

References

1. Batah SS, Fabro AT. Pulmonary pathology of ARDS in COVID-19: a pathological review for clinicians. Respir Med. 2021;176 https://doi.org/10.1016/j.rmed.2020.106239.
2. Berry J, Black P, Smith R, Stuchfield B. Assessing the value of silicone and hydrocolloid products in stoma care. Br J Nurs. 2007;16(13) https://doi.org/10.12968/bjon.2007.16.13.24243.
3. Hermans MHE. Hydrocolloid dressing versus tulle gauze in the treatment of abrasions in cyclists. Int J Sports Med. 1991;12(6):581–4. https://doi.org/10.1055/s-2007-1024738.
4. Zenda S, Ryu A, Takashima A, et al. Hydrocolloid dressing as a prophylactic use for hand-foot skin reaction induced by multitargeted kinase inhibitors: protocol of a phase 3 randomised self-controlled study. BMJ Open. 2020;10(10):1–6. https://doi.org/10.1136/bmjopen-2020-038276.
5. Bishopp A, Oakes A, Antoine-pitterson P, Chakraborty B, Comer D. The preventative effect of hydrocolloid dressing on nasal bridge pressure ulceration in acute non-invasive ventilation. Ulster Med J. 2019;88(1):17–20.
6. Walker J, Dolly S, Ng L, Prior-Ong M, Sabapathy K. The role of CPAP as a potential bridge to invasive ventilation and as a ceiling-of-care for patients hospitalized with Covid-19—An observational study. PLoS One. 2020;15(12 December):1–15. https://doi.org/10.1371/journal.pone.0244857.
7. Radovanovic D, Rizzi M, Pini S, Saad M, Chiumello DA, Santus P. Helmet CPAP to treat acute hypoxemic respiratory failure in patients with COVID-19: a management strategy proposal. J Clin Med. 2020;9(4):1191. https://doi.org/10.3390/jcm9041191.
8. Nightingale R, Nwosu N, Kutubudin F, et al. Is continuous positive airway pressure (CPAP) a new standard of care for type 1 respiratory failure in COVID-19 patients? A retrospective observational study of a dedicated COVID-19 CPAP service. BMJ Open Respir Res. 2020;7(1):8–10. https://doi.org/10.1136/bmjresp-2020-000639.
9. Ashish A, Unsworth A, Martindale J, et al. CPAP management of COVID-19 respiratory failure: a first quantitative analysis from an inpatient service evaluation. BMJ Open Respir Res. 2020;7(1) https://doi.org/10.1136/bmjresp-2020-000692.
10. Tran K, Cimon K, Severn M, Pessoa-Silva CL, Conly J. Aerosol generating procedures and risk of transmission of acute respiratory infections to healthcare workers: a systematic review. PLoS One. 2012;7(4) https://doi.org/10.1371/journal.pone.0035797.
11. World Health Organization. Rational use of personal protective equipment for coronavirus disease 2019 (COVID-19) and considerations during severe shortages. Updated March 19, 2020. Accessed June 6, 2021. https://apps.who.int/iris/handle/10665/331695.
12. Barker J, Oyefeso O, Koeckerling D, Mudalige NL, Pan D. COVID-19: community CPAP and NIV should be stopped unless medically necessary to support life. Thorax. 2020;367(75) https://doi.org/10.1136/thoraxjnl-2020-214913.
13. Chiumello D, Pelosi P, Carlesso E, et al. Noninvasive positive pressure ventilation delivered by helmet vs. standard face mask. Intensive Care Med. 2003;29(10):1671–9. https://doi.org/10.1007/s00134-003-1825-9.
14. Ferioli M, Cisternino C, Leo V, Pisani L, Palange P, Nava S. Protecting healthcare workers from SARS-CoV-2 infection: practical indications. Eur Respir Rev. 2020;29(155):1–10. https://doi.org/10.1183/16000617.0068-2020.

Chapter 25
Collaborations and Accomplishments Among the Bridge Ventilator Consortium Teams

Amir A. Hakimi, Govind Rajan, Brian J. F. Wong, Thomas E. Milner, and Austin McElroy

The Bridge Ventilator Consortium's (BVC) swift advancement from brainstorming design specifications to the development of several bridge ventilator prototypes can be largely attributed to our grassroots in academic medicine. The COVID-19 pandemic highlighted the unique ability of academic medical centers to foster collaboration among distinct specialties and mobilize the private sector that would have been otherwise siloed in their own industries. Within days, we were able to recruit and guide motivated teams of physicians, engineers, scientists, respiratory therapists, manufacturers, and legal advisors among others. Our teleconference platform made meetings easily accessible and allowed us to make tangible change at an international level. We have all learned a tremendous amount about ventilators, prototype development, device testing, and regulatory processing. The following pages highlight some of the contributions made by the BVC team. It is our sincerest hope

A. A. Hakimi (✉)
Department of Otolaryngology – Head and Neck Surgery, Medstar Georgetown University Hospital, Washington, DC, USA

Beckman Laser Institute & Medical Clinic, University of California - Irvine, Irvine, CA, USA
e-mail: Amir.a.hakimi@medstar.net

G. Rajan
Department of Anesthesiology and Perioperative Care, University of California – Irvine, Orange, CA, USA

B. J. F. Wong
Beckman Laser Institute & Medical Clinic, University of California - Irvine, Irvine, CA, USA

Department of Biomedical Engineering, University of California - Irvine, Irvine, CA, USA

Department of Otolaryngology – Head & Neck Surgery, University of California – Irvine, Orange, CA, USA

T. E. Milner
Beckman Laser Institute & Medical Clinic, University of California - Irvine, Irvine, CA, USA

A. McElroy
University of Texas at Austin, Austin, TX, USA

© The Author(s), under exclusive license to Springer Nature Switzerland AG 2022
A. A. Hakimi et al. (eds.), *Mechanical Ventilation Amid the COVID-19 Pandemic*,
https://doi.org/10.1007/978-3-030-87978-5_25

that the information included in this textbook will help guide ambitious minds to think outside the box and advance this field.

VentiVader (University of California, Irvine): Marc Madou, Horacio Kido, Ehsan Shamloo, Alexandra Perebikovsky, Amit Rao, Nick DiPatri, Yujia Liu, Dian Song, Alberto Mota, Luisa Mota, Eros Marcello, Sean Marquez

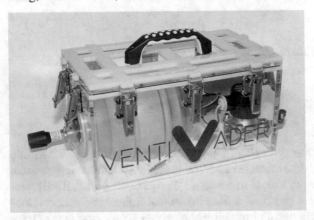

The VentiVader is a pneumatic ventilator that uses the compressed air available in hospitals, along with two solenoid valves and simple electronics, to pressurize a manual resuscitator and control oxygen delivery to a patient. A Raspberry Pi is used as a controller to automate opening and closing of the inhale and exhale solenoid valves and read the pressure sensor. To learn more, go to www.ventivader.com.

CPAP-to-Ventilator (University of California, Irvine): Bernard Choi, Elliot Botvinick, Cody Dunn, Christian Crouzet, Mark Keating, Thinh Phan, Matthew Brenner

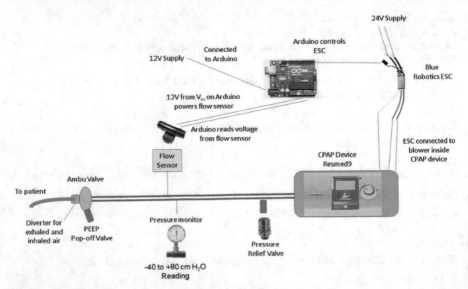

The team led by Dr. Bernard Choi and Dr. Elliot Botvinick converted a ResMed S9 AutoSetTM CPAP machine into an emergency resuscitator capable of achieving a peak inspiratory pressure of 40 cmH$_2$O.

Automatic Bag Breathing Unit "ABBU" (University of Texas at Austin): Thomas Milner, Aleksandra Gruslova, Nitesh Katta, Andrew Cabe, Scott Jenney, Jonathan Valvano, Tim Phillips, Austin McElroy, Van Truskett, Nishi Viswanathan, Marc Feldman, Richard Wettstein, Stephen Derdak

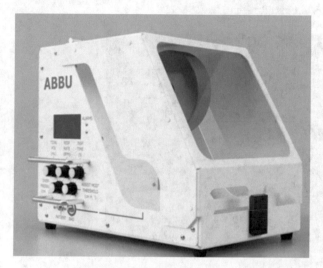

The ABBU uses a windshield wiper motor to power a small caster wheel that pushes down on a bag-valve mask to control oxygen flow. Potentiometers control the respiration rate, volume of oxygen given to patients, inspiratory/expiratory times, and maximum pressure. The device also has a "patient assist" ventilation mode, wherein the device can determine whether or not the patient is attempting to breathe on their own. It is currently under review for the Food and Drug Administration's (FDA) Emergency Use Authorization (EUA).

OxyGEN (Protofy.xyz): Philip Vazquez, Lucas Alavedra, Alex Fiestas, Ferran Caceres, Marc Watine, Joan Cuasch, David Priego, Jose Carlos Norte, Javier Meseguer, Georgia Stewart, Lluis Rovira, Noemi Blazquez, Arnau Solanellas, Ignasi Plaza, Eliane Guiu

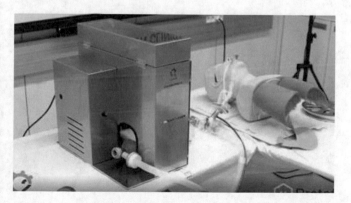

The OxyGEN is a device that automates the process of manual ventilation through cam-based actuation. It is an open-hardware project that can be readily downloaded from www.oxygen.protofy.xyz.

Virgin Orbit Ventilator (Virgin Orbit): Dan Hart, Tom Soto, Nick Fox, Scott Macklin, Kevin Zagorski, Victor Radulescu, Mike Yates

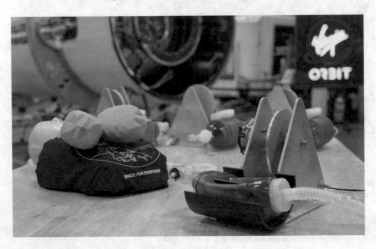

Virgin Orbit was quick to fabricate a ventilator with a cam-based actuation arm similar to that of the OxyGEN team in Barcelona. The device was granted FDA EUA.

Kahanu "The Breath" (Hawaii): Jeffrey Hayashida, Peter How, Olin Kealoha Lagon, Kai Matthes, Blair Stultz, Ryan Kawailani Ozawa

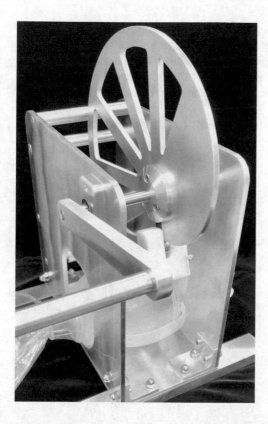

The Kahanu is built upon prior innovation of the OxyGEN team in Barcelona, using a cam-based actuation mechanism. It is solely based on mechanical respiration and does not require software or microcontrollers. The device is currently under EUA review by the FDA.

Team Marvel (Field Ready Ventilator Challenge): Ishmacl Asare, Patience Nortey, Monorvi Asampong, Nelly Appertey

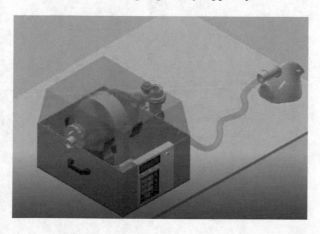

Several leaders among the Bridge Ventilator Consortium served as judges and mentors for the Field Ready Ventilator Challenge. The Marvel Team from Ghana won the challenge for their simple, practical, and scalable ventilator. When the competition started, there were only 75 ventilators in Ghana. Siemens has since partnered with the winning team to refine their design and to manufacture a prototype.

Conflicts of Interest   The authors have no relevant conflicts of interest to disclose.

Funding   This work was not funded.

Index

© The Author(s), under exclusive license to Springer Nature Switzerland AG 2022
A. A. Hakimi et al. (eds.), *Mechanical Ventilation Amid the COVID-19 Pandemic*,
https://doi.org/10.1007/978-3-030-87978-5

Printed in the United States
by Baker & Taylor Publisher Services